Personality Disorder Interview–IV: A Semistructured Interview for the Assessment of Personality Disorders

Personality Disorder Interview-IV:

A Semistructured Interview for the Assessment of Personality Disorders

Thomas A. Widiger, PhD
University of Kentucky
Lexington, KY

Steve Mangine, PhD
Lexington, KY

Elizabeth M. Corbitt, PhD
Western Psychiatric Institute & Clinic
Pittsburgh, PA

Cynthia G. Ellis, MA
University of Kentucky
Lexington, KY

Glenn V. Thomas, MA
University of Kentucky
Lexington, KY

PAR Psychological Assessment Resources, Inc.
P.O. Box 998/Odessa, Florida 33556

Published in 1995 by Psychological Assessment Resources, Inc., Odessa, FL 33556 USA

Library of Congress Cataloging-in-Publication Data
Personality disorder interview–IV: a semistructured interview for the assessment of personality disorders/Thomas A. Widiger…[et al.].

p. cm.

Includes bibliographical references.
ISBN 0-911907-21-1
1. Personality disorders—Diagnosis. 2. Interviewing in psychiatry. I. Widiger, Thomas A. [DNLM: 1. Personality Disorders—diagnosis. 2. Personality Disorders—classification. 3. Interview, Psychological. 4. Psychiatric Status Rating Scales. WM 190 P4663 1994]
RC554.P37 1995
616.85'8—dc20
DNLM/DLC
for Library of Congress 94-43676
CIP

9 8 7 6 5 4 3 2 1 Reorder #RO-2970 Printed in the U.S.A.

Table of Contents

Acknowledgments

The Personality Disorder Interview-IV is the result of years of empirical research, clinical experience, influence and advice from others, and reflection. It is difficult to acknowledge all those who deserve recognition and appreciation. Foremost would be the persons to whom the current and prior versions of this interview have been administered. Much of what we have learned has been offered by them.

We also express substantial appreciation to those who have been involved in the pilot administration of prior versions of this interview, including Seth Axelrod, Becky Bailey, Carey Bluhm, Katherine Freiman, Hal Rogers, Timothy J. Trull, Lynn Warner, and Kristopher West. Each has provided many useful and insightful suggestions. Charles Peterson was instrumental in the field application. Appreciation is also extended to the University of Kentucky, particularly Michael T. Nietzel and Shirley Jacobs, and to Psychological Assessment Resources (PAR), particularly Bob Smith and Serje Seminoff, for their encouragement, support, and facilitation of our efforts. Travis White, of PAR, warrants particular consideration for his many helpful suggestions and contributions.

It is difficult to give adequate credit to those who have provided invaluable influence, advice, suggestions, and support over the years. However, we would like to mention, in particular, Allen J. Frances, Leonard G. Rorer, John C. Clarkin, Paul T. Costa, Roger K. Knudson, and Karen Maitland-Schilling. We also give thanks and credit to the members of the *DSM-IV* Personality Disorders Work Group: Roger Blashfield, Susan Fiester, Robert Hirschfeld, Theodore Millon, Bruce Pfohl, Tracie Shea, Larry Siever, and, especially, John G. Gunderson, for their wisdom and friendship. Finally, we express our sincere appreciation to Cynthia Sanderson, Marcia Landsman, and Lisa Chat for having tolerated, for as long as they could, the personality disorders of the coauthors of this interview.

Preface

The Personality Disorder Interview-IV (PDI-IV) is a semistructured interview for the assessment of the 10 personality disorders given official recognition in the fourth edition of the American Psychiatric Association's (APA) *Diagnostic and Statistical Manual of Mental Disorders* (*DSM-IV*; APA, 1994) (i.e., the antisocial, avoidant, borderline, dependent, histrionic, narcissistic, obsessive-compulsive, paranoid, schizoid, and schizotypal personality disorders), and the two proposed disorders that are presented in the appendix to *DSM-IV* as criteria sets provided for further study (i.e., the depressive and passive-aggressive personality disorders). The purpose of the PDI-IV is to facilitate reliable and valid interview assessments of these personality disorders. Toward this end, it presents questions for the assessment of each of the 94 individual diagnostic criteria for these 12 personality disorders presented within *DSM-IV* (the antisocial conduct disorder criterion is counted as one item). More importantly, however, we also provide the history and rationale for each of these 94 criteria and discuss issues and problems that are typically encountered in their assessment. A valid diagnosis of a personality disorder cannot be done simply through the administration of a series of questions, the responses to which are mindlessly recorded and scored. One must also understand the rationale for each personality disorder criterion and the difficulties involved in its assessment.

One should not consider the PDI-IV to be a validated instrument for the diagnosis of the *DSM-IV* personality disorders. As we discuss further in the subsequent chapters, the validity of a semistructured interview depends substantially upon the interviewer. Any personality disorder semistructured interview can be administered in an unreliable and invalid fashion. There is also no gold standard to establish the validity of a personality disorder interview and only a limited amount of data on the convergent validity of the PDI-IV with respect to alternative instruments.

What the PDI-IV attempts to do is to facilitate a more systematic, replicable, and informed interview assessment of the *DSM-IV* personality disorders through the provision of a consistent set of questions that we have found to be useful in the assessment of these disorders and through instruction as to the history, the rationale, and specific difficulties that we have found with each personality disorder criterion. There are no data to document that the *DSM-IV* borderline criterion of "impulsivity in at least two areas that are potentially self-damaging (e.g., spending, sex, substance abuse, reckless driving, binge eating)" (APA, 1994, p. 654) is assessed validly by the following PDI-IV questions (assessed across time and independent of an Axis I disorder): Did you ever spend so much money that you had trouble paying it off? Did you ever go on a drinking or eating binge? Have you ever taken any major chances or risks with drugs? Did you ever do anything impulsive that was risky or dangerous? Have you ever become sexually involved with someone in a risky or dangerous way?

The relationship of these questions to the borderline criterion is perhaps self-evident, but there are differences among the alternative semistructured personality disorder interviews with respect to the questions they provide for the assessment of each criterion, and there are data to indicate that the alternative interviews will not always agree on the diagnoses that would be provided to a person (Skodol, Rosnick, Kellman, Oldham, & Hyler, 1988). However, it is not yet clear which interview is more valid (or reliable) than another, nor is it even clear that the different findings provided by each interview are due to differences in questions and scoring criteria. Each semistructured interview, including the PDI-IV, also encourages the interviewer to ask for examples and to provide additional questions for clarification and further inquiry. Variation in findings could then be due, in part, to variability in the way any particular interview is administered (as well as to variability in the way the subject responds to the questions). The various alternative personality disorder interviews are semistructured, not structured. They allow for some lattitude in how they are administered and scored.

Because the reliability and validity of a PDI-IV interview depends, in part, on the conscientiousness of the interviewer, researchers should not assume that prior success with the PDI-IV indicates that a current application will be equally successful. The reliability obtained by one research program will not necessarily generalize to another research program or to another time by the same program. The PDI-IV, like any of the other semistructured interviews, can be administered in an unreliable fashion. The interrater reliability of the administration of the PDI-IV should be documented in each study in which it is included.

What a semistructured interview does provide is a set of questions to assess each personality disorder criterion, and guidelines for the scoring of that criterion. This degree of structure will facilitate the obtainment of replicable and valid assessments. The diagnosis of personality disorders can be very difficult, particularly in cases where the interviewee is agitated, depressed, defensive, or withholding; traits that are inherent to the presence of a personality disorder. In such cases, much of the validity will depend upon the interviewer. Nevertheless, we do believe that a consideration of the material and suggestions provided herein with respect to the history and rationale of the *DSM-IV* personality disorder criteria and the issues that commonly occur in their assessment, along with the PDI-IV questions themselves, will help clinicians and researchers obtain replicable and valid diagnoses.

The first three chapters serve as an introduction and overview for this text. Chapter 1 provides an overview of the history, format, and administration of the PDI-IV. Chapter 2 discusses the many issues that bedevil the assessment of a personality disorder and how these issues are addressed by the PDI-IV. Chapter 3 presents an overview of the development of and the major revisions included within *DSM-IV*, and how these have been incorporated within the PDI-IV. Chapters 4 through 13 provide the questions and ratings for each of the 80 personality disorder criteria included within the 10 officially recognized diagnoses, a discussion of the history and rationale for each of the revisions that were made for *DSM-IV*, and a discussion of issues that commonly occur in the assessment of each criterion.

Note that the chapter order in which the diagnoses are presented does not conform to the order in which they appear in *DSM-IV*. The personality disorders in *DSM-IV* are organized with respect to three groups or clusters: (a) odd-eccentric (paranoid, schizoid, & schizotypal); (b) dramatic-emotional-erratic (antisocial, borderline, histrionic, and narcissistic);

and (c) anxious-fearful (avoidant, dependent, and obsessive-compulsive) (APA, 1994). The PDI-IV presents the disorders in alphabetical order to discourage the reification of these three clusters (see chapter 2 for further discussion) and for convenience (i.e., it is easier to find them when they are alphabetized).

Chapter 14 provides an overview and discussion of the often-used diagnosis, "Personality Disorder, Not Otherwise Specified," as well as a discussion of the general criteria for a personality disorder that have been added to *DSM-IV* (APA, 1994). Chapters 15 and 16 provide the discussion for the two proposed personality disorders (depressive and passive-aggressive, respectively) and their 14 criteria that are presented in the appendix to *DSM-IV* as criteria sets provided for further study (APA, 1994). Chapter 17 summarizes the practical instructions for the administration and scoring of the PDI-IV.

1
Introduction

In this chapter, we provide an introduction to the PDI-IV, including its history and the rationale for the material provided for each criterion, policies with respect to administration, alternative formats for administration, usage by researchers and clinicians, and recommended training and expertise of interviewers.

HISTORY

PIQ-I

The Personality Disorder Interview–IV (PDI-IV) is the fourth version of a semistructured interview. Its predecessors were the Personality Interview Questions-I (PIQ-I), PIQ-II, and PIQ-III. The impetus for the first version, the PIQ-I (Widiger, 1985), was the need within research for a systematic and replicable interview method for the assessment and diagnosis of the *DSM-III* personality disorders. The advantages of a semistructured interview had been made readily apparent by prior research on the antisocial personality disorder (Spitzer, Endicott, & Robins, 1978), psychopathy (Hare, 1980), and the borderline personality disorder (Gunderson, Kolb, & Austin, 1981). However, at the time the PIQ-I was being developed in 1983, a semistructured interview for all of the *DSM-III* personality disorders (PDs)was not yet readily available. The first published study reporting data from a *DSM-III* (APA, 1980) PD semistructured interview appeared in the *Journal of Affective Disorders* in 1984 (Pfohl, Stangl, & Zimmerman, 1984). This study used the newly developed Structured Interview for *DSM-III* Personality Disorders (SIDP; Pfohl, Blum, Zimmerman, & Stangl, 1989). Other semistructured interviews such as the Personality Disorder Examination (PDE; Loranger, 1988) were still in development. The first published report on the SIDP was in 1985 (Stangl, Pfohl, Zimmerman, Bowers, & Corenthal, 1985), the first published study using PIQ-I data was in 1986 (Widiger, Frances, Warner, & Bluhm, 1986) and the first published data using the PDE was in 1987 (Loranger, Susman, Oldham, & Russakoff, 1987).

Kappa for the interrater reliability in the diagnosis of the presence versus absence of each *DSM-III* PD assessed by the PIQ-I ranged from .52 (dependent) to .83 (antisocial), with a median kappa of .71 (Widiger et al., 1986). Interrater reliability for the assessment of the number of *DSM-III* criteria that were present for each PD ranged from .72 (schizotypal) to .90 (antisocial), with a median reliability of .80 (Widiger, Trull, Hurt, Clarkin, & Frances, 1987). Correlations of the respective scales from the PIQ-I and the Millon Clinical Multiaxial Inventory (MCMI; Millon, 1983) ranged from –.32 (compulsive) to .64 (dependent) (Widiger & Freiman, 1988).

PIQ-II

The PIQ-II (Widiger, 1987) was developed to incorporate the revisions of *DSM-III-R*. Kappa for the interrater reliability in the diagnosis of the presence versus absence of each PD ranged from .45 (schizotypal) to .92 (passive-aggressive), with a median kappa of .72 (Widiger, Freiman, & Bailey, 1990). Interrater reliability for the assessment of the number of *DSM-III-R* criteria that were present for each *DSM-III-R* PD ranged from .75 (histrionic) to .96 (dependent), with a median reliability of .88 (Bailey, West, Widiger, & Freiman, 1993).

PIQ-III & PDI-IV

The PIQ-III (Widiger, Corbitt, Ellis, & Thomas, 1992) was developed to incorporate the proposals for *DSM-IV* (Task Force, 1991), and the PDI-IV was then developed in 1993 to incorporate the final version of *DSM-IV*. Kappa for the interrater reliability in the diagnosis of the presence versus absence of *DSM-III-R*/*DSM-IV* PDs ranged from .37 (histrionic) to .81 (antisocial), with a median kappa of .65 (Corbitt, 1994). Interrater reliability for the assessment of the number of PD criteria ranged from .74 (histrionic, narcissistic, and schizotypal) to .90 (obsessive-compulsive and passive-aggressive) and .91 (sadistic), with a median reliability of .84.

The name was changed from the PIQ to the PDI for a variety of reasons. Personality Interview Questions was a poor choice descriptively, as the PDI-IV is concerned with and confined to the assessment of maladaptive (disordered) personality, not personality in general. We are currently in the process of developing a different interview for the assessment of normal personality traits (Widiger & Trull, 1992). In addition, the PIQ acronym is readily confused with the acronym for the popular Personality Inventory for Children (PIC) (Lachar, 1982; Wirt, Lachar, Klinedinst, & Seat, 1984). As an alternative, we considered the Personality Disorder Interview Questions, but this title seemed rather cumbersome and the acronym undesirable. It was decided, therefore, to simply shorten the title to Personality Disorder Interview-IV (PDI-IV), referring to its fourth revision, as well as to the fourth edition of the *DSM* (APA, 1994).

MATERIAL PROVIDED FOR EACH PD CRITERION

The following chapters on each PD diagnosis begin with a brief overview of the disorder's definition, history, and the revisions to its diagnosis that were provided by the *DSM-IV* (APA, 1994). Each criterion is then reviewed in some detail (we will, at times, refer to a diagnostic criterion as an item). For each criterion, we present (a) an overview of its history, rationale, and *DSM-IV* revisions; (b) the PDI-IV rating; (c) the PDI-IV interview questions; and (d) a discussion of common problems and issues in its assessment. Each of these sections is described below.

Overview of History and Rationale for Criterion

The initial overview of the criterion is included because we have found that interviewers and raters provide a much better assessment when they understand the history and rationale for the item. The assessment of an item taken out of the context of the purpose or intention of its inclusion within the criteria set can result in a misleading and misinformed assessment. For example, items should not be interpreted literally when such an interpretation is inconsistent with the rationale or purpose of the item (unless, of course, the purpose of the assessment is to study empirically the performance of items when they are literally interpreted without reference to the original intention of the wording, an issue that is discussed further below). It is particularly helpful to understand the rationale for the *DSM-IV* revisions, as these revisions have been informed by difficulties in the interpretation, clinical utility, positive predictive power, sensitivity, or specificity of the respective *DSM-III-R* versions.

In most cases, we also provide a brief history of the criterion. We may describe not only how it was phrased in *DSM-III-R* (APA, 1987) and *DSM-III* (APA, 1980), but also how it was phrased in drafts for *DSM-IV* (Task Force, 1991, 1993), drafts for *DSM-III-R* (Work Group, 1985, 1986), and drafts for *DSM-III* (Task Force, 1978). We may also compare how it is phrased in the World Health Organization's (WHO) *International Classification of Diseases* (WHO, 1992; see chapter 3 for a further discussion of this nomenclature), as well as other research criteria sets (e.g., Feighner et al., 1972).

PDI-IV Ratings of Criterion

The PDI-IV ratings are on a 3-point scale that ranges from 0 to 2, where 0 equals not present, 1 equals present according to the *DSM-IV* definition of the item, and 2 equals present to a more severe or substantial degree. A rating of 1 is virtually equivalent to and usually synonymous with the presence of the respective *DSM-IV* criterion. We have, at times, failed to reproduce the item verbatim, but this was only to simplify or shorten the presentation of the item. A number 1 rating is intended to mean the presence of the *DSM-IV* item as it appears in *DSM-IV*. The only exception to this rule occurs for the first depressive PD item (see DPS-1 in chapter 15).

The PIQ-I and PIQ-II items were rated on a scale from 0 to 9. The PIQ-III and PDI-IV have used a 3-point scale. The 10-point scale used by the PIQ-I and PIQ-II was helpful in providing more detailed distinctions (Widiger, Frances, & Trull, 1989). A limitation of the PDI-IV is that it no longer provides an assessment of maladaptive personality traits that are subthreshold to a respective *DSM-IV* PD criterion. A trait is considered in the PDI-IV to be simply absent (a score of 0) or present at either a clinically significant level (a score of 1) or a more severe level (a score of 2). One will, at times, observe maladaptive PD traits that are below the threshold for a *DSM-IV* criterion (Widiger & Corbitt, in press-b), and these cannot be coded using the PDI-IV. For example, one may observe a maladaptive impulsivity that is below the threshold for the BDL criterion of impulsivity (which requires the presence of impulsivity in at least two areas that are potentially self-damaging; see chapter 6). However, this is consistent with the constraints provided by the *DSM-IV* itself (which recognizes only the presence vs. absence of each PD criterion). The PDI-IV, moreover, can provide a more detailed description than the *DSM-IV* of clinically significant maladaptive personality traits that are below the threshold of a PD diagnosis (i.e., the presence of some of the PD diagnostic criteria but not enough to be given a respective diagnosis). This issue is discussed further in chapter 3.

A limitation of the PIQ-I/II 10-point scale was that it resulted in judgments, distinctions, and rater disagreements that were not particularly important or crucial to a diagnostic decision or an empirical finding. However, the major reason for the shift to a 3-point scale was to provide a closer relationship to the scoring format used in most other PD interviews, such as the SIDP-R (Pfohl, Blum, Zimmerman, & Stangl, 1989) and the PDE (Loranger, 1988). The use of a common metric will facilitate a comparison among these instruments and may improve their convergence.

PDI-IV Questions

The PDI-IV questions are ones that we have found to be especially useful to make the PDI-IV 0, 1, and 2 ratings. We also provide additional optional questions if the interviewer and interviewee have sufficient time and motivation for their consideration.

Administration of questions

The questions that are provided should be administered in the assessment of each respective item. Interviewers are, of course, free to implement minor revisions in the phrasing of a question for ease in administration (e.g., to be consistent with a particular style of speech). We also encourage the interviewer to ask all additional questions that might be necessary to render a confident assessment of a particular item. It would not be realistic to suggest that the questions that are provided will always be fully sufficient. Follow-up questions for clarification and for the request of examples will almost always be necessary (see chapter 2).

It is difficult to exaggerate the importance of asking for examples. Whenever a person states that he or she feels insecure (DEP-1, see chapter 7), has special talents or abilities (NAR-1, chapter 9), or feels rather empty much of the time (BDL-7, chapter 6), the interviewer should ask for examples or illustrations of what he or she means by this attribution. In prior versions of the PDI, we noted the specific interview questions for which the request for examples was especially important and helpful. However, this was, at times, interpreted as indicating little need to ask for examples for items where the suggestion was not explicitly provided. We have, therefore, deleted such specific suggestions among the interview questions to emphasize that a request for examples should be considered for every item and provided for most of them.

A deviation from the PDI-IV questions may be necessary at times to provide an optimal assessment. The questions provided by the PDI-IV are hardly infallible. What is important is to provide a valid and replicable (reliable) assessment. If a more valid assessment would be provided by a deviation from the questions and guidelines provided herein, then one should not adhere rigidly to the PDI-IV. However, to ensure replication and reliability, the interviewer should document explicitly the nature and extent of any deviation. An advantage of a semistructured interview is that everyone who uses it will presumably be providing consistent, uniform assessments. Deviations may be necessary at times, but they will also undermine these advantages of using a semistructured interview. When deviations do occur, their presence should be recorded so that a person who wishes to replicate this particular assessment will be aware of the variation in administration.

At times, one will find that responses to subsequent questions seem to contradict answers to prior questions. The interviewer should then return to the prior question and ask for clarification. An advantage of a semistructured interview over a self-report inventory is the opportunity to resolve such inconsistencies and to obtain clarification. This opportunity should be used as much as possible (see chapter 2).

All of the questions for a particular criterion need not be administered if the interviewer is confident that no additional questions are necessary. The motivation and cooperation of the interviewee can be strained by the presence of unnecessary and pointless questions. However, we discourage interviewers from skipping an entire criterion on the basis of an impression or presumption that the criterion is absent (or present). One will, at times, find a history of criminal acts in a seemingly timid and meek subject or severe feelings of insecurity in an aggressive, hostile subject. One does not really know until one asks. Presumptions and untested impressions can also be a major source of gender, cultural, and other stereotypes and biases. The major advantage and purpose of a semistructured interview is to ensure and document a systematic and comprehensive assessment; this is negated when the interview is neither comprehensive nor systematic. The failure to complete a systematic and comprehensive assessment of the PDs is one reason that (unstructured) clinical interviews tend to provide substantially fewer PD diagnoses than are obtained by semistructured research interviews. (However, in defense of the unstructured clinical interview, additional reasons for this discrepancy are discussed in the next two chapters.)

One clear exception to the rule that all questions must be administered occurs when the responses to earlier questions have clearly provided the answers to subsequent questions. There is considerable overlap among the PD criteria. A systematic and comprehensive assessment of all of the PD items will result in considerable repetition and redundancy. Rapport is substantially compromised when the interviewer keeps asking what are essentially the same questions, as if he or she is not paying any attention to what the interviewee has been saying Given the length of a PD interview, this can become quite annoying to the subject.

Alternative interview formats

The PIQ-I, PIQ-II, and PIQ-III were organized by thematic content rather than by disorder in order to minimize redundancy and repetition across the diagnoses (Widiger & Frances, 1987). Items from different diagnoses that covered similar territory were placed together (e.g., "no close friends" from the schizoid PD, "reluctance to confide in others" from the narcissistic PD, and "feels uncomfortable or helpless when alone" from the borderline PD, followed each other in the PIQ-III). This approach was also useful to avoid halo effects, wherein the interviewer develops diagnostic impressions that bias the ratings of subsequent items (Widiger & Frances, 1987). This approach is also taken by many of the other PD semistructured interviews (e.g., the PDE and SIDP-R). However, this approach is not user-friendly to the practicing clinician who has neither the time nor the need to assess all of the *DSM-IV* PD items in every patient. A diagnostic question or issue may be confined to a particular PD or subset of PDs, making the rest of the interview irrelevant, unnecessary, and wasteful of time. It was, perhaps, for this reason that the Structured Clinical Interview for *DSM-III-R* Personality Disorders (SCID-II; Spitzer, Williams, Gibbon, & First, 1990) and the Diagnostic Interview for Personality Disorders (DIPD; Zanarini, Frankenburg, Chauncey, & Gunderson, 1987) are organized with respect to each *DSM-III-R* PD. Because there are advantages and disadvantages to each approach, the PDI-IV is organized both ways. One version is organized with respect to the *DSM-IV* PD disorders; the other version with respect to thematic content. For research purposes or other occasions when all of the PDs will be assessed, we generally prefer the thematic content format. However, for studies that are confined to one or more of the PDs, the format organized by disorder will be more suitable. Clinicians will likely prefer the organization by disorder.

The two formats (organized by disorder and by thematic content) provide the same questions, with only one exception. The question that asks if the person ever felt warm, tender, or sentimental toward someone was deleted from the thematic content assessment of the schizoid item of emotional coldness (item 7) because it was very inconsistent with the other questions being asked at that time. Also, by the time the interviewer reached this item (i.e., item 86 in the thematic content format), there would have been more than enough material to answer this question.

It will become apparent to anyone administering the PDI-IV within the thematic content format that there will be less need than in the case of the organization by disorder to administer all of the questions. The redundancy and overlap among the PD criteria become quite apparent when one assesses similar criteria at the same time. We considered simplifying the thematic content format by deleting all of the overlapping questions. However, this would substantially prejudge the overlap and differentiation among the items. By controlling which questions are used in what manner for each item, the interview would not allow the clinician or researcher to reach his or her own judgments with respect to this overlap and differentiation. We do provide our own recommendations for how the items can be differentiated, but we do this in the discussion of the issues and problems in the assessment of each item (presented below).

The thematic content areas include (a) Attitudes Toward Self, (b) Attitudes Toward Others, (c) Security or Comfort with Others, (d) Friendships and Relationships, (e) Conflicts and Disagreements, (f) Work and Leisure, (g) Social Norms, (h) Mood, and (i) Appearance and Perception. In one important respect, this thematic organization should not be taken too literally. The items have been organized and ordered across and within these sections to maximize a consistent and smooth flow to the interview, (i.e., we begin with attitudes toward oneself, followed by attitudes toward others, and end with items that require the observation of the person being assessed). As a result, one will find that some items do not fit conceptually well within the title for that section. For example, the borderline item of inappropriate or intense anger (BDL-8) is included within the Conflicts and Disagreements section (item 55 in the thematic content format), but one could argue that borderline rage is more of an issue of mood than of interpersonal conflict. We would not disagree. It was placed within the Conflict and Disagreement section because its assessment smoothly follows the antisocial item concerned with irritability and aggressiveness (ATS-C4) that does fit well within the section on Conflict and Disagreement. Likewise, "Appearance and Perception" does not really describe adequately all of the items included within this section (e.g., schizotypal "odd beliefs" and "magical thinking," or obsessive-compulsive "inability to discard worn out or worthless objects").

We do not consider our thematic content reorganization of the PD items to be random or entirely arbitrary, but it is very important not to take the reorganization too literally. A difficulty can arise when interviewers or raters who are unfamiliar with the *DSM-IV* PD criteria sets interpret the item with respect to the thematic content section in which it appears or with respect to the items that preceded it. An item taken out of its context and placed within a new context can have its meaning lost or significantly altered. For example, we include the obsessive-compulsive item concerned with the failure to discard worn out or worthless objects (OBC-5) within the section on Appearance and Perception (thematic content item 89). This section concerns unusual, odd behaviors (as well as physical appearance). However, the item is sandwiched between the two schizotypal items of odd beliefs (item 88) and unusual perceptual experiences (item 90). Both the interviewer and the subject may then misinterpret the obsessive-compulsive item as referring to an eccentric collection of peculiar, strange, or weird objects, rather than simply worn out, worthless objects. The only way to avoid this problem completely is to administer all of the items for a particular PD at the same time, the organization by disorder used in the other PDI-IV interview format. Contextual distortion of the meaning of an item is unavoidable when the criteria sets are reorganized. The interviewer who uses the thematic content format should remain sensitive to this issue during the administration and scoring of the respective items. One final note with respect to the thematic content format is that the total number of sets of questions (93) does not correspond to the total number of *DSM-IV* PD items (94) because two of the PD items were collapsed into one set of thematic questions (i.e., the item "lacks close friends" is virtually identical for the schizotypal and schizoid criteria sets).

The amount of time it takes to administer the PDI-IV varies substantially, depending primarily on the level of interest and manner of speech of the interviewee. Some persons will provide very perfunctory answers; others will provide extensive descriptions, discussion, and details for every single item. It has been our experience that the length of an interview will vary from 1 hour to 3 hours, with the majority of interviews requiring approximately 2 hours. However, this assumes an interviewer who has had extensive experience with the interview. As one becomes more experienced with the interview, one will become more fluent with the questions and more comfortable with skipping questions and/or scoring items on the basis of responses to prior questions.

As a final note with respect to the administration of the questions, we recommend that each interview begin with a general request for a description of the major events, issues, or incidents the person has experienced since late childhood or adolescence. The administration of any semistructured PD interview can degenerate into a superficial symptom count that provides only a fragmented, piecemeal description of isolated behaviors, attitudes, and affects (Perry, 1992; Widiger & Sanderson, in press-a). The clinician or researcher administering a semistructured interview might then simply obtain a long list of PD symptoms without any appreciation or even any awareness of their historical development, interrelationship, or social/environmental context. The request for a brief summary of the major events, issues, or incidents can lengthen an interview. However, it will also alert the interviewer to key incidents and issues that should be covered during the systematic questioning and assessment of individual PD items and provide a developmental or historical context for the individual PD items.

Problems and Issues in Assessment

The final section for each criterion discusses problems and issues we have often experienced in the assessment of the respective item. All of the *DSM-IV* PD criteria require some degree of judgment in their assessment, and there are many issues that complicate PD assessments. We discuss some of these issues in the next chapter (e.g., mood state distortions, differentiation of a PD from an Axis I mental disorder, and gender bias), but it is also useful to consider their impact and relevance to the assessment of individual items. This section is usually the longest and we expect the reader will find it is often the most useful.

RESEARCH AND CLINICAL APPLICATION

As noted above, the PDI-IV was constructed for use by both clinicians and researchers. However, as we discussed in the preface, the PDI-IV is a tool that will facilitate a reliable and valid assessment. It will not ensure that such an assessment will, in fact, be obtained.

We also wish to discuss here an additional, potential limitation of particular importance when the PDI-IV is used for research purposes. In the interest of providing the most valid assessment of a PD, we have, at times, provided more differentiation among PD items (across different PDs or within the criteria set for one PD) than is provided by the *DSM-IV* itself. If this increased differentiation is included within a study, the study would not be testing a literal application of each *DSM-IV* PD criterion.

Our provision of further specification and clarification with respect to the differentiation among items is no different than providing further clarification and specification of each individual item. For example, it is both a purpose and a benefit in a semistructured interview to specify what is meant by "lacks close friends" (a criterion for the schizoid PD). To the extent that this was unnecessary (i.e., the interpretation and application of this item was self-evident and consistent across all clinicians), there would be no need for a semistructured interview. A PD semistructured interview may define "lacks" as having only one or two friends; it may define "close" as providing personal or confidential information; and it may define "friends" as excluding colleagues at work (cf. DIPD, PDE, SCID-II, or SIDP-R). Any person that uses a semistructured interview is assessing a more specific version of the *DSM-IV* PD criteria than is provided by the *DSM-IV* itself. The PD semistructured interviews provide somewhat different results, partly because of the variations in how they operationalize each of the PD criteria (Clark, 1992; Skodol, Oldham, Rosnick, Kellman, & Hyler, 1991; Zimmerman, 1994).

A major focus of the *DSM-III-R* PD revisions (Widiger, Frances, Spitzer, & Williams, 1988) and the *DSM-IV* PD revisions (Gunderson, in press-b) has been to facilitate the differentiation among the personality disorders. This is accomplished primarily through revising the criteria so that they will be more specific or unique to each PD (Gunderson, in press-b). This will be readily apparent in the PDI-IV discussion of the rationale for each item's revision. *DSM-III*, *DSM-III-R*, and *DSM-IV* also include a differential diagnosis section in the text discussion of each PD to facilitate further differentiation among the individual PDs. The PDI-IV provides this type of discussion and recommendation at the item level. That is, we often note how an item should be assessed to maximize differentiation between particular PDs and between the items within a criteria set for a single PD.

For example, the avoidant item, being "inhibited in new interpersonal situations because of feelings of inadequacy" ([APA, 1994, p. 665] AVD-5), overlaps substantially with other avoidant items (e.g., AVD-2, "is unwilling to get involved with people unless certain of being liked" [APA, 1994, p. 665]). We, therefore, indicate how these items can be differentiated (e.g., AVD-2 would concern inhibitions with respect to the initiation of new relationships, whereas AVD-5 would concern inhibitions that might occur during a new relationship). Redundancy and overlap among items within the same criteria set should be minimized to ensure that the assessment is not confined to a narrow range of behavior and is, indeed, assessing a pervasive behavior pattern (Millon, 1986, 1991b). Each item should assess a different aspect of the personality and/or behavior pattern.

Similarly, we discuss how the avoidant PD item, being "preoccupied with being criticized or rejected in social situations" ([APA, 1994, p. 665] AVD-4), may be endorsed, at times, by dependent persons because they, too, will be preoccupied with concerns about being rejected. However, we also note that the intention of the item was to assess for preoccupations with being criticized or rejected in everyday social situations, rather than with the loss of a major source of nurturance and support (e.g., preoccupation with fears of a divorce). We then discourage the coding of this avoidant item as present if the interviewee's preoccupation concerns the fear that a current (sexual) relationship is failing.

These suggestions will be helpful both to the clinician who wishes to identify the PD diagnosis that is most descriptive or accurate in characterizing a patient and to the researcher who wishes to obtain relatively homogenous samples of a particular PD. However, they will be problematic to the researcher who wishes to assess the degree of overlap and confusion among the PD criteria. The PDI-IV attempts to minimize this overlap and confusion by providing further instruction. However, this "limitation" is readily addressed by simply ignoring these additional instructions. This would be comparable to not using a semistructured interview in order to provide a more exact test of the (lack of) specificity or clarity within the *DSM-IV* PD criteria. As noted above, any study that uses a semistructured interview is assessing a more specific version of the *DSM-IV* PD criteria. It is for this reason that we placed the word limitation within quotation marks. We do not really consider the advice on how to differentiate among the PD items a limitation; it simply reflects another advantage and purpose of using a semistructured interview.

TRAINING AND EXPERTISE

The first version of the PDI-IV (i.e., the PIQ-I) was administered by lay persons (i.e., undergraduate college seniors). This has since been misinterpreted as suggesting that the

PIQ was constructed to be administered by lay (nonprofessional) interviewers. The PIQ-I was not constructed to be used by lay interviewers; it was used by lay interviewers for the special advantages to research that they provided. An interview constructed to be administered and scored by lay persons would have to require little to no clinical (professional) judgment (this issue is discussed further in the next chapter), and this has not been the case with the PIQ-I or the PDI-IV. The PIQ-I was administered by lay interviewers in a series of empirical studies (e.g., Widiger et al., 1986) because these interviewers had the advantage of lacking assumptions, experience, and prior knowledge that would substantially bias the findings of the study (Widiger & Frances, 1987). However, the employment of these interviewers required substantial training and continuous supervision, much more than would have been necessary if experienced or knowledgeable interviewers had been employed. It has been our experience that lay interviewers do not really save research time and effort, given their considerable training and supervision needs. It is our opinion that the PDI-IV could also be administered by lay interviewers if the advantages of such interviewers outweighed the disadvantages, but they would still need substantial training and supervision. In such cases, the final scoring of each item should always be provided by an experienced clinician, as was the case with the original PIQ-I studies.

The PDI-IV can be administered and scored by an experienced clinician without additional specialized training. Ideally, the PDI-IV would be administered and scored by a professional clinician trained and experienced in the diagnosis and assessment of mental disorders. However, in research we have often used graduate students with a master's degree in clinical or counseling psychology who have received close training in its administration and scoring (e.g., Widiger, Freiman, et al., 1990). No matter who is used, the successful administration and scoring of the PDI-IV depends substantially upon the skills and abilities of the interviewer. The more talented, dependable, and insightful the interviewer, the better the results. And, frankly, these traits are difficult to assess objectively in oneself. A limitation we have found with experienced clinicians is that some will have strong opinions regarding how a particular PD should be diagnosed that will be at variance with the *DSM-IV* criteria or with the interpretation of these criteria by the PDI-IV. It can be easier to train the less experienced clinician than the more experienced clinician. It is our impression that the most important variable may not be the amount of experience, but, rather, the open-mindedness of the trainee.

In sum, we are not suggesting that only the most insightful, experienced, or knowledgeable clinicians should use the PDI-IV. We are making the point that one cannot assume that an administration of the PDI-IV will ensure the obtainment of a reliable and valid finding. The administration of the PDI-IV can facilitate reliable and valid assessments but, as we have indicated before, it will not ensure that a reliable and valid assessment will be obtained. The purpose of the PDI-IV is to inform and to help guide the clinician making PD assessments. The PDI-IV will be helpful to any clinician who wishes to make PD assessments. (It would, in fact, be most helpful to those with the least familiarity with PD assessments.) The discussion of the rationale for each item as well as common issues or problems in their assessment will be helpful in assessment.

Again, it should also be acknowledged that a clinician may provide a more valid assessment by rejecting a specific PDI-IV instruction or guideline. The PDI-IV is not the final word. The same point, of course, applies to the *DSM-IV* itself. Nowhere in the *DSM-IV* is it stated that the clinician must adhere to all the diagnostic criteria that are provided. "The specific diagnostic criteria included in *DSM-IV* are meant to serve as guidelines to be informed by clinical judgment and are not meant to be used in a cookbook fashion" (APA, 1994, p. xxiii). There will be times when it is wise and proper to deviate from the diagnostic manual. On the other hand, it is obvious that the clinician at least should be informed by the *DSM-IV* criteria, given the experience and research that informed the development of the *DSM-IV* criteria and their acceptance by most organizations and institutions (Frances, Pincus, Widiger, Davis, & First, 1990; Widiger, Frances, Pincus, Davis, & First, 1991). Likewise, we also believe that the clinician will be informed by the PDI-IV given the experience and research that informed its development (presented within this text).

It is also noted within the same paragraph in *DSM-IV* as the above quotation that "lack of familiarity with *DSM-IV* or excessively flexible and idiosyncratic application of *DSM-IV* criteria or conventions substantially reduces its utility as a common language for communication" (APA, 1994, p. xxiii) and that "the diagnostic categories, criteria, and textual descriptions are meant to be employed by individuals with appropriate clinical training and experience in diagnosis" (APA, 1994, p. xxiii). "The proper use of these criteria requires specialized clinical training that provides both a body of knowledge and clinical skills" (APA, 1994, p. xxvii). Clinicians and researchers who stray from the guidelines provided in *DSM-IV* or the PDI-IV may, indeed, obtain a more valid assessment but, again, such deviations should be explicitly noted. As we indicated earlier, an advantage of a semi-structured interview is not only to facilitate the obtainment of replicable and reliable assessments through the adherence to the instructions and guidelines provided therein, but also to facilitate the awareness and documentation of any deviation from a uniform, standard, or accepted approach. Because the approaches taken by the PDI-IV are explicit, any deviation from the approach is readily noticed and documented.

Interview trainees should have already completed formal training in the diagnosis and assessment of mental disorders (e.g., within a graduate program of psychology or a psychiatric residency training program). Our training of PDI-IV interviewers typically begins by having each interviewer (e.g., master's level graduate students in clinical or counseling psychology, psychiatric residents, or psychiatric social workers or nurses) first study (a) the *DSM-IV* (APA, 1994), (b) recent articles on the diagnosis or assessment of PDs (a sample of some of the more recent articles and chapters on assessment or diagnosis include: Benjamin, 1993; Blashfield, 1984; Clark, 1992; Clark, Watson, & Reynolds, in press; Costa & McCrae, 1992a; Grove & Tellegen, 1991; Gunderson, 1992; Hirschfeld, 1993; Kaelber & Maser, 1992; M. H. Klein, 1993; Livesley, 1991; Livesley, Schroeder, Jackson, & Jang, 1994; Loranger, 1992; Millon, 1991b; Oldham, 1987; Perry, 1992; Reich, 1985, 1987, 1989; Shea, 1992; Skodol, 1989b; Tyrer, 1988; Widiger, Frances, & Trull, 1989; Widiger & Sanderson, in press-a; Zimmerman, 1993b, 1994), and (c) the PDI-IV interview and this manual. We meet for two to three sessions to discuss issues and questions raised by this literature. Interviewers then conduct pilot interviews with each other or with volunteers (e.g., hospital staff or college students), each of which is taped in order to be scored by the other raters and/or interviewers and to be reviewed by the principal investigator (or clinical supervisor). We then review all items for which there was some disagreement in scoring, as well as any additional items or responses that an interviewer or rater found problematic. Next, the interviewers conduct pilot interviews with 5 to 10 patients; each interview is again taped, scored, and reviewed in detail. We also recommend that the taping and item reviews continue throughout any data collection. Idiosyncratic drift may develop during data collection, and it is impossible to anticipate all possible problems, issues, and questions during the training (or within this manual). The problems and issues discussed within this manual were based on our experiences in interviewing hundreds of persons, but we expect that the reader will discover a failure to address an important issue. We encourage readers to send us, in care of the publisher, any suggestions they might have for improving the interview or the manual in future editions.

2

Issues in Assessment and the PDI-IV

There are many PD semistructured interviews that assess all of the *DSM-IV* PDs, including the DIPD (Zanarini et al., 1987), PDE (Loranger, 1988), SCID-II (Spitzer et al., 1990), SIDP-R (Pfohl et al., 1989), and the Personality Assessment Form (PAF; Shea, Glass, Pilkonis, Watkins, & Docherty, 1987). There are also some interviews that are confined to individual *DSM-IV* PDs, including the DIB-R (Zanarini et al., 1989), the Diagnostic Interview for Narcissism (DIN; Gunderson, Ronningstam, & Bodkin, 1990), and the Diagnostic Interview for Depressive Personality (DIDP; Phillips & Gunderson, 1990). (Most of these citations concern the *DSM-III-R* versions; it is anticipated that each will have been revised for *DSM-IV*.) There have also been many reviews of these instruments and overviews of the assessment of personality disorders (e.g., Benjamin, 1993; Clark, 1992; Klein, 1993; Oldham, 1987; Perry, 1992; Reich, 1985, 1987, 1989; Standage, 1989; Tyrer, Casey, & Ferguson, 1991; Widiger & Frances, 1987; Widiger et al., 1989; Widiger & Sanderson, in press-a; Zimmerman, 1994). The number of semistructured interviews that are now available and the number of overviews and reviews of their assessment is itself a testament to the importance as well as the complexity of personality disorder assessment. Most patients will have clinically significant maladaptive personality traits (Widiger & Corbitt, in press-b; Widiger & Rogers, 1989), but their diagnosis is fraught with many issues and problems. We believe it is important for the clinician and the researcher to be cognizant of these issues when administering the PDI-IV. Therefore, this chapter provides a brief overview of some of these issues, including mood state distortions, Axis II versus Axis I, traits versus situations, distortions in attributions, age of onset and duration, multiple diagnoses, self versus informant ratings, self-report inventories, and gender, culture, and ethnicity.

MOOD STATE DISTORTIONS

The effect of a person's mood state on his or her self-description is one of the better-documented problems in the assessment of maladaptive personality traits (Widiger, 1993b). No overview of the assessment of PDs fails to address this issue. Persons who are depressed, anxious, angry, manic, hypomanic, or even simply agitated for some specific reason are unlikely to provide an entirely accurate self-description; indeed, they may provide a very distorted and inaccurate self-description. For example, persons who are depressed will tend to describe themselves as being more dependent, introverted, self-conscious, vulnerable, and pessimistic than they would have prior to the onset of their depression (Barnett & Gotlib, 1988). Low self-esteem, hopelessness, and negativism are common features of depression, and they will naturally affect a person's self-description.

Distortions will continue even after remission of the more obvious, florid symptoms of depression (Hirschfeld et al., 1989).

The distortions provided by extreme mood states are particularly problematic for self-report inventories or, to put this in a more positive light, they are less problematic for a clinical interview (Perry, 1992; Reich, 1985, 1989; Widiger & Frances, 1987). Interviewers may be able to judge whether a self-description is being distorted by a subject's depressed, anxious, manic, or angry mood (Loranger, Lenzenweger, et al., 1991). To this end, it is useful and important to remind subjects continually that the questions refer to their typical or everyday functioning prior to the onset of whatever disorder or issue is currently troubling them (e.g., prior to becoming depressed or prior to a current divorce). Subjects will often forget this point as the interview progresses, and they will readily slide back into a self-description that reflects primarily their current mood.

However, it is also important to realize that semistructured interview assessments are not immune to the distortions of current mood states (Ames-Frankel et al., 1992; O'Boyle & Self, 1990; Ricciardi et al., 1992; Stuart, Simons, Thase, & Pilkonis, 1992). They will generally be more resilient than a self-report inventory, but they will not be immune. An interviewer can easily fail to appreciate the extent to which a person's current mood is affecting the self-description. For this reason, it is particularly important to ask for concrete examples or illustrations of the PD items. For example, depressed or anxious persons may describe themselves as having rapidly shifting emotions (HST-3) or feeling helpless when alone (DEP-6), but it can become apparent from the examples they provide of these traits that the behaviors are secondary to their mood disorder or clearly demonstrate a confusion between how they are currently feeling and how they have typically felt throughout much of their adult life.

It is also helpful to verify one's assessments of a subject by interviewing someone who knows the person well or has observed the person prior to the onset of the current mood (e.g., relatives, spouse, lover, friend, or colleague). These "informants" (as they are commonly referred to in the PD research literature) may even have a clear perception of the change in the person's behavior pattern that occurred with the onset of an Axis I disorder or situational episode.

AXIS I VERSUS AXIS II

The mood state distortion issue raises a related problem, the confusion of an Axis I mental disorder (e.g., mood, anxiety, or schizophrenic disorder) with an Axis II personality disorder. These are not always the same problem. Both can involve, for example, the confusion of a depression with a borderline PD, but the mood state issue would concern the (pathoplastic) effect of a depressed mood on the subject's description of borderline traits, whereas the Axis I issue would concern the interviewer's confusion of a symptom of depression with a symptom of a personality disorder. An example of a mood state distortion would be a manic person (inaccurately) denying the presence of any feelings of ineptness, inadequacy, or inferiority (AVD-6); an example of the Axis I confusion would be a clinician (inaccurately) diagnosing the presence of narcissistic grandiosity (NAR-1) on the basis of this expression of manic denial. The distinction between the two errors will, at times, be subtle. For example, a depressed person may say that he or she has always experienced chronic feelings of emptiness. If this statement is false due to the depressed mood, then it is a mood state distortion. However, the statement could be true and still not represent the borderline trait, "chronic feelings of emptiness," (APA, 1994, p. 654) if these feelings were secondary to a chronic (or episodic) depression.

The differentiation of Axis I versus Axis II disorders is itself a controversial and unresolved issue (Clark, Watson, & Mineka, 1994; Livesley et al., 1994; Oldham & Skodol, 1992; Widiger, 1989; Widiger & Shea, 1991). As just one example, consider the distinction between Axis I generalized social phobia and avoidant PD (Herbert, Hope, & Bellack, 1992; Holt, Heimberg, & Hope, 1992; Turner, Beidel, & Townsley, 1992; Widiger, 1992a). We will present the issues regarding this particular distinction in some detail to demonstrate the difficulties with the conceptual distinction between Axis I and Axis II that will, in turn, have a substantial impact on their differential diagnosis.

Social phobia is an anxiety disorder that involves "a marked and persistent fear of social or performance situations in which embarrassment may occur" (APA, 1994, p. 411). The person fears that he or she will act in a way that will be embarrassing or humiliating (APA, 1994). If the person fears, or becomes anxious within most social situations, this is considered to represent a "generalized" subtype of social phobia (APA, 1994). The avoidant PD, on the other hand, involves a pervasive pattern of social inhibition, feelings of inadequacy, and hypersensitivity to negative evaluations (APA, 1994). It is, perhaps, self-evident that fearing to act in a way that will be embarrassing or humiliating within most social situations will often overlap with feelings of social inhibition, inadequacy, and hypersensitivity to negative evaluations. The distinction between avoidant PD and generalized social phobia (GSP) is tenuous at best, particularly since GSP is said to be chronic and evident since childhood, "emerging out of a childhood history of social inhibition or shyness" (APA, 1994, p. 414).

In the earlier editions of the *DSM*, there was a much more confident and clear distinction between the social phobic anxiety disorder and the avoidant personality disorder. Social phobia was a new diagnosis to the *DSM-III* (Spitzer, Williams, & Skodol, 1980). In its original formulation, there was no generalized subtype, and it was considered to be quite circumscribed in its presentation. "Examples of Social Phobias are fears of speaking or performing in public, using public lavatories, eating in public, and writing in the presence of others. Generally, an individual has only one Social Phobia" (APA, 1980, p. 227). *DSM-III* excluded the diagnosis of social phobia in the presence of an avoidant PD because it was recognized that the social phobic behavior in such persons would represent expressions or manifestations of their avoidant personality traits. Just as antisocial persons tend to be reckless and to use drugs, borderline persons tend to be emotionally unstable and impulsive, narcissistic persons tend to be arrogant, and avoidant persons tend to become anxious and nervous when attention is focused upon them. However, it became apparent to anxiety disorder researchers and specialists that the phobic behavior of many of their patients would often fail to be circumscribed. Many of the persons who sought treatment from anxiety disorder specialists had much more generalized and pervasive patterns of social inhibition than was described within *DSM-III* (Spitzer & Williams, 1985). In our opinion, many of these persons probably did have an avoidant PD but they would enter or be referred to anxiety disorder clinics because their fear and anxiety was a prominent and/or immediate concern (just as many persons with antisocial PD will seek treatment for a substance use disorder, and borderline PD for a mood disorder). In any case, the generalized social phobia diagnosis was then developed in *DSM-III-R* to adequately describe these patients from the perspective of the anxiety disorder specialist (Spitzer & Williams, 1985).

Anxiety disorder specialists argued that it was best to consider these persons as suffering from an anxiety disorder rather than from a personality disorder because their symptoms would often diminish (but never be fully treated or cured) by pharmacologic interventions. Liebowitz (1992), the chair of the *DSM-IV* Anxiety Disorders Work Group, expressed this position well. "One may have to rethink what the personality disorder concept means in an instance where 6 weeks of phenelzine therapy begins to reverse long-standing interpersonal hypersensitivity as well as discomfort in socializing" (p. 251). Liebowitz was purportedly concerned that a personality disorder diagnosis would result in poor or inadequate treatment. "The danger…is that, in my experience, practitioners tend to regard Axis II conditions as amenable to psychoanalytic psychotherapy rather than pharmacotherapy or behavioral approaches" (Liebowitz, 1992, p. 251).

However, there are a number of difficulties with this argument. Indeed, one will observe a misbegotten and mistaken assumption that an Axis II disorder implies the presence of a psychosocial rather than a biogenetic etiology and an intervention using an insight-oriented psychotherapy rather than a pharmacotherapy (Gunderson & Pollack, 1985). However, we would suggest that this misleading and inaccurate stereotype is being expressed and endorsed by Liebowitz (1992), rather than by any particular practitioner. Such false distinctions should be discouraged because personality disorders do, indeed, have a substantial biogenetic component and will be responsive to pharmacologic interventions (Siever & Davis, 1991). But, the misleading distinction will not be corrected by revising the nomenclature so that conditions that respond to the pharmacology that is commonly used to treat anxiety disorders are considered to be an anxiety disorder. This would only encourage, condone, and affirm the false distinction.

Responsivity to the pharmacology that is commonly used to treat anxiety disorders does not necessarily suggest the presence of an anxiety disorder. The average person who has no anxiety disorder will experience relief from antianxiety medications. As Liebowitz has acknowledged elsewhere, "anxiety reactions are ubiquitous phenomena of normal human life" (Gorman, Liebowitz, & Shear, 1992, p. 1). Gorman et al. (1992) also suggest that "all patients with psychiatric illness experience pathologic anxiety" (p. 1). All patients and all persons would experience relief from this anxiety through anti-anxiety medications and would then presumably have anxiety disorders.

In addition, these medications do not always treat (let alone cure) the pathology of an anxiety disorder or any other mental disorder in which anxiety is present. They block, inhibit, or impair the neurochemistry that results in the experience of anxiety. They can be very effective in blocking the experience of anxiety, but the basis or source for the neurochemistry may not be treated at all. This is one reason that the treatment is rarely comprehensive in its effects and must often be sustained to maintain its effects (Gorman et al., 1992). Many of the features of a generalized social phobia and an avoidant PD (e.g., shyness, insecurity, and inhibition) do not reflect simply the dysregulation of the neurochemistry of anxiety. Altering this neurochemistry to help control or minimize feelings of anxiety will indeed be helpful to the person with an avoidant personality disorder or with GSP, but it may not resolve or even address the actual cause or source of the shyness, insecurity, and feelings of anxiousness.

The mistaken assumption that responsivity to treatment implies the presence of a disorder (and a particular disorder at that) has led to a further broadening of social phobia in *DSM-IV*. Liebowitz (1992) has been critical of the term "phobia" because it implies the presence of a circumscribed stimulus. Phobia is defined in the *DSM-IV* as a "persistent, irrational fear of a specific object, activity, or situation (the phobic stimulus)" (APA, 1994, p. 770). It is the specificity of the fear that distinguishes the phobia from other anxiety disorders, such as the (nonspecific) generalized anxiety disorder. It is then somewhat paradoxical to have a generalized subtype for a phobia. Given that the anxious, inhibited, and avoidant behavior of persons with generalized social phobia will often pervade most, if not all, social situations, and that pharmacology can reduce all forms of social anxiety, Liebowitz (1992) recommended replacing the label of social phobia with "social anxiety disorder" (p. 251). This proposal was partially approved by the *DSM-IV* Task Force in that the label of social anxiety is now placed in parentheses after social phobia in *DSM-IV* (APA, 1994, p. 411). Full approval of this proposal was rejected partly because of concerns for unanticipated repercussions that may arise from the suggestion that any and all experiences of social anxiety represent an anxiety disorder (e.g., Kramer, 1993).

The *DSM-IV* PD Work Group attempted to help differentiate AVD PD from GSP through item revision. The *DSM-III-R* criteria for avoidant PD had included items that explicitly described GSP symptomatology (e.g., fears being embarrassed by blushing or showing signs of anxiety in front of other people; APA, 1987). The deletion of such items might be helpful in reducing artifactual co-occurrence and in improving their differentiation (Millon, 1991a), but it is also quite important to recognize that the criteria that were deleted were and still are characteristic of persons with an avoidant PD. They were not deleted because they were not commonly seen in persons with avoidant PD; they were deleted because they were also characteristic of persons with GSP. No clear distinction between avoidant PD and GSP may actually be possible, at least for those cases that are sitting on the nebulous and overlapping boundary between GSP and avoidant PD (Herbert et al., 1992; Holt et al., 1992; Turner et al., 1992; Widiger, 1992a).

The personality disorders are not alone with respect to this problem. There is no clear boundary between many mental disorders (Blacker & Tsuang, 1992; Clark, Watson, & Reynolds, in press; Widiger & Trull, 1991). Is schizoaffective disorder a schizophrenic or a mood disorder; is *DSM-IV* mixed anxiety-depression a mood or an anxiety disorder; is hypochondriasis an anxiety or a somatoform disorder; is conversion disorder a somatoform or a dissociative disorder; and are posttraumatic stress and acute stress disorders an anxiety or a dissociative disorder (Clark et al., in press)? It would be preferable for these diagnoses to be given hybrid codes that would indicate that they contain features of both types of disorders. For example, it would be informative to consider hypochondriasis as involving both an anxiety and a somatoform disorder, and post-traumatic stress disorder as involving both symptoms and pathology of anxiety and dissociation. However, due to the ICD-10 and *DSM-IV* coding restraints, such hybrid conditions cannot be recognized. We must consider the condition to be either an anxiety or a dissociative disorder, not both. Thus, we must then make distinctions that are often inaccurate and misleading.

The issues and problems we have noted above with respect to the distinction between AVD PD and GSP also apply to the distinction between early onset dysthymia and depressive PD (Akiskal & Akiskal, 1992; Keller, 1989; Phillips, Gunderson, Hirschfeld, & Smith, 1990), substance related disorders and antisocial PD (Alterman & Cacciola, 1991; Gerstley, Alterman, McLellan, & Woody, 1990), impulse or mood disorders and borderline PD (Gunderson & Phillips, 1991; Widiger, 1989), and schizophrenia and schizotypal PD (Siever & Davis, 1991; Widiger & Shea, 1991). We will discuss these (and other) Axis I versus Axis II differential diagnoses throughout the PDI-IV as they become relevant in the assessment of individual PD items. In most cases, we provide suggestions to facilitate a differential diagnosis (e.g., see the discussion for ATS-A6, AVD-1, BDL-4, and SZT-1). Whenever possible, it is important and useful to provide a differential diagnosis. One general rule of thumb is to determine whether the behavior pattern has, indeed, been evident since late childhood, and not to assume that the way the person appears now has been the way the person has been throughout much of his or her adult life. On the other hand, one should also avoid the assumption that a differential diagnosis must be possible, thereby forcing a misleading distinction that does not, in fact, occur. We do indicate when no clear differentiation may be possible for individual PD items (e.g., ATS-A5). One will often find that it is best to simply provide both diagnoses, thereby retaining the information that both a specific Axis I disorder and chronic, pervasive maladaptive personality traits are present.

TRAITS VERSUS SITUATIONS

People tend to act in a consistent manner across a wide variety of situations (Digman, 1990; McCrae & Costa, 1990; Wiggins & Pincus, 1992), and persons with a personality disorder tend to be even less flexible than most other persons (Millon, 1981). However, this is not to say that persons, including those with a *DSM-IV* personality disorder, are unresponsive to the influence, press, or demands of a particular situation. Antisocial persons may restrain their impulsivity and aggressivity during therapeutic sessions, paranoid persons may suppress their suspicious antagonism when speaking to a police officer, and dependent persons may, at times, rebel against their exploitation. What tends to be more problematic in the assessment of PDs, though, is the attribution of maladaptive personality traits in persons who are primarily reacting to a situational demand, pressure, or context (Widiger & Frances, 1987, 1988).

The two *DSM-III-R* PDs for which this had been most problematic have been the self-defeating and the passive-aggressive (Widiger et al., 1989), and it is no coincidence that both were demoted in *DSM-IV*. Passive-aggressive PD was transferred from the set of officially recognized PDs to the appendix of criteria sets provided for further study, and self-defeating PD was deleted entirely from the manual. These decisions were due, in large part, to the concern that their attribution has or would reflect a confusion of situational reactions with enduring personality traits. To illustrate this problem, we will discuss the concerns regarding the passive-aggressive PD. Our attention will focus on the passive-aggressive rather than the self-defeating as the former is still included within the manual. We will briefly discuss the decision concerning the self-defeating PD diagnosis in the next chapter.

Passive-aggressive PD was included in the very first edition of the *DSM* (APA, 1952). However, this first edition of the *DSM* was influenced heavily by the nomenclatures developed within the Armed Forces and the Veterans Administration, and it was within the Armed Forces nomenclature that the passive-aggressive PD obtained its initial recognition and support (Millon, 1981). This is not meant as a denigration of these early nomenclatures, but it is quite possible that passive-aggressive behavior was not an uncommon situational reaction to the extreme discipline and deference to authority that is necessary within the armed services. It would not be surprising to find that many persons fight, oppose, or rebel against military authority in subtle, indirect, or passive ways that are not evident in their relationships prior or subsequent to their military service. Overt, direct, and obvious rebellion within such settings would only elicit more burden and trouble. Persons will, therefore, express their resistance indirectly by dawdling, procrastinating, "forgetting," or other expressions of intentional inefficiency and incompetency (i.e., the *DSM-III* criteria for passive-aggressive PD; APA, 1980). Passive-aggressive PD was, in fact, said to account for 6% of all psychiatric admissions to army hospitals in World War II, the largest percent for any character behavior disorder (Malinow, 1981).

It is a common error to mistakenly attribute the behavior of others to personality traits and to neglect or miss the contribution of situational factors (Mischel, 1984). The other person provides the figure that captures our attention, and we miss the contextual or situational ground that may have been the primary factor in determining the person's behavior. It is then quite possible that the preponderance of passive-aggressive PD diagnoses during World War II was excessive. The same difficulties with this diagnosis may occur today. One will also observe a substantial amount of passive-aggressive resistance to the authority, rules, and demands within inpatient, forensic, prison, and other institutional settings wherein the population has lost the authority, freedom, or power they held prior to their admission. These persons may be acting consistently in a passive-aggressive manner, but this apparent consistency could be confined largely to their behavior within the institution. They may not be passive-aggressive at work, at home, or within other settings and situations.

The confusion of situational reactions with personality traits is not confined to the passive-aggressive PD. It is important in the assessment of all of the PDs to verify the presence of the behavior patterns across a variety of situations, a point we often note in our discussion of individual PD items. For example, we indicate how PND-1 concerns relationships with friends or associates, whereas PND-7 concerns sexual relationships or lovers, and suggest that manifestations of paranoid ideation with respect to relatives be considered for other paranoid PD items. Similar suggestions are made for the avoidant PD criteria to maximize not only the independence of their assessment but the extent to which the assessment considers a full range of situations and contexts (cf. discussion for AVD-5).

Complicating this issue, however, is the fact that some situations may serve to potentiate or highlight personality trait dispositions. A personality trait is the disposition to respond in a particular manner within certain situations (Levy, 1983). Dependency, for example, will be much more evident with a spouse than with an employer. It may, indeed, be evident within the relationship with an employer, but it will be much more evident within the relationship with a spouse. Likewise, passive-aggressive negativism will be more evident with an employer than with a friend, and avoidant traits will be more evident when the person is alone than when the person is involved with someone (Trull, Widiger, & Frances, 1987). Gunderson (1987) described well how different borderline traits will vary in prominence depending upon the status of the person's current relationship (e.g., feelings of emptiness when the other person is being nurturant, anger and manipulation when the other person expresses his or her own needs, and suicidality when the other person appears to be separating). The importance of a particular situation to the assessment of an individual PD criterion is usually noted within its description (e.g., the DEP-7 can be assessed only within the context of the ending of a close relationship), but we also indicate when some situations that are not highlighted in the description of the item should still be emphasized in its assessment (e.g., lack of empathy, NAR-7).

TRAITS, ACTS, AND ATTRIBUTIONS

Replicable, reliable assessments are obtained by curtailing and minimizing clinical (informed but subjective) inference and judgment (Matarazzo, 1983; Spitzer, 1983). The extent to which individual (professional) judgment is required or allowed is the extent to which there is room for disagreement. Behaviorally specific and explicit criteria were, therefore, developed for *DSM-III* to minimize the influence of idiosyncratic judgments and opinions. "In *DSM-I* and *DSM-II*...the clinician [was] to a large degree on his or her own in defining the content and boundaries of the diagnostic categories, since explicit detailed definitions [were] not provided" (Spitzer et al., 1980, p. 154). Semistructured interviews were developed to curtail even further the occurrence of unreliable, variable, and idiosyncratic interpretations and assessments of these criteria (Spitzer, 1983; Wiens, 1990).

There is, however, some irony in this effort because a fully structured assessment is, itself, undesirable. A fully structured interview would be comparable to simply reading and recording the responses to a self-report inventory. The role of the interviewer would be confined to providing an occasional clarification. The Diagnostic Interview Schedule (DIS; Robins, Helzer, Croughan, & Ratcliff, 1981), which includes an assessment of *DSM-III* antisocial PD, is perhaps the most structured of interviews. It is highly structured because it was developed to be administered by lay persons to large numbers of subjects in the National Institute of Mental Health's (NIMH) Epidemiologic Catchment Area (ECA) study (Regier et al., 1988). If a person with little to no professional background is administering an interview, one would have to minimize the extent to which clinical (professional) judgment is necessary to interpret and code responses. However, this curtailment of clinical judgment by the DIS has received substantial criticism (Perry, 1992; Perry, Lavori, Cooper, Hoke, & O'Connell, 1987). It may provide very reliable diagnoses, but it may not provide the most valid diagnoses. Perry et al. suggested, in particular, a tendency of the DIS to overdiagnose antisocial PD because the assessments often take the statements of the subjects at face value, failing to consider extenuating circumstances or to determine whether the symptoms were clinically meaningful.

The authors of *DSM-III*, *DSM-III-R*, and *DSM-IV* have been aware of this problem, and they have acknowledged that the PD criteria cannot be constructed in fully specific, behavioral terms. In *DSM-III-R*, it was stated that "for some disorders, ...particularly the Personality Disorders, the criteria require much more inference on the part of the observer"

(APA, 1987, p. xxiii). In *DSM-IV*, it is stated more generally that "it is important that *DSM-IV* not be applied mechanically by untrained individuals. The specific diagnostic criteria included in *DSM-IV* are meant to serve as guidelines to be informed by clinical judgment and are not meant to be used in a cookbook fashion" (APA, 1994, p. xxiii).

The role of the PDI-IV interviewer is to assess for the traits or symptoms of each PD, not to mindlessly ask if each PD criterion is present and then simply record each response. The PDI-IV is a semistructured interview, not a structured interview. It is not realistic to assess each PD criterion by simply asking if the behavior pattern is present. Persons will vary substantially in their willingness to provide a forthright and honest self-description, in their self-insight and self-awareness, and in their understanding of the concepts and terms. Sometimes, this is quite obvious. For example, one would not ask interviewees if they have an identity disturbance (BDL-3). However, one will often be surprised at how much misunderstanding and misinterpretation can occur. For example, it is tempting to assess the schizoid PD criterion, "lacks close friends or confidants other than first-degree relatives" ([APA, 1994, p. 641] SZD-5), by simply asking persons if they have no close friends or confidants. But people, particularly those with a personality disorder, who are characterized, in part, by the presence of distorted views of themselves and others (Benjamin, 1993; Kernberg, 1984b; Kiesler, 1991; Stone, 1993), may have a very different understanding of what is meant by a close friend or confidant. We have found that some schizoid persons will say that they have close friends, but never visit them, never invite them over to visit, never go out with them, and never talk to them about anything personal. To some, a close friend means anyone whom they have known on a first-name basis for longer than a few years. The most extreme example was when one schizoid person said she had seven very close friends with whom she discussed and shared her personal fears and insecurities, and upon inquiry, it was discovered that she was referring to her cats.

Many narcissistic persons will likewise deny their faults and foibles, and may not be particularly aware of their grandiosity, conceit, arrogance, or lack of empathy. Histrionic, borderline, and dependent persons, on the other hand, have a tendency to exaggerate their symptomatology. Histrionic persons will be unaware of the extent to which they need to be the center of attention, or at least they would not acknowledge feeling uncomfortable when they are not the center of attention (i.e., HST-1). Antisocial persons will, at times, deceive the interviewer simply for their own amusement and pleasure.

Reliance on self-descriptions is complicated further by the fact that most, if not all, of the PD items involve traits that are undesirable and/or laden with personal, emotional significance. It is, perhaps, unrealistic to expect even the average person to be sufficiently insightful and forthright to provide an entirely valid self-description with respect to socially undesirable traits and foibles. This is why self-report inventories include validity scales (i.e., scales to detect the denial or exaggeration of traits and symptoms) (Berry, Wetter, & Baer, in press). The PDI-IV does not include a validity scale, nor does any other PD semistructured interview. (There is, however, a structured interview designed to detect malingering and other forms of feigning symptoms of psychopathology: the Structured Interview of Reported Symptoms, or SIRS, by Rogers, Bagby, & Dickens, 1993). The reason is that an assessment of the veridicality of a response is inherent in the assessment of each item. One should be skeptical and cautious in assessing each PD criterion, never simply accepting a subject's affirmation or denial of a trait at face value. One is assessing for the presence of the respective trait, not the opinions of the respondent.

A rule of thumb that will apply to almost all of the PDI-IV item assessments is to ask for examples or illustrations. It is not enough, for example, to simply ask whether the person is unable to make everyday decisions without an excessive amount of advice and reassurance from others (DEP-1). One should ask for examples or illustrations of what the interviewee meant by an "everyday" decision or "excessive" advice or reassurance. The request for examples should be almost habitual throughout the interview.

Many of the PDI-IV questions should be understood as initial inquiries. They are not intended to provide operational definitions of a criterion, such that they are always meant to be fully sufficient for an item's assessment. We have found the questions to be very helpful and effective in eliciting the most relevant and informative responses, but additional inquiry will often be necessary.

Many of the questions are also indirect. We will, at times, use probes or questions that can stimulate the expression or display of the trait (Widiger, 1993b). This often occurs when the criterion involves a patently undesirable trait. For example, we have found that it is unrealistic to ask narcissistic persons if they have a grandiose sense of their own self-importance (NAR-1). Many interviews and self-report inventories often approach this problem by asking if other persons have described or accused them of having this trait. This approach will be useful, at times, and we do use it (e.g., PAG-3), but we also find that a person who is unable or unwilling to describe himself or herself as grandiose is often unable or unwilling to inform the interviewer that others perceive or have accused him or her of being grandiose. If there is a significant other who could provide such information, and the interviewer has substantial doubts regarding the veridicality of the subject's report, then we would recommend that this other person be interviewed directly.

AGE OF ONSET, DURATION, AND CHRONICITY

Personality develops through childhood and adolescence, becoming evident by young adulthood and remaining quite stable thereafter (McCrae & Costa, 1990). However, it is difficult to provide a precise age of onset, and personality can indeed change with age.

Childhood onset. The role of PD diagnoses in persons under the age of 18 has been ambiguous (Hertzig, 1992), if not controversial (P. F. Kernberg, 1990; Shapiro, 1990). In the 1978 draft of *DSM-III*, it was stated that "maladaptive pervasive personality traits in children and adolescents may be of sufficient duration (at least one year) as to warrant the diagnosis of a Personality Disorder" (Task Force, 1978, p. K:1). In addition, there were said to be three childhood variants of adult personality disorders: (a) conduct disorder (which becomes adult antisocial PD), (b) shyness disorder (which becomes adult avoidant PD), and (c) introverted disorder (which becomes adult introverted or schizoid PD). It was also noted that cases of identity and oppositional defiant disorder of adolescence may become adult borderline and passive-aggressive PDs, respectively. And, "all of the Personality Disorders that do not have an equivalent category in the Childhood or Adolescence section may be applied to children or adolescents" (Task Force, 1978, p. K:2).

The final version of *DSM-III* was somewhat more cautious. The five childhood variants were still identified (although the name for the shyness disorder of childhood was changed to avoidant disorder, and introverted PD was changed to schizoid PD). However, the final version was more cautious with respect to the use of the other PDs in persons under the age of 18. "The other Personality Disorder categories may be applied to children or adolescents in those unusual instances in which the particular maladaptive personality traits appear to be stable" (APA, 1980, p. 306). It was also noted that "when this is done, there is obviously less certainty that the Personality Disorder will persist unchanged over time" (APA, 1980, p. 306). Nevertheless, it was also stated that personality disorders "begin in childhood or adolescence" (APA, 1980, p. 306) and that "the manifestations of Personality Disorder are generally recognizable by adolescence or earlier" (APA, 1980, p. 305).

Much of this discussion remained in *DSM-III-R*, but there were also signs of further caution regarding the use of PD diagnoses in persons under the age of 18. For example, rather than state that the age of onset was in childhood or that PDs are recognizable by adolescence or earlier, it was noted only that the PDs "are recognizable by adolescence or early adult life" (APA, 1987, p. 336). In addition, schizoid disorder of childhood was deleted from the nomenclature, and oppositional disorder was shifted from a childhood variant of PAG PD to a less severe variant of conduct disorder (APA, 1987). The only childhood variants of adult PDs listed in *DSM-III-R* were conduct disorder (antisocial PD), avoidant disorder (avoidant PD), and identity disorder (borderline PD).

This trend has continued with *DSM-IV*. Identity disorder of childhood has been moved out of the mental disorders section of *DSM-IV* to the (V-code) section for conditions that may be the focus of clinical attention (APA, 1994). It is no longer considered to be a mental disorder (nor a childhood variant of borderline PD). Many of the children and adolescents who were being given the diagnosis of an identity disorder were simply struggling (severely) with a normative developmental stage and few were likely to go on to develop a borderline PD. In addition, avoidant (shyness) disorder of childhood has been subsumed by the adult Axis I anxiety disorder of social phobia (APA, 1994). Timidity, shyness, and inhibition within childhood are considered in *DSM-IV* to represent an anxiety disorder rather than a personality disorder. The only childhood variant of a PD that has remained in *DSM-IV* is conduct disorder (for antisocial PD).

There is also less encouragement for the application of the other nine PD diagnoses in persons under the age of 18. It is now stated that this can be done "in those relatively unusual instances in which the individual's particular maladaptive personality traits appear to be pervasive, persistent, and unlikely to be limited to a particular developmental stage" (APA, 1994, p. 631). It is indicated that the behavior pattern must be present for at least 1 year, with a further caution that "it should be recognized that the traits of a Personality Disorder that appear in childhood will often not persist unchanged into adult life" (APA, 1994, p. 631).

The text discussions of each PD do attempt to provide descriptions of how the respective disorder is typically expressed or appears in childhood. However, such descriptions are included only for the antisocial PD and for the PDs from the odd-eccentric cluster (paranoid, schizoid, and schizotypal) (the SZT PD criteria set also includes a description of the childhood variant of the odd beliefs and magical ideation criterion). The discussion of age-related features for the borderline, narcissistic, avoidant, and dependent PDs is confined to cautions and skepticism regarding the application of these diagnoses in children or adolescents.

Little is known about the prevalence and stability of the *DSM-IV* PDs in persons under the age of 18 (Hertzig, 1992), and we would also discourage the application of the PDI-IV to persons below this age. We rarely provide a PD diagnosis to someone under the age of 18 because many maladaptive behavior patterns during childhood and adolescence will be situational or developmental in origin, and they will not persist into adulthood. Adolescence can be a time of tremendous turmoil and stress, and what appear to be borderline personality traits during this time may not persist much beyond adolescence. The person's reaction to this developmental period may be quite maladaptive, but also time-limited.

We would, in fact, suggest caution in the provision of PD diagnoses to young adults (e.g., ages 18 to 25). The age of 18 does represent a demarcation from adolescence to adulthood (e.g., the power to vote, graduation from high school, and leaving home), but it provides more of a legal or social definition of adulthood than a psychological development into adulthood. Some persons may appear borderline, histrionic, or antisocial at the age of 20, but not at the age of 25. They were, perhaps, within an extended developmental period of "adolescence." There are also data to suggest that some adult personality traits do not stabilize until the middle or late 20s (Costa & McCrae, 1993).

This caution becomes quite evident when one tries to document the stability or chronicity of individual PD items in young adults. As noted above, many PD items are readily confused with mood states, Axis I disorders, and situational reactions. The differentiation is typically resolved by assessing whether the behavior has been evident throughout the person's adult life, but this may not be helpful if the duration of the adult life has been, itself, quite brief. Documenting that a behavior was present since the age of 18 in someone who is 18 (19 or 20) will not be helpful when trying to distinguish between a PD and an Axis I disorder.

In such cases, we do advise the interviewer to consider the behavior pattern prior to the age of 18 (e.g., ages 15–18) but, as just indicated, this should be done with considerable caution. In addition, the PD criteria were written for persons beyond the age of 18 and may not be applicable to adolescents or children (the ATS PD criteria set and the one SZT criterion of odd beliefs are exceptions). For example, one obviously would not apply the dependent PD criteria to an infant, nor perhaps should one apply some of the criteria to an adolescent who is still under the authority, guidance, and support of his or her parents.

Adult onset. It is also questionable whether a PD must have been present since the age of 18 (i.e., onset no later than the age of 18). The convention in *DSM-IV* is that a PD must have been evident since late childhood or adolescence. It is stated at the beginning of each PD criteria set in *DSM-IV* that the behaviors are present "beginning by early adulthood" (the one exception is for ATS PD, which requires an even earlier onset prior to age 15). It is stated in the general criteria for a PD (discussed in the chapter on PDNOS) that "its onset can be traced back at least to adolescence or early adulthood" (APA, 1994, p. 633). A person may not be first diagnosed until well into adulthood but the diagnosis "by definition, …

requires an onset no later than early adulthood" (APA, 1994, p. 631). In other words, *DSM-IV* does not recognize an adult onset PD.

The 10th edition of the International Classification of Diseases (ICD-10) developed by the World Health Organization (WHO, 1992) does include two diagnoses that recognize that PDs can arise after the age of 18: enduring personality change after a catastrophic experience and enduring personality change after a psychiatric illness. These diagnoses are to be used for persons with no preexisting PD who evidence "a definite and enduring change in a...pattern of perceiving, relating to, or thinking about the environment and the self" (WHO, 1992, p. 208) that is significantly maladaptive and is in response to a catastrophic experience or a mental disorder. Both of these diagnoses were considered for *DSM-IV* (Gunderson, in press-a; Task Force, 1991) but both were ultimately rejected (Gunderson, in press-b).

We have observed apparent personality changes in persons who have suffered major mental disorders. Severe mental disorders can have a substantial effect on the personality. However, it is usually quite difficult to determine whether this change is in reaction to the occurrence of the disorder or is, instead, a manifestation of the Axis I disorder. The social withdrawal of persons who have previously suffered schizophrenia is probably best considered to represent a residual phase of schizophrenia rather than the development of an avoidant or schizoid personality disorder in reaction to having experienced the active phase. On the other hand, consider the social withdrawal that is commonly seen in persons who have experienced panic attacks. This withdrawal does not appear to be a direct expression of the panic disorder pathology, but reflects, instead, a change in behavior in reaction to experiencing the sudden, unexpected panic attacks. However, this withdrawal is currently conceptualized as an Axis I disorder (panic disorder with agoraphobia), in part, because the avoidant behavior is usually quite circumscribed without a significant change in overall personality functioning (although by the time of *DSM-V* there may be a diagnosis of panic disorder with agoraphobia, generalized type).

Some people will become dependent or avoidant, or will develop other personality changes due to the stress, difficulties, and insecurities that develop as a result of suffering from a severe depression or a psychosis (Barnett & Gotlib, 1988). These persons would be appropriately diagnosed as having maladaptive personality changes secondary to the experience of an Axis I mental disorder. However, as indicated above, the differentiation of Axis I and PD disorders is already very complicated and controversial. (See also the discussion below of the new schizophrenia exclusion criterion within the PAR, SZD, and SZT PD diagnoses.) Because there have as yet been no systematic studies to indicate that such changes can be reliably diagnosed, can be differentiated reliably from the Axis I disorder, or are, in fact, enduring thereafter (Triebwasser & Shea, in press), it was decided that the inclusion of a diagnosis of personality change due to a mental disorder in *DSM-IV* would only further complicate and confuse rather than advance clinical diagnosis (Gunderson, in press-b).

More compelling was the ICD-10 diagnosis of enduring personality change after a catastrophic experience. There has been substantial anecdotal and some systematic research to document the development of enduring personality changes following severe and/or sustained stressors, such as concentration camp experiences; prolonged kidnapping; or any other form of sustained torture, victimization, and suffering. Enduring personality changes that are commonly seen include hostile, mistrustful attitudes; social withdrawal; feelings of emptiness or hopelessness; apathy; alienation; and estrangement (Shea, in press; WHO, 1992). To the extent that some *DSM-IV* PDs result, in part, from the sustained experience of abusive, exploitative, and/or neglectful parenting, it is not surprising to find that similar experiences in adulthood would, at times, have a similar effect. However, because of the absence of systematic research on a specific set of diagnostic criteria and the potential overlap and confusion with post-traumatic stress disorder (and *DSM-IV* acute stress disorder), the final decision was not to include this diagnosis within *DSM-IV* (Gunderson, in press-b).

On the other hand, there are *DSM-IV* PDs that can arise after (and before) the age of 18. In *DSM-III-R*, they were diagnosed as an "organic personality syndrome" (APA, 1987, p. 114) and placed within the class of organic mental disorders. In *DSM-IV*, they are termed "personality change due to a general medical condition" and placed among the Axis I mental disorders due to a general medical condition (APA, 1994). Specific subtypes include the labile (affective instability), disinhibited (poor impulse control), aggressive, apathetic, and paranoid. In other words, personality change after the age of 18 is recognized when there is a clear medical condition to corroborate or authenticate the personality change (e.g., a brain tumor, injury, or epilepsy); personality change due to psychosocial experiences is not recognized. It has been our clinical experience that some persons do become avoidant, schizoid, dependent, or develop other maladaptive personality traits as they cope with difficult experiences of growing old (e.g., losing their spouse and friends, becoming disabled or vulnerable, or facing their own mortality and death). Perhaps there will be sufficient documentation of such changes by the time *DSM-V* is developed.

It should also be noted that PDs can dissipate or remit. A personality disorder does tend to be more resistant to therapeutic interventions than most Axis I disorders, but that does not mean that they are untreatable or unresponsive. In fact, most PDs tend to mellow with age. This has been most clearly documented with respect to the borderline and antisocial PDs (the latter particularly with respect to the overt acts of aggression and criminality). This gradual decrease in the severity and even presence of PD symptomatology is probably the result of accumulating experiences that reinforce the benefits of change and the costs of not changing. PDs are, by definition, maladaptive, and even without treatment, most persons will gradually develop some degree of adjustment to their environment.

Duration. In sum, the general convention in *DSM-IV* is that a PD must have been evident since late childhood or adolescence and must be present throughout adulthood. However, the assessment and documentation of this chronicity can also be problematic. On the one hand, it would be insufficient to assess whether a PD criterion had been present only within the past year but, on the other hand, it would be unrealistic to document its presence every year from the age of 18 to the present time in someone who is 53.

Each semistructured interview (and self-report inventory) has taken a somewhat different approach to the assessment of the duration of a behavior pattern (Zimmerman, 1994). The SCID-II (Spitzer, Williams, et al., 1990) and PDE (Loranger, 1988) assess each criterion over the past 5 years; the SIDP-R (Pfohl et al., 1989) asks the person to describe his or her usual self, although a 5-year time frame is also emphasized; and the DIPD (Zanarini et al., 1987) is confined largely to the past 2 years. The PDE also requires that at least one of the PD criteria (from a respective diagnosis) be present before the age of 25.

Our approach is to ask persons if the behavior has been characteristic for much of their adult life and evident since the age of 18. If the person is well beyond the age of 18, one should also ask for instances or examples of the behavior when the person was a young adult. If one finds that the behavior pattern was not present prior to a particular point in time within adulthood, then the interviewer must consider whether the behavior pattern reflects instead an Axis I disorder or situational reaction.

Complicating this assessment is the fact that some traits (or PD symptoms) will be more frequent than others in their appearance or expression. For example, feelings of emptiness (BDL-7) will have a more continuous presence than expressions of suicidality (BDL-5). All of the items should be evident since adolescence and throughout the adult life, but the frequency threshold that is necessary for this attribution will not be constant within or across items (Rorer & Widiger, 1983). For example, one may need more examples of overspending than of unsafe sex to attribute the item of borderline impulsivity (BDL-4), and one may need more expressions of borderline anger (BDL-8) to consider it present than expressions of borderline suicidality (BDL-5). In addition, even if one accepts the need for fewer suicidal acts than acts of anger, it is not clear exactly how many suicidal acts are needed. There is no need for a suicidal gesture every year since the age of 18 to attribute the presence of suicidal behavior, gestures, or threats in a 35-year-old female, but how many acts are necessary? One act every 5 years could be sufficient, but, then again, it might not.

Complicating the assessment even further is the fact that the expression or manifestation of a trait will not be unresponsive to situational factors (Gunderson, 1987). Dependent persons may appear less dependent when they are involved with an especially tolerant, nurturant, or available mate; imprisonment will constrain many antisocial PD traits; and some professions may temporarily mask the maladaptivity of narcissistic and obsessive-compulsive PD traits through the rewarding, facilitating, or perhaps exploitation of excessive achievement-striving, status-seeking, and/or workaholism.

In other words, it is not possible to provide one specific rule for how often a trait should be evident within a particular period of time. Any such rule would be arbitrary, pseudospecific, and subject to numerous qualifications and exceptions. It is necessary to address this issue on an item-by-item basis, assessing in each case whether the behavior pattern does appear to represent a personality trait that has been evident since adolescence and present throughout much of the adult life. This point is discussed explicitly for a number of the PDI-IV item assessments (e.g., BDL-5 and ATS-A4).

MULTIPLE VERSUS DIFFERENTIAL DIAGNOSIS

It is stated in *DSM-IV* (as was also the case in *DSM-III-R*) that all of the relevant PD diagnoses should be provided when a person meets the diagnostic criteria for more than one PD. However, many patients will meet the criteria for two, three, four, and even more PD diagnoses (Nurnberg et al., 1991a; Skodol, Rosnick, Kellman, Oldham, & Hyler, 1988; Widiger, Trull, Hurt, Clarkin, & Frances, 1987; Zanarini, Frankenburg, Chauncey, &

Gunderson, 1987;). Multiple PD diagnoses are inconsistent with the theory that personality disorders represent distinct clinical syndromes. It is difficult to discuss or conceptualize the comorbidity of four (or even just two) personality disorders within one person, as if each has its own independent and distinct etiology and they interact over time to complicate each other's course and treatment. People have just one personality (except, perhaps, those with an Axis I dissociative identity disorder), and it can seem odd to diagnose them with comorbid personality disorders (Lilienfeld, Waldman, & Israel, 1994). Multiple PD diagnoses are also cumbersome and confusing in both research and clinical practice, and are usually ignored in clinical practice (Gunderson, 1992). The modal number of PD diagnoses within inpatient charts is usually just one; two PD diagnoses are an exception; rarely, if ever, are there three or more PD diagnoses. However, the mean number of PD diagnoses per inpatient is around three when a systematic and comprehensive assessment of each PD criterion is conducted (Skodol et al., 1988; Widiger et al., 1987; Zanarini et al., 1987).

DSM-IV (and *DSM-III-R*) also provides a section within the text discussion of each PD that is concerned with differential diagnosis. This material indicates the more common co-occurrences among the PDs (e.g., avoidant with the schizoid, dependent, and paranoid PDs; APA, 1994) and how each PD can be differentiated from the other PDs. This material can be helpful when a patient meets the criteria for more than one PD and the clinician needs or intends to confine the diagnosis to just one PD. However, there is some inconsistency in indicating that all of the PD diagnoses should be given when a person meets the criteria for more than one, and yet also indicating how the PDs that commonly co-occur should be differentiated.

The authors of *DSM-IV* realized that multiple PD diagnoses are problematic and undesirable while recognizing that they are descriptively accurate and unavoidable. An additional recommendation implemented in *DSM-IV* is to rank multiple diagnoses in their order of importance (APA, 1994). The clinician is largely free to decide the basis on which this rank order will be made. Importance could mean relevance or need for treatment, severity of impairment, predominance of symptoms, or degree of empirical support (Gunderson, 1992; Widiger & Sanderson, in press-b). Which is the most important PD will vary across the needs, interests, and concerns of each clinician and researcher. If a personality disorder rather than an Axis I disorder is the principle reason for the interview or consultation, then the clinician is encouraged in *DSM-IV* to indicate which of the PDs is the basis or reason for the interview (APA, 1994).

A more radical proposal considered for *DSM-IV* was to provide explicit hierarchical rules whereby some PDs would trump or veto others (Gunderson, 1992, in press-b). There was some precedent for this proposal. In *DSM-III*, all of the other PDs trumped the passive-aggressive PD diagnosis, and schizoid PD contained an exclusion criterion for schizotypal eccentricity that essentially vetoed a diagnosis of schizoid PD in the presence of the schizotypal PD (APA, 1980). However, none of these hierarchical exclusion rules were retained in *DSM-III-R* because they were usually ignored, and they had little empirical or conceptual justification (Widiger et al., 1988).

Similar problems arose with the hierarchical proposals for *DSM-IV*. There are a number of possible rules for deciding which PD diagnosis would take precedence over another, including degree of empirical validation, level of functional impairment, extent of evident symptomatology, relevance to treatment, or relevance to any particular clinical decision. Because no single, simple rule was likely to be uniformly sufficient or acceptable, and any complex rule would be cumbersome and equally flawed, the PD Work Group decided not to provide a hierarchical exclusion rule that would effectively delete the recognition of potentially relevant PD symptomatology. A borderline PD may indeed be the principle reason for an intervention but the additional avoidant, dependent, or narcissistic traits may still be very important and relevant to the understanding of the person's psychopathology and treatment. A difficulty with any hierarchical exclusion rule is that it would not actually resolve the issue it was trying to address. The empirical fact is that many borderline patients have clinically significant avoidant, dependent, narcissistic, antisocial, and/or schizotypal traits (Widiger & Frances, 1989b). Providing only the borderline diagnosis to these patients would be inaccurate and misleading. In addition, most patients will not present as prototypic borderline, antisocial, dependent, or antisocial PDs. Personalities come in shades of gray (or mixtures of the 10-12 *DSM-IV* colors) rather than in tidy categories of distinct black or white. A hierarchical rule eliminates the complexity of personality only by fiat.

An additional proposal was to provide a table in the introductory section to the personality disorders that could be used to indicate the extent to which each personality disorder was present (Widiger & Sanderson, in press-b). Rather than characterize each disorder as simply present or absent, the clinician would be encouraged to indicate, for example, whether no traits were present, whether it was a subthreshold case, whether the person just barely met the criteria for the disorder, or whether the patient met all of the criteria for the disorder.

Six levels were provided: absent, traits, subthreshold, threshold, moderate, and extreme. The rating in each case was compatible with the categorical format. "Absent" meant what it implied, an absence of any of the criteria. "Traits" meant that there are simply one to three criteria (*DSM-IV* and *DSM-III-R* recommend that the clinician code personality disorder "traits" on Axis II when the patient meets some of the criteria but not enough to be given the diagnosis). "Subthreshold" meant that the person had only one symptom short of meeting the criteria for the disorder. "Threshold" meant that the person just met the threshold for the diagnosis. "Moderate" meant that the person had more than enough of the criteria, and "extreme" meant that all of the diagnostic features were present. Table 2-1 presents the proposed table (revised to be consistent with the final *DSM-IV* diagnostic criteria sets).

There were, however, a few concerns regarding this proposal (Widiger & Sanderson, in press-b). One was that the table might be too cumbersome for practical use. It is unlikely that clinicians would systematically assess all of the criteria for all of the personality disorders and then provide a tabular summary of the extent to which each personality disorder was present. However, the proposal was not to require such a comprehensive rating. The proposal was simply to make the rating available. The table would provide uniform criteria and terminology to be used when the clinician or researcher found it useful to do so. Clinicians would then be given the language and means by which to describe the extent to which each personality disorder was present.

It was also suggested that it would not be appropriate to apply diagnostic labels (e.g., "subthreshold borderline," or "schizotypal traits") to persons who did not have the

Table 2-1
Converting the DSM-IV Diagnostic Categories to Dimensional Ratings

Personality disorder	Number of criteria					
	Absent	Traits	Subthld	Threhld	Moderat	Extreme
Paranoid	0	1-2	3	4	5-6	7
Schizoid	0	1-2	3	4	5-6	7
Schizotypal	0	1-3	4	5-6	7-8	9
Antisocial[a]	0	1	2	3-4	5-6	7
Borderline	0	1-3	4	5-6	7-8	9
Histrionic	0	1-3	4	5	6-7	8
Narcissistic	0	1-3	4	5-6	7-8	9
Avoidant	0	1-2	3	4	5-6	7
Dependent	0	1-3	4	5	6-7	8
Compulsive	0	1-2	3	4-5	6-7	8
Passive-aggressive[b]	0	1-2	3	4	5-6	7
Depressive[b]	0	1-3	4	5	6	7

Note. Subthld = subthreshold; Threhld = threshold; Moderat = moderate.
[a]Conduct disorder criterion is not included. [b]Not an officially recognized personality disorder.

respective disorders. This practice was already encouraged in *DSM-III-R* (APA, 1987, pp. 16-17) and *DSM-IV* (APA, 1994) but the presence of the table would provide additional encouragement. It is our opinion that many persons who fail to meet the *DSM-IV* diagnostic thresholds do, in fact, have clinically significant maladaptive personality traits (Skodol, 1989b; Widiger & Corbitt, in press-b) but the PD Work Group felt that the encouragement of subthreshold assessments would undermine the validity and credibility of the categorical distinctions (Widiger & Sanderson, in press-b).

We are providing this table in the PDI-IV so that it is available to clinicians and researchers who might find it useful. The purpose of this table is to encourage clinicians to consider the extent to which each maladaptive personality syndrome is present rather than to simply categorize a PD as present or absent, as well as to facilitate the acknowledgment and communication of more complex personality profiles. We would encourage clinicians to acknowledge at least some of this complexity by indicating the extent to which a few of the PDs are present in any particular case (e.g., indicating that the patient presents as only a threshold borderline with avoidant traits, or as an extreme antisocial with moderate borderline symptoms and paranoid traits).

An even more radical approach is to abandon the *DSM-IV* PD diagnoses altogether in favor of a smaller set of more independent dimensions that cut across and likely define the 10 (or 12) *DSM-IV* PD diagnoses. Such a proposal was also considered for *DSM-IV* (Widiger & Sanderson, in press-b). A major difficulty with this proposal was the lack of consensus among the *DSM-IV* PD Work Group and Task Force members regarding what dimensions would be included and the absence of established or even familiar relevance of these dimensions to everyday clinical practice.

For example, one approach would be to use the three *DSM-IV* cluster constructs of odd-eccentric, dramatic-emotional-erratic, and anxious-fearful as dimensions by which to describe the personality profile of each patient. However, these three constructs are almost as problematic as the 10 PD diagnoses. There is, at times, as much co-occurrence across the clusters (e.g., borderline with schizotypal and avoidant with schizoid) as there is within. In addition, the cluster constructs do not adequately describe the PDs included within them. For example, the narcissistic PD is not captured well by the construct of dramatic-emotional-erratic; there is also clearly more to the antisocial PD than being dramatic, emotional, or erratic; and schizoid PD is more anhedonic than odd or eccentric (Schopp & Trull, 1993; Widiger & Costa, 1994).

The final decision regarding the proposal to include an alternative dimensional system in the *DSM-IV* was to simply alert the clinician to this perspective and to note the variety of dimensional models that might be considered. We would recommend, in particular, the five-factor model (FFM) of personality, which consists of the dimensions of neuroticism, introversion versus extraversion, openness versus closedness to experience, antagonism versus agreeableness, and conscientiousness (McCrae & Costa, 1990). There is considerable empirical support for the FFM classification of normal personality (Digman, 1990; Goldberg, 1990, 1993; John, 1990; Wiggins & Pincus, 1992) and for the ability of the FFM to describe, explain, and account for each of the *DSM-IV* PDs (Clark & Livesley, 1994; Clarkin, Hull, Cantor, & Sanderson, 1993; Costa & McCrae, 1990; Schroeder, Wormworth, & Livesley, 1992; Shopshire & Craik, 1994; Soldz, Budman, Demby, & Merry, 1993; Trull, 1992; Wiggins & Pincus, 1989). Widiger, Trull, Clarkin, Sanderson, and Costa (1994) indicate how each *DSM-III-R* and *DSM-IV* PD would be understood from the perspective of the FFM. An overview of the application and relevance of this model to PDs is provided in the text edited by Costa and Widiger (1994). We expect that this model, or one quite similar to it, will eventually prove to be more useful and relevant to everyday clinical practice than the categorical distinctions provided in *DSM-IV* (Costa & Widiger, 1994; Stone, 1993).

SELF AND INFORMANT REPORTS

As indicated above, it will be helpful at times (and may even be necessary) to interview someone close to the subject in order to obtain sufficient information to render a confident assessment. Some persons will be so depressed, anxious, hostile, or psychotic that a valid interview is not possible. The responses of some antisocial and paranoid persons may be so deficient and questionable that one needs independent verification. Some narcissistic, dependent, histrionic, paranoid, schizoid, and other persons may be unaware of traits that are readily apparent to those who interact closely with them. Many of the PD traits involve the person's manner of relating to others (Benjamin, 1993; Kiesler, 1991; Wiggins & Pincus, 1989), but even those that do not may be well known to friends and colleagues (e.g., traits of conscientiousness). An interview with a close friend, relative, spouse, colleague, institutional staff, or employer is rarely uninformative. It will usually generate indicators of additional maladaptive personality traits (Zimmerman, 1994; Zimmerman, Pfohl, Coryell, Stangl, & Corenthal, 1988). We indicate throughout the interview specific items where an interview with an informant may be particularly helpful (e.g., ATS-A6, HST-1, & PAR-1).

Use of the PDI-IV with an informant can be straightforward. One simply converts the questions from first-person to third-person pronouns and converts indirect inquiries to direct inquiries regarding the target subject's traits or behaviors (e.g., NAR-1). However, practicing clinicians may not always have time to administer the entire PDI-IV to an informant. We suggest first administering the PDI-IV to the identified subject, thereby identifying which criteria or responses to cross-validate with a particularly appropriate informant.

A disadvantage of this approach is not being able to double-check the informant's responses with the target subject. One may find that the informant has raised issues or provided information that should be verified or explored with the subject, requiring a second subject interview. However, the reverse situation is also possible. If one began with the informant, one might feel the need to return to the informant after having interviewed the subject. If somebody does need to be interviewed twice, it is usually easiest and most informative to interview the target subject twice.

It is also important to keep in mind that all of the problems that are inherent to a PD interview with a subject can occur in an interview with an informant. An interesting and controversial question arises regarding which person provides the most valid information (Zimmerman, 1994). We prefer to consider both as simply providing different perspectives, each having its own advantages and disadvantages. Informants are not objective observers. Their own maladaptive personality traits will distort their perceptions of others; they may also be within a mood state that may affect their description (e.g., anger or infatuation); they may even have an axe to grind with the target subject (e.g., lingering bitterness, resentment, or envy). There are data to indicate that the PD ratings of a patient by that patient's relative(s) may be correlated with the PD traits within the relatives (Zimmerman, 1993a). For example, narcissistic persons may devalue the subject, a borderline informant may idealize the subject, or a dependent person may deny the person's unreliability and irresponsibility. They may simply be limited in how well they know the person, and they may be unaware of how ignorant or how wrong they are. Informants, like the subjects themselves, are providing subjective opinions and impressions.

We are not suggesting that nobody can provide useful or valid information. Both the subject and the informant will provide useful and valid information. We are suggesting that one should not take any attribution at face value or accept uncritically every perception or opinion. The attributions of the informant should be evaluated in the same manner as the self-attributions of the subject.

SELF-REPORT INVENTORIES

We would also encourage the interviewer to supplement the administration of the PDI-IV with a self-report inventory (Widiger & Frances, 1987). We do believe that one can use the PDI-IV to provide a valid assessment of the *DSM-IV* PDs, and we would discourage clinicians from relying only upon a self-report inventory to provide their clinical PD diagnoses. Self-report inventories include validity scales because they are more susceptible to mood states, response biases, deception, and other forms of distortion and error than semistructured interviews. Semistructured interviews do not include validity scales because the consideration and assessment of such distortions are inherent to the assessment of every PD item. A self-report inventory must accept whatever response a subject provides, whereas an interviewer records his or her own professional judgments regarding the person's traits rather than the perceptions, attributions, or opinions of the person.

Nevertheless, self-report inventories will usually (if not always) provide very informative information (Widiger & Sanderson, in press-a). They have the advantage of entirely reliable administration and scoring, which allows for the obtainment of normative data and the development of empirically-based interpretive scoring systems. They are also much less expensive to administer. We especially encourage the clinician to administer and score a self-report inventory prior to the administration of the PDI-IV. If there is time for this to be done, then there is little reason for it not to be done. The results of the inventory will alert the clinician to unanticipated areas of inquiry (Widiger & Sanderson, in press-a). Self-report inventories may also be particularly helpful in the assessment of traits that are difficult for the subject to discuss openly with the interviewer (e.g., PAR-4, "reads hidden demeaning or threatening meanings into benign remarks or events" [APA, 1994, p. 637] or SZD-3, "little if any interest in having sexual experiences with another person" [APA, 1994, p. 641]).

Many clinicians may prefer not to administer the complete PDI-IV. This decision will, at times, be based on a limited need or purpose (e.g., a referral question may be confined to just one or two of the *DSM-IV* PDs). However, it may also be based upon an initial impression of the most relevant PDs. This is a useful and efficient way to administer the PDI-IV. However, we would encourage such decisions to be informed by the results of a self-report inventory. As noted above, the inventory may alert the clinician to areas of inquiry that were not originally anticipated (e.g., antisocial traits in someone who initially appeared to be dependent). Gender-biased attributions can be particularly problematic within unstructured clinical interviews. Clinicians (and researchers) may attribute histrionic traits to antisocial female subjects and antisocial traits to histrionic male subjects (Ford & Widiger, 1989; Hamilton, Rothbart, & Dawes, 1986). Self-report inventories may be less prone to such bias simply because a questionnaire item is unaware of (or at least not influenced by) the gender of the person.

Some semistructured PD interviews include a brief self-report questionnaire to be administered prior to the administration of the interview (e.g., SCID-II; Spitzer et al., 1990). These preinterview screening questionnaires are constructed to err in the direction of false positives (i.e., to overdiagnose the presence of PDs, which are then confirmed or rejected by the interview). However, it is our recommendation to administer an inventory that was constructed to stand on its own (Widiger & Sanderson, in press-a). If the subject and the clinician/interviewer are going to take the time and effort to administer, complete, and/or score an inventory, then it might as well be one that was constructed to provide comprehensive, valid PD assessments. Such inventories will not be much longer than a screening questionnaire, and they will provide much more information. In addition, given the uniform finding that self-report inventories tend to diagnose more PDs than are diagnosed by semistructured interviews, they can be considered screening questionnaires (i.e., erring in the direction of false positives) (Widiger & Sanderson, in press-a; Zimmerman, 1994).

There are a variety of such inventories to choose from, including the Personality Assessment Inventory (PAI; Morey, 1991), the Millon Clinical Multiaxial Inventory-II (MCMI-II; Millon, 1987), the Personality Diagnostic Questionnaire—Revised (PDQ-R; Hyler & Rieder, 1987), the MMPI-2 personality disorder scales developed originally by Morey, Waugh, and Blashfield (1985) and revised by Ben-Porath (1994), the Schedule for Normal and Abnormal Personality (SNAP; Clark, in press), the Dimensional Assessment of Personality Pathology—Basic Questionnaire (DAPP-BQ; Livesley, 1990), and the Wisconsin Personality Disorders Inventory (WISPI; Klein et al., 1993). All of the above citations concern the *DSM-III-R*. It is likely that all have been revised for *DSM-IV*. We would advise the clinician to become familiar with a few of them, trying each within his or her clinical practice. We have found it to be illuminating to administer more than one inventory to the same patient, thereby allowing a direct comparison of results. If multiple testing of the same patient is too demanding or expensive, we would advise administering different inventories to different patients, again allowing for some experience with more than one and a comparison of the inventory results with one's own assessment obtained through the PDI-IV or another interview.

We would also recommend the administration of the Revised NEO Personality Inventory (NEO PI-R; Costa & McCrae, 1992b) which is a self-report inventory for the assessment of "normal" personality traits. We believe that the diagnosis of personality disorders will ultimately be coordinated with the assessment of personality in general, and the most compelling locus of this integration will be within the five factor model (FFM) of personality (Costa & Widiger, 1994; Widiger, 1993a; Widiger & Costa, 1994), consisting of the personality trait dimensions of neuroticism, introversion versus extraversion, openness versus closedness to experience, antagonism versus agreeableness, and conscientiousness (Digman, 1990; Goldberg, 1993; John, 1990; McCrae & Costa, 1990). The NEO PI-R is the best self-report instrument for the assessment of the FFM (Widiger, 1992b), and clinicians will find that assessment of the *DSM-IV* PDs and the FFM personality traits provides a particularly comprehensive assessment (Costa & Widiger, 1994).

GENDER, CULTURE, AND ETHNICITY

One of the most controversial issues in the diagnosis of the *DSM-II*, *DSM-III*, *DSM-III-R*, and one that will likely remain for the *DSM-IV* PDs has been the question of gender (sex) bias. A complete discussion of this difficult issue is beyond the scope of this manual, but any person who diagnoses females with a dependent personality disorder or a histrionic personality disorder should become familiar with the various perspectives and positions on this controversy. We would recommend, in particular, papers by Caplan (1991), Kaplan (1983), Walker (1994), Widiger, Corbitt, and Funtowicz (1994), Widiger and Spitzer (1991), and Williams and Spitzer (1983). The major thrust of the issue is whether the *DSM* PD diagnoses that occur more often in women (e.g., HST, DEP, and BDL) reflect a gender bias. Concerns regarding this issue are quite understandable. Sexism, sex-role stereotyping, and sex bias are not difficult to find, and it would be naive to think that they have not influenced to some extent the development (mostly by males) of diagnostic criteria sets for disorders that involve, at least in part, maladaptive variants of stereotypically feminine traits (Kaplan, 1983). On the other hand, to the extent that the PDs involve maladaptive variants of common personality traits, it is to be expected that one would find maladaptive variants of stereotypically feminine and masculine traits (Widiger & Spitzer, 1991).

It has been well documented that clinicians (and likely researchers) overdiagnose the histrionic PD in females and (to a lesser extent) the antisocial PD in males (e.g., Ford & Widiger, 1989; Hamilton et al., 1986). Antisocial symptomatology within female patients is often misperceived as histrionic symptomatology. This confusion is understandable. The histrionic PD symptomatology involves, to some extent, maladaptive and extreme variants of stereotypically feminine traits (just as the antisocial and obsessive-compulsive PD criteria sets involve to some extent maladaptive and extreme variants of stereotypically masculine traits). The prototypic histrionic patient will be female, and the prototypic antisocial patient will be male (Sprock, Blashfield, & Smith, 1990; Widiger & Spitzer, 1991). As a result, interviewers will tend to perceive antisocial females as being histrionic, and histrionic males as being antisocial. This is a problem of assessment, and needs to be addressed within the process of applying the *DSM-IV* PD criteria.

A semistructured interview that encourages a systematic assessment of each antisocial (and histrionic) criterion in female subjects will help to minimize the occurrence of this gender bias (Ford & Widiger, 1989). However, it is important to be sensitive to the question of gender bias when assessing individual items (Widiger, Corbitt, & Funtowicz, 1994). Consider, for example, the *DSM-III-R* histrionic criterion of overconcern with physical attractiveness (APA, 1987). This item involved, by definition, excessive and maladaptive concern with physical attractiveness because it specified *overconcern*. However, it is not really clear what constitutes an overconcern, and it would not be surprising to find that male clinicians had a lower threshold for this attribution than female clinicians or that normal females were being assessed with an overconcern by both male and female clinicians (Widiger, Corbitt, & Funtowicz, 1994). The *DSM-IV* revision of this item addressed this concern but, as we indicate in its discussion within chapter 8 (HST-4), similar problems may still occur. We discuss throughout the PDI-IV, and particularly with respect to items from the dependent and histrionic criteria sets, issues with respect to gender bias (e.g, DEP-3 & DEP-5, and HST-2 & HST-4).

Systematic research on cultural and ethnic bias has received much less attention than gender bias within the PD literature (Alarcon & Foulks, in press; Landrine, 1992), with only a few exceptions (e.g., Blackburn, 1988; Loring & Powell, 1988). However, we suspect that the issue of ethnic and culture bias may receive more attention in the future because the problems here are as problematic and as controversial. Consider, for example, the possibility that there is a PD criterion that is relatively normative within a particular cultural group. That is, most members of this cultural group have been encouraged to develop a particular behavior pattern that is considered to be maladaptive within a *DSM-IV* PD criteria set. Would it then be appropriate to consider the behavior pattern to be symptomatic of a PD in a person from this culture? On the one hand, one might say "no," because it would be arbitrary to consider what is normal (i.e., adaptive) within one setting to be abnormal (i.e., maladaptive) within another. On the other hand, perhaps it might be correct to consider the behavior pattern to be maladaptive within any setting (in an absolute sense), including the culture in which it was encouraged. Perhaps it was normative within the original culture, but still maladaptive.

For example, aggressive and even criminal behavior may be considered to be adaptive within a tough, urban environment, and some have suggested that such behavior patterns should not be diagnosed as antisocial (Alarcon & Foulks, in press; Blackburn, 1988). One would then be providing a diagnosis of a mental disorder in someone who had, in fact, developed a behavior pattern that was adaptive to the environment. On the other hand, others have argued that one is confusing etiology with pathology here. Many mental disorders are the result of pathogenic environments (e.g., physical and sexual abuse, or inadequate and inconsistent parenting), and such persons may be adapting to a pathogenic environment. The position taken by *DSM-IV* with respect to this particular example is not really clear. On the one hand, it is stated that ATS PD is "associated with low socioeconomic status and urban settings" (APA, 1994, p. 647) but when "assessing antisocial traits, it is helpful for the clinician to consider the social and economic context in which the behaviors occur" (APA, 1994, p. 647) because "the diagnosis may, at times, be misapplied to individuals in settings in which seemingly antisocial behavior may be part of a protective survival strategy" (APA, 1994, p. 647).

Consider an equally, if not more problematic, case in which submissive behavior within females is being encouraged by a particular group. Some cultures may encourage submissiveness in females and assertiveness in males (Brown, 1986). The submissiveness may be considered excessive and maladaptive within modern western culture, but not for females within a more traditional western or nonwestern culture (Alarcon & Foulks, in press). The *DSM IV* indicates that the behavior pattern should be one that "deviates markedly from the expectations of the individual's culture" (APA, 1994, p. 633). Considering submissiveness to be undesirable or maladaptive may be confusing a liberal, political (e.g., feminist) judgment with a professional, clinical judgment. On the other hand, one may observe clear indications of the maladaptivity of the submissiveness (e.g., tolerance and acceptance of physical abuse). Complicating the assessment even further is the fact that the apparently dependent female from the traditional or conservative background may feel quite satisfied, willing, or comfortable with the submissiveness. She might (justifiably) argue that the clinician is confusing a value judgment with a clinical judgment. The same issues apply in the assessment of other traits, including devotion to work and productivity, aggressiveness, and suspiciousness.

These are clearly very difficult and sensitive issues (American Psychological Association, 1993). We are not attempting here to argue for one position over another, although by developing a PD interview, we demonstrate our belief in the validity of the construct of a personality disorder diagnosis. We also believe that some persons develop maladaptive behavior patterns as a result of their familial and cultural environment. On the other hand, one must be very careful, cautious, and informed in the assessment and diagnosis of a PD in such persons. Therefore, this issue is discussed repeatedly throughout the PDI-IV with respect to items that may be particularly susceptible to cultural, ethnic, gender, or other forms of bias, as well as in chapter 14 where the general criteria for a personality disorder are considered.

3

DSM-IV and the PDI-IV

It is helpful when providing a diagnosis of a *DSM-IV* personality disorder to understand the process and nature of its development for *DSM-IV*. Therefore, this chapter presents an overview of the process by which the personality disorder section of *DSM-IV* was developed, as well as an overview of the revisions that affected most of the PDs.

In May of 1988, the Board of Trustees of the American Psychiatric Association (APA) appointed a Task Force to begin work on *DSM-IV* (Frances, Widiger, & Pincus, 1989). Thirteen Work Groups were then developed, one of which was devoted to the personality disorders. Dr. John Gunderson chaired this PD Work Group, whose ultimate membership consisted of Drs. Roger Blashfield, Susan Fiester, Robert Hirschfeld, Theodore Millon, Bruce Pfohl, Tracie Shea, Larry Siever, and Thomas Widiger. A draft of the recommended proposals for the personality disorders was published by the APA in 1991 (Task Force, 1991), and the final recommendations were published in 1993 (Task Force, 1993). The *DSM-IV* itself was published in 1994 (APA, 1994). The recommendations by the PD Work Group were based primarily upon four considerations: (a) empirical research, (b) compatibility with the international nomenclature, (c) clinical utility, and (d) clinical theory. The nature and extent of each of these considerations will be discussed in turn.

BASES FOR REVISION

Empirical Data

A consistent criticism of the decisions that were made for the *DSM-III* and *DSM-III-R* PD criteria sets was the absence of supportive data (e.g., Perry, 1990). The primary justification for a revision in *DSM-IV* was the indication through empirical research of an apparent problem with a *DSM-III-R* criteria set and/or the likelihood of an improvement with a particular revision (Frances, Pincus, Widiger, Davis, & First, 1990). A substantial amount of empirical data was made available to the PD Work Group (Gunderson, in press-a, in press-b). These data were obtained through (a) systematic reviews of the literature, (b) studies solicited by the Work Group, and (c) a field trial (Widiger, Frances, Pincus, Davis, & First, 1991).

The purpose of the literature reviews was to provide a comprehensive and neutral summary of the empirical and clinical literature that was relevant to a particular issue or proposal for a respective PD (Widiger, Frances, Pincus, & Davis, 1990). Abbreviated versions of 13 of these literature reviews were published in the *Journal of Personality Disorders* (Gunderson & Shea, 1991; Shea, 1993; Widiger, 1991). More extensive versions will be published in the second volume of the *DSM-IV Sourcebook* (Gunderson, in press-a;

Widiger et al., 1991), along with the two PD reviews that were concerned with the adult onset proposals discussed in chapter 2 (Shea, in press; Triebwasser & Shea, in press). These reviews have also been published in a text edited by Dr. W. J. Livesley (in press), accompanied, in most cases, by a critical commentary. We will refer to these reviews in the following chapters as we discuss each of the PDs and their diagnostic criteria.

A major concern of the PD Work Group was the extent, direction, and source of the co-occurrence and overlap among the personality disorder diagnoses. The PD Work Group wanted to revise the criteria sets to maximize the differentiation among the PDs, thereby facilitating the effort of the clinician to identify which PD is most important or relevant to the understanding of a particular patient's personality disorder pathology (Gunderson, in press-a, in press-b). As noted earlier, the research had indicated substantial co-occurrence among the PDs (e.g., Blashfield & Breen, 1989; Fyer, Frances, Sullivan, Hurt, & Clarkin, 1988; Morey, 1988b; Nurnberg et al., 1991a; Oldham et al., 1992; Pfohl, Coryell, Zimmerman, & Stangl, 1986; Widiger & Rogers, 1989). Many patients would meet the *DSM-III-R* criteria for more than one PD, some for as many as five or more (Skodol et al., 1988; Widiger, Trull, et al., 1987; Zanarini et al., 1987). The *DSM-IV* PD Work Group intended to revise the *DSM-III-R* criteria to increase its specificity.

The reviews, however, indicated a dearth of relevant data in the published literature. Most of the published research prior to 1990 concerned the borderline and/or the schizotypal PD criteria sets, with little or nothing on the other PDs. For example, there was substantial research concerning the antisocial PD that used the *DSM-III-R* or *DSM-III* criteria sets (Widiger & Corbitt, 1993), but very little data on the antisocial PD criteria set itself. However, it was apparent that any research program that had administered a semistructured interview would have obtained a substantial amount of data on the performance characteristics for all of the *DSM-III-R* PD criteria. Therefore, researchers who had published data on performance characteristics for one or more of the PDs and the authors of the major semistructured interviews were solicited to provide (a) the co-occurrence rates for all of the *DSM-III-R* PDs, and (b) the sensitivity, specificity, positive and negative predictive power, and phi coefficients for every *DSM-III-R* PD criterion. Freiman and Widiger (1989), Millon and Tringone (1989), Morey and Heumann (1988), Pfohl and Blum (1990), Skodol (1989a), and Zanarini, Frankenburg, Chauncey, and Gunderson (1989) provided these data for all of the *DSM-III-R* PDs (the Zanarini et al. data were based on the *DSM-III* criteria sets). First and Spitzer (1989), Freiman and Widiger, Millon and Tringone, Morey and Goodman (1989), Pfohl and Blum, Skodol, and Zanarini et al. also provided these same statistics with respect to the relationship of each *DSM-III-R* PD criterion to every other *DSM-III-R* PD diagnosis (the Zanarini et al. data were again based on the *DSM-III* criteria). Blashfield (1988) also provided unpublished face validity data for all of the PDs, and Dubro (1988), Malow and Donnelly (1988), McGlashan and Fenton (1988), and Reich (1988) provided data on the performance characteristics of a subset of the personality disorders. In sum, the *DSM-IV* PD revisions were based, in part, on data obtained from four different semistructured interviews, including the PIQ-II (Widiger, 1987), the SCID-II (Spitzer et al., 1990), the SIDP-R (Pfohl et al., 1989), and the DIPD (Zanarini et al., 1987), as well as two surveys of findings from practicing clinicians (Millon & Tringone, 1989;

Morey & Goodman, 1989). These efforts were funded, in part, by a grant from the John D. and Catherine T. MacArthur Foundation (Frances et al., 1990), and are referred to hereafter as the *DSM-IV* MacArthur studies.

The performance characteristic data were helpful in determining which criteria should be revised and/or deleted (Morey, 1988a; Widiger & Trull, in press). These data were also used to order the criteria in terms of their diagnostic power. In *DSM-IV*, the first item is considered to be the most diagnostic, with decreasing effectiveness as one moves down the list. This does not mean that the last item is weak, unhelpful, or not diagnostic. If this was the case, such items would have been deleted.

In most cases, the rank order was based on the correlation of the item to the presence versus absence of the diagnosis, as provided by the *DSM-IV* MacArthur studies (and additional data, when available). However, in some cases emphasis was given to specificity values (i.e., the extent to which the item was unique to that diagnosis) and/or clinical theory (e.g., the placement of "frantic efforts to avoid real or imagined abandonment" [APA, 1994, p. 654] at the top of the list for the borderline PD diagnosis). One important limitation of this rank order is that it was based on data using the *DSM-III-R* criteria. It is not certain that the same rank order would be obtained with the *DSM-IV* revisions that have been made to each item (cf. AVD-1) (Blashfield, Blum, & Pfohl, 1992; Zimmerman, 1988).

Two additional *DSM-IV* PD studies were also funded, in part, by the MacArthur Foundation. One was a reanalysis of the extensive data obtained by Dr. Hare and his colleagues with the original and revised Hare Psychopathy Checklist (HPCL; Hare, 1992) to develop a shorter, simplified criteria set for use within the *DSM-IV* antisocial PD field trial (Hare et al., in press). The other was a pilot test of proposed revisions to the schizotypal criteria set (Silverman et al., in press).

An extensive field trial, funded, in part, by the National Institute of Mental Health (NIMH), was conducted on the proposed revisions to the antisocial PD criteria set (Widiger et al., in press). The field trial considered, in particular, the proposals to include more traditional traits of psychopathy and to reduce and simplify the criteria set for easier use in general clinical practice (Widiger & Corbitt, 1993). It would have been desirable to have obtained field trial data for all of the PDs, but this was not realistic given the limited funding.

ICD-10 Compatibility

A second source of input and basis for change was the criteria developed by the World Health Organization (WHO) for the 10th edition of the International Classification of Diseases (ICD-10; WHO, 1992). The impetus for the development of *DSM-IV* was the desire and need to coordinate the *DSM* with the development of ICD-10 (Frances, Widiger, & Pincus, 1989). Congruency with the ICD-10 nomenclature is quite important for international communication and for the comparison of findings across societies and cultures. The success of the recently developed International Society for the Study of Personality Disorders is due, in part, to the presence of a common, mutual nomenclature. The *DSM-IV* Task Force and PD Work Group also had a substantial impact on the development of ICD-10 (e.g., the recognition of the borderline PD in ICD-10) that was facilitated, in part, by the receptivity of the *DSM-IV* PD Work Group to input from representatives of ICD-10 (Drs. Alv Dahl, Armand Loranger, and Charles Pull).

Some of the *DSM-IV* revisions were obtained from the ICD-10 (e.g., OBC-8, "rigidity and stubbornness" [APA, 1994, p. 673]; and the PND-5, "persistently bears grudges" [APA, 1994, p. 63]). The ICD-10 influence is particularly noteworthy with respect to the revisions for the schizoid PD. This influence was problematic at times, as the ICD-10 criteria were not based upon or informed by systematic research. Data were being obtained on the ICD-10 criteria (Loranger, Hirschfeld, Sartorius, & Regier, 1991) but only after the criteria sets had been completed (Loranger, Sartorius, et al., 1994). In addition, the rationale and source for the ICD-10 criteria were not always known. Their source was, at times, the *DSM-III-R* or the *DSM-III* criteria sets. There is some irony in obtaining international compatibility by adopting a criterion for *DSM-IV* that was obtained from the 1980 edition of the *DSM* (e.g., the HST-6, "self-dramatization, theatricality, and exaggerated expression of emotion" [APA, 1994, p. 658]).

On the other hand, there was little cost in accepting a wording used in the ICD-10 that did not have a major effect on the meaning or intention of the criterion. In addition, the ICD-10 would, at times, provide a version that appeared to address a problem or issue identified within a literature review. In our summary of the revisions of each item, we identify revisions based in large part on ICD-10 compatibility.

Clinical Utility

A third basis for change was clinical utility (Frances et al., 1990). *DSM-III* and *DSM-III-R* were constructed largely for the benefit and use of the researcher (Frances et al., 1990; Spitzer, Endicott, & Robbins, 1975, 1978; Spitzer, Williams, & Skodol, 1990). This is particularly evident in the lengthy, complex, and detailed criteria sets. Researchers are quite willing and able to take 2 to 4 hours to diagnose the personality disorders. Researchers may devote months and even years to studying a particular PD. Extended, detailed assessments are not unusual nor particularly burdensome to the researcher. It is part of the nature of research to be extremely, if not excessively, exact, precise, and detailed in their assessments. The amount of time it takes to obtain a diagnosis is not a major concern. Practicing clinicians, on the other hand, must often make immediate decisions based upon their diagnoses. They do not have the luxury to devote hours and perhaps days of their attention to the assessment of a very limited domain of psychopathology. They must be able to consider any or all disorders that might apply, and they must reach a decision for a particular patient within a limited period of time.

The WHO also recognized the conflicting needs and demands of the clinician and the researcher and, therefore, published two versions of the ICD-10: a clinician's version and a researcher's version (Sartorius, 1988; Sartorius et al., 1993). The researcher's version resembles *DSM-IV* in its provision of specific and explicit diagnostic criteria. The clinician's version provides more narrative descriptions, at times using the format of earlier versions of the ICD and resembling, in this respect, the format of *DSM-II* (APA, 1968). The descriptions of each disorder are intended to be congruent across the two formats, but the WHO felt that clinicians would find detailed, specific criteria and algorithms too cumbersome and impractical. (There was also a concern that one could not gain acceptance of very specific criteria sets across the diverse cultures, perspectives, and experiences of the WHO membership.)

The *DSM-IV* Task Force also considered the option of providing different versions for the researcher and the clinician (Frances et al., 1990). However, it was decided that this would complicate the relevance of research findings to clinical practice and the relevance of clinicians' experiences to research. It would be odd, to say the least, to conduct research on disorders, the diagnoses of which were different within clinical practice. The WHO clinician's version would also represent a regression to the unreliability of *DSM-II* (Spitzer et al., 1980). A narrative format encourages persons to develop and apply their own interpretations and rules for how a disorder should be diagnosed, thereby compromising substantially the validity, and certainly the reliability, of clinical diagnoses as well as the ability of clinicians to communicate effectively with each other (Matarazzo, 1983; Spitzer et al., 1980). The *DSM-IV* Task Force, therefore, decided to retain the specific and explicit format that was, indeed, a major innovation of *DSM-III* but, at the same time, to attempt to simplify the criteria sets whenever possible (Frances et al., 1990).

The best example of the effort at simplification with respect to the PDs involved the antisocial PD criteria set. The *DSM-III-R* antisocial criteria were the longest and most complex of the PD criteria sets, consisting of 10 adult items, 1 child item, and 23 subcriteria. The detail of the antisocial PD criteria set was due, in large part, to its origin in the influential research criteria sets developed by Spitzer et al. (1978), Feighner et al. (1972), and Robins (1966). However, converting the antisocial PD criteria set to the more general format used for the other PDs might have compromised significantly the reliability of its diagnosis (Widiger & Corbitt, 1993, in press-a). Antisocial is the only PD with consistently reliable diagnosis in clinical practice. The PD Work Group did not want to undermine the only diagnostic criteria set that had consistently performed well (at least with respect to reliability). Therefore, the Work Group obtained data from the antisocial field trial on whether the criteria set could be shortened without significantly changing diagnostic results. It was conceivable that one or more of the criteria could be deleted without substantially affecting the diagnosis. The *DSM-IV* MacArthur and field trial studies indicated that two of the adult criteria could be deleted: "lacks ability to function as a responsible parent" (APA, 1987, p. 345) and "has never sustained a totally monogamous relationship for more than one year" (APA, 1987, p. 346) (Widiger et al., in press; Widiger & Corbitt, in press-a).

Clinical Theory

The final source of revision was clinical theory. Clinical theory was not a primary influence. Priority was given to empirical data, ICD-10 compatibility, and clinical utility. If priority had been given to clinical theory, then it is likely that each criteria set would reflect the particular theoretical orientation or perspective of the primary author of that revision (e.g., Dr. Millon for the avoidant PD, Dr. Gunderson for the borderline, and Dr. Widiger for the antisocial). The end result would have been inconsistent and idiosyncratic content.

Members of the *DSM-IV* PD Work Group have a theoretical perspective which guides and informs their recommendations. To each person, this perspective is useful and even illuminating, but to those with a different perspective, it is often perceived as an a priori bias. In fact, one restraint on the impact of each member's theoretical perspective was the diverse perspectives represented within the Work Group. It was difficult for any one particular perspective to have a substantial influence, given the opposition from at least one other perspective. However, an additional and even more severe constraint was the general process by which *DSM-IV* was developed, wherein emphasis was given to empirical support for a proposed revision, the presentation of these data within documents that required a specific format to maximize critical review of the rationale and empirical support for the proposed revisions, the circulation of these documents to numerous advisors and critics of the proposals, the presentations of the proposals at meetings and conventions, and the publication of the proposals for critical review in the 1991 *DSM-IV Options Book* (Task Force, 1991) and the draft of the final version in the 1993 *DSM-IV Draft Criteria* (Task Force, 1993). Initial proposals were continually abridged and narrowed as time passed, with the final decision representing a substantially curtailed version.

Nevertheless, some degree of influence from clinical theory was inevitable and necessary. This was most evident with respect to item revision. The empirical research was very helpful in indicating which items were most problematic (e.g., poor reliability, sensitivity, or specificity) but not necessarily how the item should be revised. There was research to guide a few of the item revisions. For example, the new borderline criterion of transient, stress-related paranoid ideation or severe dissociative symptoms was informed by a substantial amount of prior research (Gunderson, Zanarini, & Kisiel, 1991). Research was also available on alternative items for the narcissistic PD (Gunderson, Ronningstam, & Smith, 1991; Ronnigstam & Gunderson, 1990) and for the antisocial PD (Hare, Hart, & Harpur, 1991).

However, there was little or no data on new or alternative items for the other PDs. The research indicated which items required substantial revision or even deletion, but the revision was often guided by clinical theory with respect to the disorder and its diagnostic criteria, such as the emphasis given in *DSM-IV* dependent PD for the need to be taken care of (Hirschfeld, Shea, & Weise, 1991), the new histrionic PD criterion of considering relationships to be more intimate than they really are (Pfohl, 1991), and the new passive-aggressive PD criterion of alternating between hostile defiance and contrition (Millon, 1993). Many item revisions, however, were relatively straightforward, involving minor clarifications or a consensus resolution of an obvious problem that had been identified in the research.

One additional area of clinical theory impact that is worth noting concerns the *DSM-IV* text discussion of each PD. The *DSM-IV* text was based, for the most part, on documented research. This resulted in the deletion of some statements from *DSM-III-R* that were potentially controversial and had little or no systematic empirical support, such as the statement that persons with a paranoid PD "may be overrepresented among leaders of cults and other fringe groups" (APA, 1987, p. 338). However, one instance in which it was advisable for theory to veto research in *DSM-IV* concerned the prevalence rates for each disorder within various clinical settings. The prevalence rates that were obtained through systematic empirical studies were usually based on literal applications of the *DSM-III-R* criteria. These studies are very useful in providing data on the performance of the criteria sets, but they may not be providing realistic estimates of the actual prevalence rates for the disorders. These studies were providing prevalence rates of the disorders' diagnostic criteria, not necessarily the prevalence rates of the disorders. A goal of the *DSM-IV* PD Work Group was to revise the criteria sets to increase their specificity, thereby decreasing the prevalence rate obtained by the criteria set. It would then be somewhat inconsistent to provide a prevalence rate based upon the literal applications of criteria sets that were revised, in part, because this same research was indicating that the criteria set lacked specificity and resulted in an excessive prevalence rate.

OVERVIEW OF DSM-IV REVISIONS

Subsequent chapters of this manual will discuss the rationale for the deletion, revision, or replacement of each *DSM-III-R* PD criterion. However, it may also be helpful to provide a broad overview of the extent of the revisions and to briefly discuss revisions that affected all of the PDs.

PD Diagnoses Added, Deleted, or Moved

DSM-III-R included 11 officially recognized PDs (i.e., paranoid, schizoid, schizotypal, antisocial, borderline, histrionic, narcissistic, avoidant, dependent, obsessive-compulsive, and passive-aggressive) and two within the appendix of proposed diagnostic categories needing further study (i.e., self-defeating and sadistic). The self-defeating and sadistic PDs have been deleted entirely from the manual in *DSM-IV*, passive-aggressive PD has been shifted (or demoted) from an officially recognized PD to the appendix of criteria sets provided for further study, and depressive PD has been added to this appendix. The passive-aggressive and depressive PDs are listed within the PD diagnostic category of personality disorder not otherwise specified (PDNOS). The rationale for the demotion of the passive-aggressive PD and for the addition of the depressive PD will be presented in subsequent chapters.

Self-defeating (SDF) PD was deleted because there was insufficient data to document its validity and its misdiagnosis had the potential to cause harm, particularly to female victims of abuse, discrimination, or harassment (e.g., blaming the victims for their victimization; Walker, 1987). One might argue that there is insufficient data to document the validity for many of the officially recognized PDs but none of the other PDs have as much potential to do harm. Maintaining the self-defeating PD within the appendix would have provided the diagnosis with at least a quasiofficial recognition that was perhaps unwarranted (Widiger, in press).

Similar concerns were raised for the sadistic (SDS) PD proposal. A national survey of forensic psychiatrists was conducted to assess its (presumed) support among clinicians who evaluate persons that abuse their spouses and/or children. This survey found that only 11% of the specialists believed that the SDS diagnosis would be very useful, and 66%

indicated that it had considerable potential for misuse, particularly to mitigate criminal responsibility (Spitzer et al., 1991). There was some data to suggest that it may represent a valid diagnosis (Gay, in press) but the support was too preliminary and insufficient to provide recognition to a diagnosis that had substantial potential for harmful consequences and social misuse. A more detailed presentation of the history of the SDF and SDS proposals and the rationale for their deletion is presented elsewhere (Widiger, in press).

Table 3-1
Overview of Revision to DSM-III-R Personality Disorder Criteria Sets

	Number of criteria						
	In *DSM-III-R*	Unchanged	Minor revision	Signfcant revision	Deleted	Added	In *DSM-IV*
Paranoid	7	0	2	5	0	0	7
Schizoid	7	2	1	4	0	0	7
Schizotypal	9	2	4	3	0	0	9
Antisocial[a]	11	0	3	6	2	0	8[b]
Borderline	8	2	3	3	0	1	9
Histrionic	8	2	1	3	2	2	8
Narcissistic	9	1	2	5	1	1	9
Avoidant	7	1	0	5	1	1	7
Dependent	9	0	0	8	1	0	8
Obs-Compulsive	9	0	5	2	2	1	8
Pas-Aggressive[c]	9	0	0	8	1	3	7[b]
Total number	93	10	21	52	10	9	87[d]

Note. Signfcant = significant; obs-compulsive = obsessive-compulsive; pas-aggressive = passive-aggressive. [a]Conduct disorder criterion counts as one item. [b]Sum of items unchanged, receiving minor revision, receiving significant revision, and added does not equal number in *DSM-IV* because some *DSM-III-R* items (coded as significantly revised) were collapsed into one item. [c]Passive-aggressive is not an officially recognized personality disorder in *DSM-IV*. [d]Does not include depressive personality disorder, which contains seven additional items.

Criteria Set Revisions

Table 3-1 presents an overview of the extent to which the *DSM-III-R* PD criteria were revised. *DSM-III-R* included 93 criteria across the 11 officially recognized PDs (the *DSM-III-R* antisocial PD conduct disorder criterion, with 15 subitems, is counted as one item). Only 10 criteria (11%) remained virtually unchanged. The rest (89%) received at least some revision.

However, it should be noted that this revision varied in consequence. We classified the extent of revision into five categories: unchanged, minor revision, significant revision, deleted, or added. Unchanged means that there was, indeed, no change (except perhaps with respect to typing). Minor means that the revision involved simply changes to grammar, the deletion of examples, and/or minor clarification in wording, all of which had no intended or likely effect on the content, meaning, or interpretation of the item (e.g., the deletion of the example of describing one's mother as a beautiful person from the histrionic impressionistic speech item [HST-5]; and the change in wording from "impulsiveness" to "impulsivity" for BDL-4). Significant revisions included any changes that had the intention or likely effect of altering the interpretation or meaning of the item. This typically involved a revision in the wording of an item (e.g., the *DSM-III-R* schizotypal criterion of no close friends or confidants, or only one, other than first-degree relatives, became "lack of close friends or confidants other than first-degree relatives" in *DSM-IV* [APA, 1994, p. 645, item 8]), but it could also include the deletion of examples when this deletion would have the effect of changing the meaning or interpretation of an item (e.g., the deletion of the examples of driving while intoxicated and recurrent speeding from the antisocial recklessness criterion [item 6]). Deleted meant that the item and its content were deleted from the criteria set (or the item was replaced with a new item that provided a significant change in content). For example, the *DSM-III-R* antisocial PD item of parental irresponsibility was deleted entirely from the criteria set. On the other hand, the *DSM-III-R* antisocial PD items of "unable to sustain consistent work behavior" and "fails to honor financial obligations" (APA, 1987, p. 345) were collapsed into one *DSM-IV* item of consistent irresponsibility (item 6). These two *DSM-III-R* ATS items were, therefore, classified as significantly revised rather than deleted because their content was retained in the collapsed version. Added means that an item with new content was added (e.g., the avoidant PD criterion [AVD-6] of a belief that one is socially inept, personally unappealing, or inferior).

In other words, items classified as unchanged or receiving only minor revision could be considered essentially unchanged. However, even with this more liberal classification, we would consider 67% of the items as having received at least a significant revision (i.e., a deletion, or a change in meaning, content, or interpretation). The following chapters on each PD will discuss the nature and extent of each item's revision.

Text Revision

DSM-III-R provided a description of each PD, in addition to the diagnostic criteria. This description included a (narrative) explication of the diagnostic criteria, and (when known) a presentation of associated features, age at onset, impairments, complications, predisposing factors, prevalence, sex ratio, familial pattern, and differentiation from other mental disorders (APA, 1987). This text discussion has been modified and expanded in *DSM-IV*. The major revisions for the PDs are an expansion of the explication of the diagnostic criteria and inclusion of a discussion of specific culture, age, and gender features (APA, 1994).

The text discussion of the diagnostic criteria sets has been expanded substantially in *DSM-IV*. In *DSM-III-R*, this section of the text was confined largely to a narrative reiteration of the diagnostic criteria. In *DSM-IV*, this section provides examples and illustrations of the criterion, as well as a further clarification of its meaning. Many of the examples in the *DSM-IV* text discussion had been examples provided within the *DSM-III-R* criteria for the diagnosis. For instance, included within the *DSM-III-R* criterion of impressionistic speech was the example of describing one's mother simply as a beautiful person (APA, 1987). Driving while intoxicated or recurrent speeding were included within the criterion for antisocial recklessness. These examples were often helpful in illustrating concretely what was meant by the criterion, but their presentation within the criteria set was also problematic. Specific behavioral examples are rarely adequate for defining precisely what is meant by a particular personality trait (Widiger & Trull, 1987). One must usually note the presence of many qualifications or exceptions. For example, there are many reasons other than the presence of histrionic impressionistic speech for describing one's mother as being a beautiful person. Because one or two concrete examples are never sufficient to define exactly what is meant by a personality trait, the authors of *DSM-III* and *DSM-III-R* had to continually expand the criteria to include additional examples or to note qualifications and exceptions. However, any such expansion would then necessitate further expansion, resulting in lengthy, complex, and cumbersome criteria sets that remained inadequate. For example, the *DSM-III-R* antisocial parental irresponsibility item contained six examples (some with further specification) that were still inadequate (e.g., the failure to consider custody responsibilities, drug usage in presence of children, or involvement of offspring in crimes as additional examples of antisocial parental irresponsibility). In addition, clinicians and researchers have, at times, reified the examples as providing the operational definitions for the trait, as if driving while intoxicated or recurrent speeding were necessary and sufficient for determining the presence of antisocial recklessness. There is clearly much more to the trait of antisocial recklessness than simply the reckless use of a car.

Therefore, in *DSM-IV*, many of these examples have been moved out of the criteria set and into the text discussion (within the first section, now titled "diagnostic features," APA, 1994). This shift also allowed the *DSM-IV* PD Work Group to provide additional examples and further commentary without expanding the criteria set itself. Clinicians and researchers are then advised to consider the text discussion closely when applying the criteria sets.

An argument against the shifting of examples to the text and the expansion of the text itself is that some clinicians and researchers may not read or consider the text discussion, relying solely upon the criteria set provided within the *DSM-IV* table. However, the *DSM-IV* Task Force decided that clinicians and researchers should and will consider the text discussion, particularly when it becomes clear that it does, in fact, provide additional and useful information.

The text discussion in *DSM-IV* also includes a new section concerned with specific culture, age, and gender features (APA, 1994). This section will be particularly useful for the diagnosis of personality disorders. It provides a discussion of each PD across different ages, gender, and cultures. The diagnosis of a personality disorder can be quite problematic and even controversial when adequate consideration is not given to the influence of gender, age, and culture on the behavior of the subject and the perceptions of the diagnostician (Alarcon & Foulks, in press; Landrine, 1992; Widiger & Spitzer, 1991). For example, histrionic traits are, at times, overdiagnosed in female patients; criminal acts are less apparent in antisocial persons as they age; and excessive deference to authority may be normative within some cultural groups. These issues will be discussed in more detail in the following chapters as they become relevant to individual PD items.

4

Antisocial Personality Disorder

Overview: Antisocial (ATS) personality disorder was defined in *DSM-III-R* as "a pattern of irresponsible and antisocial behavior" (APA, 1987, p. 345). However, the ATS PD involves much more than simply being irresponsible, and the inclusion of the trait of being "antisocial" was not particularly helpful in describing these additional traits, as it simply repeated the name of the disorder. In *DSM-IV*, antisocial PD is described as "a pervasive pattern of disregard for, and violation of, the rights of others" (APA, 1994, p. 645).

The *DSM-III* and *DSM-III-R* criteria for ATS were derived from the Research Diagnostic Criteria (RDC) developed by Spitzer, Endicott, and Robins (1978), which were, in turn, derived from the Feighner et al. (1972) criteria for ATS PD and the Robins (1966) criteria for sociopathic personality. One of the issues for *DSM-IV* was whether the *DSM-III-R* placed too much emphasis on these research criteria and not enough emphasis on the more traditional traits of psychopathy (Stone, 1993; Sutker, 1994; Widiger & Corbitt, 1993), such as lacks empathy, glib and superficial charm, and inflated, arrogant self-appraisal (Hare et al., 1991). However, the *DSM-IV* ATS field trial indicated that some of these traits of psychopathy (derived from the Psychopathy Checklist developed by Hare, 1992) were difficult to assess reliably. In addition, the field trial indicated that the *DSM-III-R* ATS items performed as well as the more traditional traits of psychopathy, except within the prison setting (Widiger et al., in press). The criminal, delinquent, and irresponsible behaviors that are emphasized in the *DSM-III-R* and *DSM-IV* criteria for ATS PD are relatively specific to the ATS/psychopathic disorder within most clinical settings. However, within prison and forensic settings, they will be quite nonspecific. This issue will be discussed further below.

An additional issue for *DSM-IV* was the length and complexity of the *DSM-III-R* criteria set (Widiger & Corbitt, 1993). The *DSM-III-R* ATS criteria set consisted of one childhood item (age 15 or younger) and 10 adulthood items (age 18 or older). The childhood item included 12 subitems, and 3 of the 10 adult items included subitems (parental irresponsibility contained 6 subitems). The total number of items and subitems was 30.

The *DSM-IV* MacArthur and field trial studies indicated that two of the adult items could be deleted without affecting the diagnosis (Widiger et al., in press). Two items were also collapsed into one item (i.e., inconsistent work behavior and failure to honor financial obligations). Three of the remaining adult items were revised, and three received only minor revision. The threshold for diagnosis was revised from 4 of the 10 adult items to 3 of 7 to maximize agreement with the *DSM-III-R* threshold for diagnosis (Widiger et al., in press). The childhood conduct disorder item was also revised significantly by the *DSM-IV* Child and Adolescent Disorders Work Group. However, this criteria set was not simplified. It was, in fact, expanded (see discussion below). In sum, the *DSM-IV* criteria for ATS PD consists of one child and seven adult items.

The two items that were deleted were "lacks ability to function as a responsible parent" (APA, 1987, p. 345) and "has never sustained a totally monogamous relationship for more than one year" (APA, 1987, p. 346). Parental irresponsibility was the least prevalent, most unreliable, and least diagnostic item in the *DSM-IV* MacArthur and field trial studies (Widiger & Corbitt, 1993; Widiger et al., in press). It was also the most complex item, consisting of seven subitems. Its infrequency was due, in part, to requiring that the person be a parent in order for the item to be considered. It was also difficult to assess. Many antisocial persons are quite willing to acknowledge a history of assaults, thefts, and extortion but not a failure to care for a dependent child. Deletion of the item changed the diagnosis in only 2 of the 507 field trial subjects (Widiger et al., in press).

"Has never sustained a totally monogamous relationship for more than one year" (APA, 1987, p. 346) performed almost as poorly as parental irresponsibility in the *DSM-IV* MacArthur and field trial studies. It is characteristic of antisocial persons to fail to be faithful and reliable in their sexual relationships, but the *DSM-III-R* characterization of this trait (as a failure to sustain a totally monogamous relationship for more than one year) was perhaps too narrowly defined. Many antisocial persons, particularly those within middle age, will have been able to sustain a monogamous relationship for at least one year, whereas the reverse is often true for many nonantisocial adolescents and young adults. The earlier Feighner et al. (1972) version of this item was much broader, requiring the presence of "marital difficulties manifested by any of the following: deserting family, two or more divorces, frequent separations due to marital discord, recurrent infidelity, recurrent physical attacks upon spouse, or being suspected of battering a child" (p. 60). Deletion of this *DSM-III-R* item, along with parental irresponsibility, changed the diagnosis in less than 2% of the 507 subjects in the *DSM-III-R* field trial (Widiger et al., in press).

A final point with respect to the ATS criteria set is the exclusion criterion, that the behaviors have not occurred exclusively during the course of schizophrenia or a manic episode (APA, 1994). This exclusion criterion was present in *DSM-III* and *DSM-III-R* (*DSM-III*, however, also excluded severe mental retardation; APA, 1980). It is indeed important to exclude instances in which a failure to plan ahead is due to schizophrenia or a reckless disregard for the safety of oneself or others is due to a manic episode. However, it has been our experience that such occurrences are usually quite apparent (cyclothymic hypomania will be more problematic). What is usually more difficult is the differentiation of ATS PD from a substance related (substance use) disorder (Alterman & Cacciola, 1991; Widiger & Corbitt, 1993). Many antisocial acts can be the immediate and direct result of a substance dependence (e.g., thefts to pay for drugs, drug dealing, acts of violence involved with or during drug usage, or the illegal drug usage itself). The RDC criteria for ATS had specified that only those ATS acts that could not be clearly attributed to a substance use disorder would qualify (Spitzer et al., 1978). However, *DSM-III*, *DSM-III-R*, and *DSM-IV* have taken a quite different approach. The *DSM* recognizes that the causal relationship between substance usage and antisocial personality is often mutually interactive. Substance use, including abuse and dependence, will often be the result of antisocial personality traits. In addition, the *DSM* requirement that ATS PD be diagnosed only when there has been a history of ATS behavior prior to age 15 will usually date the onset of ATS prior to the onset of a substance dependence. Therefore, the *DSM* has indicated (within the section on differential diagnosis) that both diagnoses should be given when the criteria for both are met, regardless of the extent to which some of the antisocial behaviors may appear to be a consequence of a substance related disorder (APA, 1987, 1994).

It will, at times, be difficult, arbitrary, and perhaps even meaningless to determine when a particular adult ATS act is due to a substance related disorder rather than to an antisocial personality trait (e.g., childhood antisocial traits can contribute to the development and escalation of drug usage which, in turn, contributes to antisocial behaviors). A proposal considered for *DSM-IV* was to include substance related disorder within the exclusion criterion (along with schizophrenia and manic episodes), but the final decision was to retain the *DSM-III-R* guideline because the exclusion criterion would probably have had the effect of rarely diagnosing ATS PD in persons with a substance dependence even when the substance use was independent of or, in fact, a direct manifestation of antisocial traits. However, in the PDI-IV interview, we do highlight the differentiation of a substance related disorder and ATS PD in the instances in which it is often problematic (i.e., ATS-A1, -A2, -A4, -A5, & -A6). Table 4-1 presents the complete *DSM-IV* criteria set for the diagnosis of ATS PD.

Criterion ATS-C

Evidence of Conduct Disorder, as indicated by a repetitive and persistent pattern of behavior in which the basic rights of others or major age-appropriate societal norms or rules were violated, as manifested by the presence of three (or more) of the following criteria over a 12-month period of time prior to the age of 15: (1) often bullied, threatened, or intimidated others (2) often initiated physical fights (3) used a weapon that can cause serious physical harm to others (e.g., a bat, brick, broken bottle, knife, gun) (4) stolen while confronting a victim (e.g., mugging, purse snatching, extortion, armed robbery) (5) physically cruel to people (6) physically cruel to animals (7) forced someone into sexual activity (8) often lied to obtain goods or favors or to avoid obligations (i.e., "cons" others) (9) often stayed out at night despite parental prohibitions, beginning before age 13 (10) stole items of nontrivial value without confronting victim (e.g., shoplifting, forgery) (11) deliberately engaged in fire setting with the intention of causing serious damage (12) deliberately destroyed others' property (other than by fire setting) (13) ran away from home overnight at least twice while living in parental or parental surrogate home (or once without returning for a lengthy period) (14) often truant from school, beginning before 13 years of age or (15) broke into someone else's house, building, or car.

Revisions and Rationale: Antisocial PD is one of only two *DSM-IV* PDs to include criteria during childhood, and the other instance involves only illustrations for a subset of the adult items (e.g., SZT-2). This childhood conduct disorder criterion is very useful in documenting the presence and stability of the behavior pattern prior to the age of 15.

Revision of the criteria set was managed by the *DSM-IV* Childhood and Adolescent Disorders Work Group (Lahey et al., in press). They were not as concerned with a simplification of the criteria set as the PD Work Group, and, in fact, expanded the set from 13 to 15 items (the threshold for diagnosis remains at 3, which could have the effect of increasing its prevalence, although this effect may be offset by individual item revisions). Seven of the original 13 items were unchanged from *DSM-III-R* (items 2, 4, 5, 6, 7, 12, and 15); six

Table 4-1

DSM-IV Criteria for Antisocial Personality Disorder

A. There is a pervasive pattern of disregard for and violation of the rights of others occurring since age 15 years, as indicated by at least three (or more) of the following:

(1) failure to conform to social norms with respect to lawful behaviors as indicated by repeatedly performing acts that are grounds for arrest

(2) deceitfulness, as indicated by repeated lying, use of aliases, or conning others for personal profit or pleasure

(3) impulsivity or failure to plan ahead

(4) irritability and aggressiveness, as indicated by repeated physical fights or assaults

(5) reckless disregard for safety of self or others

(6) consistent irresponsibility, as indicated by repeated failure to sustain consistent work behavior or honor financial obligations

(7) lack of remorse, as indicated by being indifferent to or rationalizing having hurt, mistreated, or stolen from another

B. The individual is at least age 18 years.

C. Evidence of Conduct Disorder, as indicated by a repetitive and persistent pattern of behavior in which the basic rights of others or major age-appropriate societal norms or rules were violated, as manifested by the presence of three (or more) of the following criteria over a 12-month period of time prior to the age of 15:

Aggression to people and animals

(1) often bullies, threatens, or intimidates others
(2) often initiates physical fights
(3) has used a weapon that can cause serious physical harm to others (e.g., a bat, brick, broken bottle, knife, gun)
(4) has been physically cruel to people
(5) has been physically cruel to animals
(6) has stolen while confronting a victim (e.g., mugging, purse snatching, extortion, armed robbery)
(7) has forced someone into sexual activity

Destruction of property

(8) has deliberately engaged in fire setting with the intention of causing serious damage
(9) has deliberately destroyed others' property (other than by fire setting)

Deceitfulness or theft

(10) has broken into someone else's house, building, or car
(11) often lies to obtain goods or favors or to avoid obligations (i.e., "cons" others)
(12) has stolen items of nontrivial value without confronting a victim (e.g., shoplifting, but without breaking and entering; forgery)

Serious violation of rules

(13) often stays out at night despite parental prohibitions, beginning before age 13 years
(14) has run away from home overnight at least twice while living in parental or parental surrogate home (or once without returning for a lengthy period)
(15) is often truant from school, beginning before age 13 years

D. The occurrence of antisocial behavior is not exclusively during the course of schizophrenia or a manic episode.

Note. From *Diagnostic and Statistical Manual of Mental Disorders* (4th ed., pp. 90-91, 649-650), by American Psychiatric Association, 1994, Washington, DC: Author. Copyright 1994 by American Psychiatric Association. Adapted with permission.

were revised significantly (items 3, 8, 10, 11, 13, and 14); and two were added (items 1 and 9). However, to facilitate the use of the criteria, the items were reorganized within the areas of aggression to people or animals, destruction of property, deceitfulness or theft, and serious violation of rules, as presented in Table 4-1 (APA, 1994). The order presented above reflects their descending order of diagnostic value (discussed further below).

The two new items are "often stays out at night despite parental prohibitions, beginning before age 13 years" (APA, 1994, p. 90), and "often bullies, threatens, or intimidates others" (APA, 1994, p. 90). These two items were found to be very diagnostic of conduct disorder (CD) in the *DSM-IV* disruptive behavior disorder field trial (APA, 1994), although the bullying item was, in fact, originally proposed for the diagnosis of oppositional defiant disorder (Task Force, 1991). These items were added, in part, to help address a potential sex bias within the *DSM-III-R* CD criteria (Goodman & Kohlsdorf, 1994). Some of the *DSM-III-R* CD criteria may apply mostly, if not only, to boys with conduct disorder (e.g., forcing someone into a sexual activity). Intimidating others and staying out at night are more indicative of CD in girls than the physically aggressive and assaultive items that were emphasized in *DSM-III-R*.

Additional items considered for inclusion were "onset of alcohol or other substance use before age 13 and recurrent use during past six months" (Task Force, 1991, p. C:20) and "has engaged in sexual activities in order to obtain money, goods, or drugs" (Task Force, 1991, p. C:21). The latter item was considered because it might provide a behavior that would be particularly diagnostic of CD in girls. Neither item, however, performed sufficiently well in the *DSM-IV* disruptive behavior disorder field trial (Lahey et al., in press), although it is now noted in the *DSM-IV* text discussion of CD that "females with...Conduct Disorder are more likely to exhibit lying, truancy, running away, substance use, and prostitution" (APA, 1994, p. 88) (whereas boys are more likely to exhibit fighting, stealing, vandalism, and school disciplinary problems). The substance use item would also have complicated even further the differentiation of ATS PD from a substance related disorder by including the onset of substance dependence prior to the onset of the adult antisocial behaviors.

The (six) CD item revisions were largely for clarification and to increase their threshold for attribution. The *DSM-III-R* item of "used a weapon in more than one fight" (APA, 1987, p. 55) was revised to emphasize that the weapon can cause serious physical harm (e.g., a bat, brick, broken bottle, knife, or gun). The *DSM-III-R* item of "often lies" (APA, 1987, p. 55) was revised to "often lies to obtain goods or favors or to avoid obligations" (APA, 1994, p. 90) in order to emphasize that it involves an explicit effort to con others (comparable to the adult item) rather than simply failing to tell the truth (e.g., excluding lies that are simply to avoid telling on someone or to spread gossip or rumors). The *DSM-III-R* item of stealing (without confrontation) was revised to emphasize that the items involve a nontrivial value (e.g., excluding petty shoplifting that is primarily done for excitement). An additional proposal for this item was to include thefts (of nontrivial value) within one's own home (Task Force, 1993) but this was not included in the final version of the item (APA, 1994). The *DSM-III-R* item of deliberately engaging in fire setting was revised to require an intention of causing serious damage (e.g., excluding accidental fires or fires that were set for fun or excitement rather than to deliberately cause damage). The *DSM-III-R* item of running away from home was revised to indicate that it could occur only once (*DSM-III-R* required twice) if there was a failure to return after a lengthy period of time. And, finally, the *DSM-III-R* item for being truant from school was revised to specify that the truancy has to begin prior to age 13.

The order of the items has also changed. The order provided in *DSM-III-R* reflected their descending order of diagnostic value, based on the *DSM-III-R* field trial (APA, 1987; Spitzer, Davies, & Barkley, 1990). In the published draft for *DSM-IV* (Task Force, 1993), this order was revised to be consistent with the results obtained from the *DSM-IV* disruptive behavior disorders field trial (Lahey et al., in press). The order given on page 49 is consistent with the field trial findings and the 1993 draft version of *DSM-IV*. The change in order is substantial and significant, as it reflects a change in the discriminating power of the respective items. For example, the new item of "bullies, threatens, or intimidates others" (APA, 1994, p. 90) that was originally considered for inclusion within the criteria for oppositional defiant disorder (Task Force, 1991) is placed at the top of the list because it was found to be the most diagnostic item for Conduct Disorder, and the item that was previously at the top of the list (stealing without confrontation of a victim on more than one occasion) is now within the bottom third of the list (item 10).

However, the order in which the items appear in *DSM-IV* and in Table 4-1 does not reflect their diagnostic value. The final decision was to reorganize the items with respect to thematic content (aggression to people and animals, destruction of property, deceitfulness or theft, and serious violation of rules) to facilitate the understanding and retention of this lengthy criteria set.

Rating:

0) Absent
1) Conduct disorder: 3 to 7 of the behaviors listed below
2) Conduct disorder: 8 to 15 of the behaviors listed below

Questions:

I am now going to ask you questions about things you might have done prior to the age of 15. It is important to emphasize that these things must have happened <u>before</u> you were <u>15</u> years old.

a. <u>Prior to the age of 15</u>, did you deliberately destroy others' property (other than by fire setting), deliberately engage in fire setting with the intention of causing serious damage, or break into someone else's house, building, or car?
b. Did you often initiate physical fights, use a weapon that can cause serious physical harm to others (e.g., bat, brick, broken bottle, knife, gun), or often bully, threaten, or intimidate others?
c. Did you ever steal things of nontrivial value without actually confronting the victim, such as shoplifting, burglary, or forgery?
d. Did you ever steal with a direct confrontation of your victim, such as mugging, purse snatching, extortion, or armed robbery?

e. Did you often lie to obtain goods or favors or to avoid obligations, or run away from home overnight at least twice while living in your parents' home (or once without returning for a lengthy period)?

f. Prior to the age of 13, did you often stay out at night despite parental prohibitions, or were you often truant from school? [*if employed, absent from work*]

g. Again, prior to age 15, were you ever physically cruel to people, physically cruel to animals, or did you ever force someone into a sexual activity?

[*Note that the set of conduct disorder behaviors that are present must together span at least 12 months.*]

Issues and Problems: The assessment of the 15 childhood CD items can be as complex and time-consuming as assessing all seven adulthood items. There are twice as many items to assess in childhood (15) as there are to assess in adulthood (7). A proposal considered for *DSM-IV* was to require only the presence of "evidence" of conduct disorder, without suggesting that the specific *DSM-IV* criteria for a CD diagnosis had to be met. This would be more consistent with the ICD-10 criteria for a dissocial personality disorder, as it does not require that a conduct disorder be present in order to diagnose the adult personality disorder. The ICD-10 only notes that the presence of a conduct disorder during childhood or adolescence "may further support the diagnosis" (WHO, 1992, p. 204). Given that only 3 of 15 criteria are necessary for a CD diagnosis, it was felt that a less specific requirement of documenting only the evidence for a conduct disorder would simplify the assessment without actually changing any diagnostic result. Most clinicians and researchers would likely interpret "evidence" to mean some CD criteria (rather than none, just one, or even just two CD criteria). On the other hand, ATS PD has been the only PD disorder to be diagnosed reliably in everyday clinical practice due, in part, to its very specific diagnostic criteria (Widiger & Corbitt, 1993). The final decision was to require only the "evidence" of a conduct disorder (rather than the known presence of a conduct disorder), but the clinician is also explicitly referred to p. 90 of the manual wherein the *DSM-IV* CD criteria are provided. We interpret this to mean that the person should have met the *DSM-IV* criteria for a conduct disorder prior to the age of 15 in order to be given the adult diagnosis of antisocial PD.

If the purpose of the assessment is only to determine whether the person would meet the *DSM-IV* criteria for ATS PD, then one can save considerable time by confining the assessment of the CD items only to those persons who meet the threshold for the adult criteria (they cannot be given the diagnosis of ATS PD if they fail to have 3 of the 7 adult criteria, no matter how many of the child CD criteria are present). Administering the childhood criteria after the adulthood criteria is also helpful in highlighting the presence of adult ATS features in the absence of a history of CD features within childhood (which would meet the ICD-10 criteria for dissocial PD).

Additional time can be saved by desisting from further assessments once the person has met at least 3 of the 15 childhood criteria. To facilitate this approach, we begin this section of the interview with what we have found to be the more straightforward and simpler items to assess (e.g., items 12, 11, & 15), followed by the more complex or difficult items (e.g., items 1, 4, 10, & 8), and ending with the more provocative, sensitive, or difficult items (i.e., items 5, 6, & 7). We also placed together the two items that involve a different age requirement (i.e., items 9 & 14). We find this order to be helpful in the assessment.

However, we also acknowledge that this can become rather confusing because one now has three different ways in which the CD criteria are organized: (a) by thematic content, as in *DSM-IV* (APA, 1994) and Table 1; (b) by descending order of diagnostic value, as in the draft version of *DSM-IV* presented above (Task Force, 1993), and (c) by ease in assessment, as presented in the PDI-IV interview.

We do advise assessing for the presence of at least four CD items in case any doubts or questions arise later concerning the presence of any one of the items that were considered to be present. In addition, it should also be emphasized that failing to assess for all 15 will prohibit a full description of the extent and breadth of the antisocial history. It will also prohibit the *DSM-IV* distinction between mild, moderate, or severe CD that is based on the extent to which the behaviors are harmful toward others (APA, 1994) and our own rating of 1 (three to seven items) versus 2 (eight or more items).

It is also important to emphasize the age requirements. All of the CD items must be present prior to the age of 15. The person should be reminded of this requirement during the assessment of each item, as it is often forgotten. In addition, items 9 and 14 have an age requirement of 13, rather than 15 (their insertion among items that have the age 15 requirement can be confusing, but it also helps to remind the interviewer and the subject of the specific age requirement). Note, as well, that although the person must be at least 18 at the time of the assessment the adulthood items may have occurred since the age of 15.

In the 1993 draft version of *DSM-IV*, it was specified that the total set of CD items (i.e., three or more) must span a period of at least 6 months. The purpose of this requirement was to ensure that the antisocial acts did not involve a temporary situational event. However, any one item could have a duration of less than 6 months. Many of the items (e.g., items 3, 4, 5, 6, 7, 10, 11, 12, and 15) require the occurrence of only one act or instance to be considered present (e.g., one needs to have used a gun only once to qualify for item 3). The others specify that the behavior has occurred often or at least twice (e.g., item 1 indicates that one has often bullied, threatened, or intimidated others). The requirement for a total span of 6 months across three or more items was not included in the final version. It is simply noted in *DSM-IV* that three or more of the criteria must have occurred "in the past 12 months, with at least one criterion present in the past 6 months" (APA, 1994, p. 90). If one was assessing a child or adolescent, this would effectively require at least 6 months duration across the set of items. However, the final version of this wording is not applicable if one is interviewing an adult and assessing the items retrospectively. Therefore, we use the wording provided in the 1993 draft, but indicate that the total set of CD items that are present must span at least 12 months.

The individual items are very specific. This is quite helpful in a retrospective assessment. For example, it is much easier to assess whether a person ever mugged or robbed someone prior to age 15 than to assess whether the person often bullied or intimidated people many years ago. Nevertheless, it is also apparent that considerable clinical judgment is still necessary, even for the seemingly specific items. It may be impossible to have items so specific that no clinical judgment is necessary. For example, many of the items indicate that the behavior was "often" present or that the period of time was "lengthy," but there is no indication of what is meant by often or lengthy. In addition, some judgment is necessary to determine what constitutes "bullies" (item 1), being "cruel" to animals (item 6), or "avoiding an obligation" (item 8). Reliability is improved if each item is interpreted literally, but we advise some common sense and clinical judgment to maximize validity. For example, one should consider what is normative behavior for that person's setting and culture, and the intention or spirit of the item (i.e., to describe a child with a conduct disorder that eventually becomes an antisocial personality disorder). For example, pulling the tail of a cat is being physically cruel to an animal, and lying to avoid taking out the garbage when it is one's turn is lying to avoid an obligation, but these acts are relatively minor and inconsistent with the intention of the items. Setting a cat on fire and selling phony magazine subscriptions to one's neighbors are more consistent with a conduct disorder.

One should also consider what is normative within the particular culture, setting, or time in which the child was raised (Goodman & Kohlsdorf, 1994; Sutker, 1994). Intimidation, for example, may be more common in some settings than in others. It is noted in the text discussion of this disorder that the diagnosis "may at times be misapplied to individuals in settings where patterns of undesirable behavior are...viewed as protective (e.g., threatening, impoverished, high-crime)" (APA, 1994, p. 88). This point is well taken, particularly when the assessment concerns a child rather than an adult who has continued to engage in criminal, antisocial acts. However, one should also be careful not to err in the opposite direction of dismissing, ignoring, or excusing what is perhaps the development of an antisocial personality disorder. Some acts, such as burglary, assaults, or rape, should be considered as present even if they are common to a person's particular setting, neighborhood, or peer group. In such cases, we might consider the setting to be providing a sociocultural contribution to the etiology of the antisocial behavior pattern.

Criterion ATS-A1

Failure to conform to social norms with respect to lawful behaviors as indicated by repeatedly performing acts that are grounds for arrest.

Revisions and Rationale: This item was essentially unchanged from *DSM-III-R*. The only revision was to move the examples (destroying property, harassing others, stealing, and pursuing an illegal occupation) from the criteria set to the text. A history of repeatedly performing acts that are grounds for arrest is a prototypic symptom of an antisocial PD. It was the most diagnostic criterion in the *DSM-IV* MacArthur studies, and the most diagnostic criterion in four of the five sites in the *DSM-IV* antisocial PD field trial (Widiger et al., in press). It would be very unusual for an antisocial or psychopathic person not to have repeatedly committed acts for which he or she could have been arrested.

There has been some controversy regarding the apparent emphasis placed on criminal acts within the *DSM-III* and *DSM-III-R* criteria for ATS PD (Hare et al., 1991; Robins et al., 1991; Sutker, 1994). It is of interest to note, in this regard, that in the 1978 draft of the *DSM-III* ATS PD criteria set, three of the eight ATS items involved different criminal activities (i.e., three or more nontraffic arrests or a felony conviction; repeated thefts, whether caught or not; and illegal occupation; Task Force, 1978). These three different criminal acts were subsequently subsumed within the one item in the final version for *DSM-III* (APA, 1980).

Rating:

0) Absent
1) Failure to conform to social norms with respect to lawful behavior as indicated by repeatedly performing acts that are grounds for arrest
2) Primary source of income has been through the pursuit of criminal acts

Questions:

[*Emphasize that the rest of the questions now return to when the person was at least 15 years of age.*]

a. Ever been arrested? (*If yes:*) How often and for what?

b. Ever steal anything, or commit extortion?

c. Ever destroyed someone's property or threatened someone?

d. Ever swindle, embezzle, commit a fraud, launder money, or bribe someone?

e. Ever do anything against the law? (*If yes:*) What, and how often?

f. How do you make most of your income?

g. Would you describe yourself as being a criminal, or as someone who often breaks the law?

Issues and Problems: It is important to emphasize in the assessment of this item that the act need only be in violation of the law (i.e., grounds for arrest). Many antisocial and psychopathic persons may have no history of arrests, but the item refers to acts that are grounds for arrest. No actual arrest record is necessary.

An issue in the assessment of this item is that there is wide variation in the acts that can qualify. The examples provided in *DSM-III-R* were destroying property, harassment, stealing, or an illegal occupation (e.g., pimping, prostitution, fencing, or drug dealing). However, these examples may have contributed to a neglect of "white-collar" crimes (fraud, embezzlement, swindling, bribery), and an overemphasis on "blue-collar" crimes. Some antisocial (psychopathic) persons may never have committed the more directly confrontational, aggressive crimes, confining their activities instead to the more exploitative and manipulative crimes.

The Feighner et al. (1972) version of this criterion provided a hierarchy of acts depending upon the seriousness of the crime (i.e., four or more were necessary for tickets or arrests for moving traffic violations, two or more for nontraffic arrests, and only one act if it was a felony conviction). Robins (1966) simply specified three or more non-traffic arrests. We also use an informal hierarchy, placing more emphasis on acts that explicitly involve egregious harm to, exploitation of, abuse of, or a violation of the rights of others, and less emphasis on acts that directly involve drug usage (e.g., public intoxication, driving while intoxicated, or drug dealing), a questionable violation of the rights of others (e.g., prostitution), or acts that are relatively minor or common (e.g., traffic violations and tax evasion). We would also exclude arrests for acts that directly involve political or religious protests or demonstrations, even when they involve harm to others or violation of the rights of others. In addition, some criminal acts will be more appropriately included within subsequent ATS items, such as irritability and aggressiveness (e.g., assault), impulsivity (e.g., a spur of the moment decision to commit a particular crime), recklessness (e.g., driving while intoxicated or reckless driving), deceitfulness (e.g., fraud), and irresponsibility (e.g., failure to provide alimony or defaulting on debts). The issue of the overlap among the ATS items is discussed in the material provided for these respective items.

Note as well that there must be a history of repeated acts. One act, no matter how egregious, would not be sufficient. It is important to exclude acts that were committed as a result of an emotional or drug-induced state, or a situational event (e.g., economic deprivation, homelessness, or a social protest). The purpose of the item is to assess for a disposition to commit such acts, not simply for the presence of the acts themselves. A personality trait disposition to engage in such acts should not be inferred if there is no history of repeatedly engaging in such acts.

It is noted in the *DSM-IV* text discussion of ATS PD that the diagnosis may, at times, be misapplied to persons within inner city neighborhoods where antisocial behavior can be part of a protective survival strategy (APA, 1994). The commission of crimes (e.g., presence of formal or informal gangs) may even appear to be common or normative within some settings. On the other hand, an impersonal, violent urban setting may also be providing environmental factors that facilitate, if not nurture, the development of antisocial tendencies.

This item is listed first among the seven adult ATS items because the repeated commission of criminal, illegal acts is highly diagnostic of ATS PD and psychopathy within most clinical settings. However, for persons within a prison or forensic setting, this item can convert from the most to the least diagnostic item, as criminal acts will be normative within such populations (Widiger et al., in press). This item, by itself, will clearly fail to differentiate a chronic, career criminal from the person with antisocial PD. Persons who qualify for this item will also qualify for the V code (conditions that may be a focus of clinical attention) for adult antisocial behavior (e.g., professional thieves, racketeers, or drug dealers; V71.01, APA, 1994, p. 683). The differentiation of antisocial PD from simple adult antisocial behavior will depend upon other ATS PD items.

One approach to the problem of the diagnostic value of the *DSM-IV* ATS PD criteria set within prison and forensic settings is to ignore it. The fact that there is a high base rate for criminal acts within a prison (i.e., 100%) indicates that there is a high base rate for ATS PD within this setting, perhaps as high as 50% (Hare, 1992; Hare et al., 1991; Robins, Tipp, & Przybeck, 1991; Widiger & Corbitt, 1993). However, the item was constructed largely for the purpose of differentiating ATS PD from other PDs within general clinical settings wherein criminal acts are more specific to ATS PD. If the ATS criteria set had been developed solely for use within forensic and prison settings, the violation of social norms would not be given as much prominence (i.e., at the top of the list) and would likely be revised.

Another approach to this problem would be to raise the threshold for the attribution of the item within a prison or forensic setting. One could raise the threshold with respect to the seriousness of the crime(s). A simple algorithm for this would be the length of the prison sentence. Or, one could raise the threshold with respect to the number of crimes committed (e.g., number of arrests) or the chronicity of the criminal history (e.g., number of years in which arrests or crimes were committed). However, one must be careful not to confuse the egregious (harmful) nature of a criminal act with the likelihood that there is a trait disposition to engage in such acts. Otherwise, there is a potential to let one's own emotional horror or moral repugnance affect one's professional judgment. However, the chronicity of the behavior pattern can provide a useful indicator of the disposition to engage in criminal acts. An antisocial, psychopathic person does have the disposition to become a "career criminal." A limitation to this indicator is that it cannot be used for young adults, who have not yet had the time to establish such a history.

A third approach to this problem is to consider other traits of psychopathy and ATS PD. We recommend, in particular, traits that have been included in the Hare Psychopathy Checklist, such as lack of empathy, inflated and arrogant self-appraisal, and glib, superficial charm (Hart & Hare, 1989), whose validation has been confined largely to prison populations. These personality traits of psychopathy will be more unique to the antisocial person within a prison or forensic setting (Widiger et al., in press). This point is also made in the *DSM-IV* text discussion of associated features of ATS PD.

These additional traits of psychopathy, however, can be difficult to assess reliably. Their assessment will often require considerable clinical judgment. Some of them are already included within the criteria for narcissistic PD (i.e., lack of empathy and arrogant self-appraisal) and a discussion of their assessment is presented in the material provided for this disorder. Glib, superficial charm will be suggested by persons acting as if they are already your "good buddy," or by slick, smooth, superficially entertaining conversation that may not really be appropriate to the situation (see Hare, 1992). One will get the impression of how easy it would be to place one's trust or faith in the person. A psychopathic person may indeed be very friendly, personable, charming, and well liked. The person will appear to have and may indeed have many friends who will testify to his or her friendliness, charm, and good will. However, this will be in stark contrast to his or her vicious, cruel, selfish, and self-centered exploitation, abuse, or victimization of others, even perhaps those who testify on his or her behalf.

A final issue in the assessment of this item is the differentiation of criminal acts that are due to an Axis I schizophrenia, manic episode, or substance-related disorder. Acts that are the result of a psychotic condition should be excluded (we also advise considering a diagnosis of a hypomanic episode of cyclothymia when the acts are atypical and particularly impulsive). Criminal acts that are directly related to substance use are not excluded (APA, 1994). However, in such cases, it is useful to assess whether and what antisocial acts were present prior to the onset of a substance dependence. This may be helpful in the eventual determination of whether the antisocial behavior preceded or followed a substance-related disorder. In addition, in our assessment of this item we exclude arrests that are confined to substance intoxication (e.g., disorderly conduct and driving while intoxicated). We also assess for further acts if the criminal history appears to be confined to substance-related behaviors (e.g., drug possession or drug dealing).

Criterion ATS-A2

Deceitfulness, as indicated by repeated lying, use of aliases, or conning others for personal profit or pleasure.

Revisions and Rationale: This item received only minor revision from *DSM-III-R*. The change was simply to replace "no regard for the truth" (APA, 1987, p. 345) with "deceitfulness" (APA, 1994, p. 650). There was no intention of changing the actual meaning or assessment of the item. Deceitfulness provides a better representation of this psychopathic personality trait (Hare, 1992), whereas no regard for the truth has a somewhat moralistic, pejorative connotation. It is, by most persons' standards, immoral to lie and con others, but explicit and implicit condemnation or moral repudiation of the act should be kept separate from a clinical identification of the act's presence.

Perhaps, the more substantial revision was moving the item up to second within the list. This placement is in recognition of the finding within the *DSM-IV* ATS field trial that deceitfulness is very diagnostic of ATS PD, second only to acts of criminality (Widiger et al., in press). Everybody, including George Washington, has lied to someone, but lying, deceit, conning, and manipulation is an everyday act for antisocial, psychopathic persons. A review of their history will indicate that they cannot be trusted, including their proclamations of remorse, guilt, and desire for change and treatment.

This item is also one of only two *DSM-III-R* (and *DSM-IV*) items to load on the interpersonal/affective factor of the Hare Psychopathy Checklist (HPCL), which consists of such items as glibness, superficial charm, grandiosity, proneness to boredom, lack of remorse or guilt, shallow affect, lack of empathy, and failure to accept responsibility for one's actions, along with pathological lying and manipulative conning (Hare et al., 1991). The HPCL makes a further distinction between pathological lying and conning/manipulation. This distinction is, at times, useful, but it can also be subtle. Conning and manipulation refer to deception for the explicit purpose of cheating, defrauding, swindling, or bilking someone or some institution. Pathological lying refers to chronic and continual, everyday, face-to-face acts of lying that have no apparent or obvious material gain. The classic examples of pathological lying involve elaborate and fantastic fabrications that are patently false and have no clear benefit or purpose. In such cases, lying appears to have an intrinsic value or pleasure, rather than being a means for obtaining some material benefit. Pathological lying was the original Robins (1966) criterion for sociopathy, defined as "fantastic history given which does not apparently serve the function of omitting or whitewashing reports of antisocial behavior" (p. 343). However, in the subsequent versions of this item in the RDC, *DSM-III*, *DSM-III-R*, and *DSM-IV*, both forms of deceit are considered to be diagnostic of ATS PD.

Rating:

0) Not present
1) Deceitfulness, as indicated by repeated lying, use of aliases, or conning others for personal profit or pleasure
2) Deceitfulness, including repeated lying, conning others, <u>and</u> pathological lying

Questions:

a. Is it often necessary to bend the rules?
b. Did you ever lie to anyone? [*Act surprised if denied "since everyone has lied to someone."*]
c. Did you ever have to deceive someone to get something from them?
d. Did you ever use an alias?
e. Did you ever con somebody out of something?
f. Have you deceived your friends or relatives to get something from them?
g. Do you often enjoy fooling, conning, or deceiving people?

Issues and Problems: A common issue in the assessment of this item is that it can involve an apparent contradiction in asking someone who is not to be trusted whether he or she has often been deceitful or dishonest. It may be unrealistic to hope that a pathological liar is being forthright and honest within a clinical interview (Hare, 1992; Stone, 1993). The psychopathic person might find the efforts of many researchers and clinicians to be rather naive. On the other hand, psychopathic, antisocial persons are also characterized by arrogance and conceit (Hare, 1992). They may have considerable pride in their successful exploits and may be quite willing to gloat and brag about their successful cons, swindles, and manipulations. The deception in such presentations may, in fact, involve an exaggeration and embellishment of the success of their dishonesty, rather than a denial.

However, one will often experience very compelling denials of any history of deception in antisocial persons. In such cases, it is important, and may even be necessary, to review past hospital, employment, court, or prison records. The manner in which one uses this information will vary. In some instances, it will be best to confront the person directly regarding what is already known; in other cases, the additional information is best kept to oneself to be used in an assessment of the extent to which the person is being dishonest within the interview.

Conning others for personal profit (or pleasure) will overlap with ATS-A1 (committing acts that are grounds for arrest). If there is a history of criminal acts beyond grifter cons and swindles, we use the swindles and cons to represent the current item (A2), as conning and swindling is a prototypic example of antisocial deceit. However, we will use a history of swindles and cons to represent ATS-A1 if there is no history of any other form of criminal behavior, because there will usually be many additional indications of deception outside of overt criminal activity. Antisocial persons will deceive and manipulate their family and friends for money, support, or just for the sport of it. Promises are often made and rarely kept. They may have many ongoing sexual affairs, telling each person whatever is necessary to keep him or her compliant. They will cheat at any game they may play, they will deceive and exploit their employers, and they will manipulate the hospital staff in whatever manner best serves their perceived interests (past medical records should always be obtained and reviewed carefully).

At times, pathological lying may be evident within the interview itself, as antisocial persons may be unable to resist the opportunity to try to deceive the interviewer. They may provide baldly exaggerated stories of fantastic exploits or grossly exaggerated accounts of their own history of suffering and being victimized. However, to be considered as a true or classic example of pathological lying, the fabrication should have no clear benefit to the person other than the interest or pleasure in providing the phony story. Elaborate lies for the purpose of an alibi, to refute an accusation from someone else, or to solicit sympathy from the interviewer, would represent instances of deceit but would not represent examples of the more classic pathological lying.

A final issue in the assessment of this item is the extent to which the deceitfulness is secondary to a substance related disorder. In the assessment of this item, we do not include lying or deceit that is directly related to substance use, such as lying to staff, employers, or family regarding the existence or extent of drug usage. Deception and denial (to others and to oneself) is a common problem in a substance related disorder. The presence of antisocial traits will further complicate and exacerbate this problem. Thus, it is important to assess the extent to which any deceitfulness can be attributed to antisocial traits that occurred prior to or independent of the substance related disorder.

Criterion ATS-A3

Impulsivity or failure to plan ahead.

Revisions and Rationale: The *DSM-III-R* version of this item was "fails to plan ahead, or is impulsive, as indicated by one or both of the following: (a) traveling from place to place without a prearranged job or clear goal for the period of travel or clear idea about when the travel will terminate [or] (b) lack of a fixed address for a month or more" (APA, 1987, p. 345). This item was then interpreted (correctly) as being confined to simply these two manifestations of wanderlust. The Feighner et al. (1972) version of this item was explicitly confined to "vagrancy or wanderlust" (p. 60). However, the original Robins (1966) criteria for sociopathy included impulsivity and vagrancy as distinct items. Vagrancy represented the wanderlust (i.e., a period of several months or more of travel around the country without prearranged employment) and impulsivity was more broadly defined. Impulsivity, as assessed by Robins, included a frequent moving from one city to another, but it also included elopement, sudden army enlistment and an unprovoked desertion of the home. In sum, the impulsivity of the antisocial person will include behaviors other than a simple wanderlust. Antisocial persons are as likely to make a sudden change in employment or relationships as they are to make a sudden change in residence (APA, 1994). Maladaptive impulsivity will also be evident in business decisions. The problem for antisocial persons is that their decisions will lack forethought or foresight with respect to their eventual consequences. Confining the item to wanderlust also contributed to a confusion of impoverishment and homelessness with antisocial personality traits. Poor migrant workers may have little idea when their travel will eventually end and may lack a fixed address for more than a month. It was, therefore, decided in *DSM-IV* to move the two wanderlust examples out of the criteria set and into the text, thereby deleting the specific requirement that the assessment of the item be confined to these two subitems. The term "impulsive" was also moved in front of "failure to plan ahead" to emphasize that the criterion refers to the general trait of impulsivity rather than simply a failure to plan ahead.

Rating:

0) Absent
1) Impulsivity or failure to plan ahead
2) Impulsive decisions with respect to residence, employment, and relationships

Questions:

a. Have you ever just taken off and traveled from place to place? (*If yes:*) How long and often?

b. Have you ever made sudden or impulsive decisions regarding your job or a criminal act?

c. Have you ever impulsively begun or ended a relationship?

Issues and Problems: We begin the assessment of this item with the specific *DSM-III-R* wanderlust criteria (provided above). This is helpful for historical continuity and to allow a determination of whether the person would (or would not) have met the *DSM-III-R* criteria for this item. However, it is important in the assessment of the original version of this item to consider the motivation or reason for the roving travel. The intention of the item was to identify a wandering grifter rather than simply an impoverished drifter.

In any case, the *DSM-IV* version of the item is broader, including sudden (impulsive) changes in relationships and employment, as well as changes in residence. A person who drifted from one job or person to another would be considered as having this trait, even if he or she failed to drift from one city to another. The intention of the item is to assess for the repeated tendency to make spur-of-the-moment decisions, such that major changes in one's life have (or could have) occurred without much forethought, reflection, or consideration of the possible negative consequences. This can include suddenly quitting one's job and moving, but it may also include impulsive sexual affairs and spur-of-the-moment criminal or business decisions. This will often be one of the areas in which antisocial persons will acknowledge the maladaptivity of their traits. The criminal acts that have resulted in their arrest will often have been impulsive and poorly planned, if planned at all.

Including impulsive criminal acts within this item will result in an overlap with ATS-A1 (failure to conform to social norms with respect to lawful behavior). However, failure to conform to the law need not involve impulsive criminal acts. The acts for ATS-A1 will often involve premeditated and even well planned crimes. However, if criminal acts are considered for the current item (ATS-A3), there should be a history of many such spur-of-the-moment criminal acts and at least some indication of impulsivity within other domains of functioning (e.g., job, residence, or relationships).

This item will also overlap with ATS-A6 (irresponsibility), particularly with respect to the work obligations. If the presence of ATS-A6 was confined to the presence of a history of impulsive changes in employment, then we would not use these same acts in the consideration of the current item (which could include impulsivity with respect to residence, relationships, or other domains of functioning).

A final issue in the assessment of this item is the differentiation of impulsivity that is due to an Axis I mental disorder. Persons within a manic episode will often make impulsive life decisions that will have disastrous consequences. It is important in the presence of such impulsivity to consider a diagnosis of bipolar mood disorder. We also advise considering cyclothymia when there is a history of such impulsive life decisions (APA, 1994). Persons suffering from schizophrenia may also display an apparent wanderlust, but, in such cases, there may also be a grossly deteriorated and impoverished functioning. Persons with a chronic history of substance dependence (e.g., alcoholism) will also display an impoverished drifting and lack of any apparent plans for the future. It is important, in such cases, to assess whether there was any impulsivity prior to the onset of the substance dependence, at least for the consideration of the presence of this particular item. However, this can be very difficult to assess in a person with a long history of substance dependence. In such cases, emphasis may then be given to ATS traits (e.g., lack of remorse) that are more clearly independent of substance dependence (Gerstley et al., 1990).

Criterion ATS–A4

Irritability and aggressiveness, as indicated by repeated physical fights or assaults.

Revisions and Rationale: This item was essentially unchanged from *DSM-III-R* and *DSM-III*. Aggressiveness has always been considered a trait of the antisocial personality disorder (Cleckley, 1941). The only revision was to move from the criteria set to the text the qualification that the aggressive acts are not required by one's job (e.g., police officer, bouncer, bodyguard, or soldier) or were taken to defend oneself or someone else. These qualifications were moved to the text because they are largely obvious, and it is not really possible to provide within the criteria set all of the possible qualifications that should be considered for each item. For example, a person with a profession of soldier or police officer would not be excluded if the profession was selected, in part, because it provided the person with the opportunity to express an aggressive disposition.

Rating:

0) Absent
1) Irritability and aggressiveness, as indicated by repeated physical fights or assaults
2) Person has assaulted friends and relatives, as well as strangers

Questions:

a. Have you ever been in a fight as an adult? (*If "yes":*) Did you start it?
b. Have you ever been arrested for assault?
c. Ever get so angry that you hit your wife or child? (*If "yes":*) How often?
d. Ever get into physical fights with relatives or friends?

Issues and Problems: This item concerns irritability and aggressiveness "as indicated by" repeated physical fights or assaults. Irritability and aggressiveness could be suggested by other acts, such as bullying, intimidating, and threats. However, the only acts of irritability and aggressiveness that qualify for this item are acts that involve physical fights or assaults. Fights within the home do qualify, including the physical abuse of a spouse or a child. The fights may be confined to only one area of the person's life (e.g., fights within the home or within bars) provided they are consistent in their occurrence. However, some persons may be involved in fights within the home that have been instigated largely by their spouse. These would then constitute fights to defend oneself and should not be included. Sexual abuse would not qualify, unless the act was assaultive in nature (i.e., a manifestation of irritability and aggressiveness). This is not meant to excuse or belie the serious nature of sexual abuse, but such behaviors might reflect other traits of psychopathy (e.g., lack of empathy or failure to conform to social norms with respect to lawful behavior) or other disorders (e.g., paraphilia).

Note, as well, that the fights and assaults must be "repeated." The earlier Feighner et al. (1972) version of this item specified that only one instance was necessary if a weapon was used (e.g., club, knife, or gun). However, never should a personality trait be considered as present based on only one instance or manifestation of its presence, no matter how intense or excessive the act. The item is assessing a personality trait of aggressiveness and irritability, not the occurrence of an isolated act of violence.

Some clinical judgment is necessary to decide whether there is a sufficient history of acts to consider them to be "repeated." What is meant by "repeated" is not explicitly or specifically defined in *DSM-IV* (APA, 1994), nor, perhaps, can it be so defined without also specifying a long list of exceptions and qualifications. If the case is ambiguous, it is helpful to keep in mind that the judgment is whether the acts appear to reflect a personality trait of irritability and aggressiveness (i.e., a disposition to engage in physical acts of aggression). Does the sum total of acts over time suggest that the person is prone or disposed to commit or engage in physical fights? For example, two major fights over a period of time might not qualify, unless they were coupled with other indicators of irritability and aggressiveness, such as overt threats, bullying, and hostile intimidation.

We will include here physical fights and assaults that occur during and may even be confined to episodes of drug intoxication, but only if there is a repeated history of such acts, and their occurrence is consistent with the person's behavior pattern when not intoxicated. The disposition toward such acts should be apparent by the presence of other indicators of aggressiveness and irritability during times in which the person is not intoxicated (e.g., bullying, intimidation, and threats).

A final issue in the assessment of this item is whether the fights and assaults are the result of an Axis I disorder, such as schizophrenia or a manic episode. One will often observe substantial irritability and aggressiveness in persons within a manic episode (although, perhaps, not to the extent of physical fights and assaults). It is important to assess the extent to which this behavior might have been confined to manic (or even hypomanic) episodes. However, in any case, it is always necessary in the assessment of any ATS criterion to determine the extent to which the behavior was present since late childhood, characteristic throughout adult life, and not confined to a discrete episode within the person's adult life.

Criterion ATS–A5

Reckless disregard for safety of self or others.

Revisions and Rationale: The *DSM-III-R* version of this item specified that the recklessness was "indicated by driving while intoxicated, or recurrent speeding" (APA, 1987, p. 345). This technically required, and was often interpreted as requiring, that the assessment of recklessness be confined to these two acts of recklessness in the use of a car (e.g., Loranger, 1988). However, there is clearly more to antisocial recklessness than recurrent speeding and driving while intoxicated. In addition, the confinement of the item to these two offenses presumes that the person possesses or often uses a car. This is a safe assumption in most, but not all, settings. And, the attribution of the presence of the behavior will depend substantially upon local enforcement practices. (Similar concerns were raised with respect to the *DSM-III* and *DSM-III-R* criteria for substance abuse and dependence [Rounsaville, Spitzer, & Williams, 1986; Widiger & Smith, 1994]). For example, many American communities have experienced substantial changes in attitudes toward and enforcement of drunken driving, and it is likely that the attribution of recklessness will have been affected by such changes in community standards.

Speeding and driving while intoxicated may occur often in persons with an antisocial PD, but persons who do not have an antisocial PD can also have numerous speeding violations or repeated episodes of driving while intoxicated (particularly those with a substance related disorder). In any case, as indicated above, antisocial recklessness is not confined to these two acts. Additional examples of antisocial recklessness include sexual behaviors and drug usage that provide a high risk for harmful consequences (APA, 1994). Antisocial persons may not be particularly concerned about "safe sex," and they may, in fact, flaunt with bravado the odds of developing AIDS. They may also use a variety of dangerous drugs, again with a careless and defiant disregard for the risks and dangers (e.g., by using dangerous combinations of drugs or old needles). Their recklessness will place not only themselves but others in danger, including any children within their care or "supervision." They are not only negligent when it comes to parental responsibilities, as indicated in the deleted *DSM-III-R* item (e.g., failure to arrange for supervision when away from home) but also reckless (e.g., exposure of a child to drugs or weapons, and the presence of a child during acts of recklessness). The reference to recklessness with respect to the safety of a child was included in the *DSM-IV* text discussion of ATS PD, in part, to emphasize antisocial acts that might be particularly evident within antisocial females.

Rating:

0) Absent
1) Reckless disregard for safety of self or others
2) Reckless disregard for safety of self <u>and</u> others

Questions:

a. Do you like to do dangerous or exciting things?

b. Did you ever drive a car while you were really drunk? [*Ask for DUIs.*]

c. Did you ever drive really fast? [*Ask about any tickets.*]

d. Did you ever take any real risks or chances with drugs or sex?

e. Have you ever almost killed or hurt someone in an accident?

f. Have your children (*if any*) been with you when you did any of these things?

g. Have people ever said that you were being unnecessarily foolish or crazy because of the chances you take?

Issues and Problems: A problem in the assessment of this item is that it will often overlap with other ATS items, particularly item ATS-A1 (failure to conform to social norms with respect to lawful behavior) and item ATS-A3 (impulsivity). For example, reckless driving and reckless drug usage is (in most cases) a violation of the law. Reckless driving may be acknowledged primarily on the basis of the person having been repeatedly cited or arrested. To the extent that the criminal act clearly reflects a reckless disregard for physical safety, we consider the behavior to represent the current item rather than the failure to conform to social norms. In our experience, the recklessness, rather than the disposition to violate the rights of others, is typically the primary source or basis for the act (e.g., driving while intoxicated, or dangerous combinations of drugs). It would also be unusual for a criminal disposition to be confined to acts that are all instances of a reckless disregard for safety. The presence of such a criminal disposition should be evident in other forms of criminal acts. Many criminal acts will involve a risk to physical safety (e.g., the burglary of a home), but to be considered as an instance of the current item, they should involve an apparent, substantial, and immediate risk for which most persons (including other persons who are quite willing to commit criminal acts) would describe as very foolish, risky, or reckless.

The physical fights of the antisocial person can convey a sense of recklessness, particularly when they occur frequently, impulsively, and without any apparent appreciation of the many injuries the person is likely to suffer. However, in this case, we typically consider such fights to reflect instances of item ATS-A4 (irritability and aggressiveness) because item ATS-A4 is confined to the specific behavior of repeated physical fights or assaults. In addition, the differentiation of a reckless versus a nonreckless fight or assault will often be very subtle, and the frequency of such acts may not be sufficient to render a confident differentiation.

The most problematic differentiation usually involves item ATS-A3, "impulsivity or failure to plan ahead." Impulsive acts will often involve a reckless disregard for physical safety, and reckless acts are often impulsive. The impulsivity of item ATS-A3 will usually involve major life decisions, such as changing a residence, employment, or relationship, but it can also include impulsive acts of criminality or sexual involvement that result in substantial physical danger. The distinction we make is that the failure to plan ahead in the impulsivity item does not involve a failure to appreciate an immediate or likely threat to physical safety. Failure to recognize or appreciate threats to physical safety should be considered as an instance of a reckless disregard for physical safety. Failure to plan ahead will involve a failure to anticipate or appreciate negative consequences, but these consequences will usually involve the likely effect on one's employment, marriage, expenses, or freedom (e.g., loss of job, divorce, debt, or arrest). In other words, one could interpret item ATS-A3 to represent a recklessness with respect to social, occupational, financial, legal, and other consequences, and item ATS-A5 to represent a recklessness with respect to physical safety or health.

A final issue in the assessment of this item is the differentiation of reckless disregard for safety that is due to an Axis I mental disorder versus antisocial PD. Persons within a manic episode will often display a careless and reckless disregard for their safety and the safety of others. It is particularly important to consider a diagnosis of a bipolar mood disorder (and cyclothymia) when the person displays impulsive and reckless acts that have not been characteristic of their previous or usual behavior (APA, 1994). Persons with a substance-related disorder will also display a reckless disregard for safety. Recurrent substance use in situations when it is physically hazardous is a *DSM-IV* criterion for substance abuse, and continued use despite a known physical problem that has been caused or exacerbated by the substance (e.g., an ulcer made worse by alcohol) is a *DSM-IV* criterion for substance dependence (APA, 1994). It is useful in such cases to assess whether there is any recklessness that is independent of or has occurred prior to the drug usage. On the other hand, recklessness with respect to drug use is a common example of antisocial recklessness. (It was one of the two subcriteria in *DSM-III-R*; APA, 1987). Therefore, we do not exclude recklessness with respect to substance use. In any case, antisocial recklessness with respect to substance use will typically go beyond the recklessness that is common or inherent in persons who have a substance dependence or substance abuse disorder. Antisocial persons will use very dangerous combinations of drugs impulsively or with a display of bravado. For example, continued use of alcohol despite the presence of an ulcer would be characteristic of persons with an alcohol dependence, whereas "chugging" dangerously large amounts of liquor (in the absence of a history of sufficient tolerance for this amount of alcohol) would be more characteristic of persons with antisocial recklessness.

Criterion ATS-A6

Consistent irresponsibility, as indicated by repeated failure to sustain consistent work behavior or honor financial obligations.

Revisions and Rationale: This item is a collapsed version of two *DSM-III-R* items: "unable to sustain consistent work behavior" and "repeatedly fails to honor financial obligations" (APA, 1987, p. 345). Antisocial persons will consistently fail to honor their obligations with respect to work and finances. It is always risky and often disappointing to rely on them.

Both of the original *DSM-III-R* items were considered for deletion, given their relatively weak performance in the *DSM-IV* field trial (Widiger et al., in press). "Unable to sustain consistent work behavior" (APA, 1987, p. 345) was also a complex *DSM-III-R* item, involving three quite specific and independent subitems (i.e., "significant unemployment for six months or more within five years when expected to work and work was available, repeated absences from work unexplained by illness in self or family, [and] abandonment of several jobs without realistic plans for others" APA, 1987, p. 345). Earlier versions were even more complex. The original Robins (1966) version of this item specified "at least six of the following: six-plus jobs within 10 years, successive jobs at less pay or less prestige, fired for incompetence or personality conflict, unemployment for more than a month at a time, quitting because of fights or arguments, much time out for illness, chronic absenteeism, job troubles from drinking, no job for as much as 3 years duration in the last 10 years" (p. 342). The *DSM-III* version was almost as complex, specifying an inability to sustain consistent work behavior, "as indicated by any of the following: (a) too frequent job changes (e.g., three or more jobs in 5 years not accounted for by nature of job or economic or seasonal fluctuation), (b) significant unemployment (e.g., 6 months or more in 5 years when expected to work), (c) serious absenteeism from work (e.g., average 3 days or more of lateness or absence per month), (d) walking off several jobs without other jobs in sight" (APA, 1980, p. 320). There are clearly a variety of ways of expressing an antisocial irresponsibility with respect to work, and it is difficult to specify each of them, even within one page. One would also need to specify the many exceptions and qualifications to each of the possible acts of irresponsibility.

The *DSM-III-R* financial obligation item was defined in such a way that it was readily confused with a more general socioeconomic impoverishment (i.e., failure to honor financial obligations "as indicated by defaulting on debts or failing to provide child support or support for other dependents on a regular basis," APA, 1987, p. 345). This was even more problematic in the original Robins (1966) version of this item, which was defined as being "totally or partially supported by relatives, friends, social agencies, or public institutions" (p. 342).

Rather than delete either item, the *DSM-IV* Personality Disorders Work Group decided that the more conservative decision would be to collapse the two items into one item, thereby retaining in *DSM-IV* the consideration of both irresponsibility with respect to work and financial obligations. However, by including both within one item, each is given somewhat less impact. The item is also defined in *DSM-IV* as a consistent irresponsibility to emphasize that it is the personality trait of irresponsibility that is being assessed, rather than *any* specific reason for failing to sustain consistent work behavior or *any* specific reason for failing to honor financial obligations.

However, a proposal considered for *DSM-IV* was to also include within this item irresponsibility with respect to parental obligations (i.e., the *DSM-III-R* item of parental irresponsibility). Parental irresponsibility does indeed represent an additional expression of antisocial irresponsibility, and its inclusion would facilitate a conservative approach to revising the nomenclature (Frances et al., 1990). However, it was decided that the item would then become too complex, and parental irresponsibility was, in any case, the worst performing item of *DSM-III-R*.

Rating:

0) Absent
1) Consistent irresponsibility, as indicated by repeated failure to sustain consistent work behavior or honor financial obligations
2) Repeated failure to sustain consistent work behavior <u>and</u> honor financial obligations

Questions:

a. Do you have a job?

b. Have you ever been unemployed? (*If "yes":*) For how long? Why? Any other times?

c. Did you ever miss a few days of work? (*If "yes":*) How often? Why?

d. Did you ever quit a job without having another one lined up? (*If "yes":*) How often has this happened?

e. What have you done when you couldn't pay back a debt?

f. Do you owe any child support?

g. Did you ever have to borrow money from friends that you couldn't pay back?

Issues and Problems: This item is defined as a consistent irresponsibility "as indicated by" repeated failure to sustain consistent work behavior or honor financial obligations. As noted above, there are other ways to express irresponsibility (e.g., failure to care adequately for a child), but they would not be included within this item. The irresponsibility considered for this item is confined to work and finances. In addition, to facilitate reliability and historical continuity, we begin the assessment of this item with the original *DSM-III-R* criteria for the two items of being unable to sustain consistent work behavior and failing to honor financial obligations (provided above). However, we also apply some clinical judgment to delete obvious cases of error. For example, some persons without antisocial traits but with a substantial history of substance (alcohol) dependence or another source of economic impoverishment will readily meet the *DSM-III-R* criteria of significant unemployment for 6 months or will default on a variety of mortgages and debts. These other sources of financial hardship should be excluded. In addition, some antisocial persons may actually never default on a debt but will repeatedly float, turn over, transfer, refinance, or otherwise manipulate their debts to continually avoid, excuse, or abdicate their financial obligations.

A difficulty that is common to most, if not all, of the ATS items is that many persons will be unwilling or resistant to admit to their presence. This will be particularly true for persons with an antisocial personality disorder, as one of the criteria for its diagnosis is deceitfulness. As we noted earlier, it is paradoxical to request antisocial persons to be forthright with respect to the "skeletons" within their legal, employment, financial, drug, marital, or sexual history. Court, employment, and other documents are usually helpful and, at times, even necessary to assess this item (Hare, 1992). Interviews with colleagues, relatives, employers, staff, and others can also be very helpful. An interviewee's awareness that the interviewer has obtained additional, independent information may, itself, be helpful in minimizing deception, but the antisocial person will often provide a very compelling and convincing denial. Actual documentation from reliable records is often necessary to provide a confident assessment of this item (and other items).

Our questions for this item are phrased in a socially desirable direction to facilitate or encourage the acknowledgment of this irresponsibility. For example, we ask if the person ever had to borrow money that he or she could not pay back, rather than asking whether he or she ever "welched" on a debt to a good friend. This phrasing should not be misunderstood to imply that any failures to pay debts would qualify for this item. Honoring financial obligations will be much more difficult for persons with many dependents or persons who have had an understandable difficulty finding adequate employment. Among those with economic hardships, responsible honoring of financial obligations might be better judged by the presence of showing good faith (e.g., by staying in contact with the lender or by efforts to pay part of the debt or make some form of restitution) rather than simply by a failure to honor a debt.

A final issue in the assessment of this item is the differentiation of a poor work or financial history that is secondary to an Axis I mental disorder, such as schizophrenia, a manic episode, or a substance related disorder (e.g., alcoholism). Persons suffering from any major Axis I disorder (e.g., major depression) will have difficulty meeting their work and, perhaps, their financial obligations. However, a more difficult differential diagnosis will concern substance-related disorders. Substance dependence may result in substantial difficulties with employment and financial responsibilities. Failure to fulfill major role obligations is also one of the diagnostic criteria for a substance abuse disorder (APA, 1994). On the other hand, drug usage will be cited by antisocial persons as an excuse for a more general and fundamental disregard for social and financial obligations. Thus, it is useful in the assessment of this item to determine whether any work or financial irresponsibility preceded a substance-related disorder. We still consider the item to be present if the substance-related disorder is only at the level of a substance abuse (i.e., a substance dependence is not present) or if there was any apparent irresponsibility prior to the onset of a substance dependence. Otherwise, we would not consider the item to be present (i.e., if the work and financial irresponsibility are readily attributed to a substance dependence).

Criterion ATS-A7

Lack of remorse, as indicated by being indifferent to or rationalizing having hurt, mistreated, or stolen from another.

Revisions and Rationale: This item was not included within the *DSM-III* criteria for ATS PD (APA, 1980). Lack of guilt concerning sexual exploits and crimes was included within Robins' (1966) original criteria for sociopathic personality, but it proved to be among the worst performing items in her influential study. Its assessment was based simply on the interviewer's impressions regarding the way the person reported his or her history. No questions or explicit criteria for its assessment were provided. "For these reasons, lack of guilt, which many authors feel to be the primary feature of the disease, was especially difficult to establish in any reliable fashion" (Robins, 1966, p. 81). Lack of guilt or remorse was not included within the subsequent Feighner et al. (1972) or RDC (Spitzer et al., 1978) criteria for ATS PD. However, because it has traditionally been considered to represent a central trait of psychopathy (Cleckley, 1941; Hare, 1992), it was added to the *DSM-III-R* criteria set (Widiger et al., 1988).

For *DSM-IV*, the definition of lack of remorse was revised from "feels justified in having hurt, mistreated, or stolen from another" (APA, 1987, p. 346) to "being indifferent to or rationalizing having hurt, mistreated, or stolen from another" (APA, 1984, p. 650). Feeling (unjustifiably) justified is indicative of a lack of remorse, but many persons who lack remorse will not say, for example, that their theft, rape, abuse, or extortion was justified.

They may indicate, instead, that they simply do not care whether it was justified or not, as they are not concerned with the pain, suffering, or costs that they inflicted. Rationalization was added for compatibility with the ICD-10 criteria for dissocial PD, which includes the criterion of a "marked proneness to blame others, or to offer plausible rationalizations, for the behavior that has brought the patient into conflict with society" (WHO, 1992, p. 204). Rationalization and blaming others are more indirect indications of a lack of remorse, although offering an (inadequate) justification is itself a form of rationalization.

Rating:

0) Absent
1) Lack of remorse, as indicated by being indifferent to or rationalizing having hurt, mistreated, or stolen from someone
2) Explicit and overt acknowledgement of an absence of remorse

Questions:

a. Why did you [*insert any prior exploitative act*]?

b. Have you tried to make it up to [*insert victim*]? (*If "no":*) Why not?

c. Have you felt guilty or remorseful for [*insert act*]? (*If "yes":*) What have you done about it?

Issues and Problems: Lack of remorse was not assessed reliably in two of the *DSM-IV* antisocial personality disorder field trial sites (Widiger et al., in press). It can be very diagnostic of ATS PD, but its assessment will often require considerable clinical judgment. One will, at times, observe a blatant expression of no regard, remorse, or guilt with respect to victims, stating, for example, that he or she "couldn't care less" about the pain or suffering they have caused. Delight, laughter, and cynical jokes regarding their victims is usually an indication of no remorse. However, even in these cases, the assessment can be mistaken. Persons who are currently angry, bitter, or resentful may appear to have no feelings of remorse or guilt, stating that their victims "can go to hell for all I care." Such angry expressions may, indeed, reflect a trait of no remorse, but they may also express a temporary mood state of anger in response to having felt mistreated, abused, abandoned, neglected, or victimized. Persons within a bitter, hostile divorce can appear and become quite vicious toward one another and act in a manner that is not indicative of their usual functioning.

Indifference toward one's victims is so clearly wrong morally that many antisocial/psychopathic persons will fake an expression of remorse or guilt. They may, in fact, be very good at presenting a compelling display of tearful regret and guilty contrition. False expressions of remorse can be very useful in the obtainment of reduced sentences, parole, and the trust of future victims. We are more convinced by what they have done than by what they say, or what they say they will do. Most persons who feel truly guilty or remorseful will do something to make amends. They might at least apologize to the person they have mistreated, slighted, victimized, or abused, and they will usually make some offer of amends or compensation. Persons who have feelings of remorse are troubled by these feelings, and they will desire to relieve this remorse through some sincere act of restitution or contrition. The antisocial person may express remorse or guilt but will never have done anything to diminish or resolve the purported feelings of remorse or guilt. He or she may instead offer a variety of excuses or rationalizations for why such an effort would not be possible, appropriate, or sufficient. A truly guilty or remorseful person, however, would try to do something, even if it would not be sufficient.

A history of criminal acts will itself suggest little remorse or guilt. If someone has robbed 100 apartments over 5 years, it is difficult to imagine that he or she has been feeling at all remorseful for the act of burglary; otherwise, the behavior would not continue. On the other hand, persons with a paraphilia or an impulse control disorder (e.g., kleptomania or pathological gambling) will often feel very remorseful and guilty but continue to perform the forbidden or destructive act. However, this driven quality is not typically present within antisocial persons nor, perhaps, within most persons who perform criminal acts. Thus, we would not infer the presence of no remorse simply from one act or a history of acts. Some persons who have committed a series of criminal acts will feel very guilty and remorseful when they are confronted with the actual pain and suffering they have caused. They may have been successful for sometime in denying or suppressing their feelings of guilt by dehumanizing their victims or by avoiding any recognition that they are doing any real harm to any particular individual.

Rationalization will be common in many persons who have committed criminal acts (e.g., "they can afford it," "they have insurance to cover it," or "everybody does it"). Such persons may, in fact, feel very ashamed and embarrassed once their acts become public knowledge, indicating the presence of feelings of guilt. They have had the capacity for feelings of remorse, but they have been successful in suppressing these feelings to the extent that was necessary to continue to benefit from their criminal acts. For this reason, we place less emphasis on rationalization and more emphasis on actual indifference. Rationalizations will often be used to try to control or suppress feelings of guilt, remorse, and shame. Psychopathic, antisocial persons would actually have little need to offer an excuse or rationalization or at least no need to control or suppress feelings of remorse. Their rationalizations may, in fact, be more for the benefit of the feelings of those around them (to try to mitigate or minimize expressions of outrage and condemnation) than for the benefit of their own feelings.

5
Avoidant Personality Disorder

Overview: Avoidant (AVD) personality disorder was a new addition to the *DSM-III* (Frances, 1980). A criticism of this inclusion was that AVD PD had little clinical relevance (e.g., Gunderson, 1983), as the proposal was derived from a particular theoretical model (i.e., Millon, 1969, 1981). However, it has been one of the most frequently diagnosed personality disorders (Widiger, 1991; Widiger & Rogers, 1989) as timid, anxious, and insecure introversion is a common social and clinical problem (Pilkonis, 1984). The major issues for *DSM-IV* were the differentiation of AVD PD from generalized social phobia (Widiger, 1992a; Widiger & Shea, 1991) and from schizoid personality disorder (Livesley & West, 1986; Livesley, West, & Tanney, 1985; Trull, Widiger, & Frances, 1987).

AVD PD was defined in *DSM-III-R* as a pervasive pattern of "social discomfort, fear of negative evaluation, and timidity" (APA, 1987, p. 352). This definition was revised in *DSM-IV* to a "pervasive pattern of social inhibition, feelings of inadequacy, and hypersensitivity to negative evaluation" (APA, 1994, p. 662). This revision was designed, in large part, to facilitate the differentiation of AVD PD from generalized social phobia. Social inhibition implies a more general self-conscious introversion rather than simply a social discomfort. Hypersensitivity may also be less readily confused with a phobia than with a fear, and pervasive feelings of inadequacy may be less characteristic of persons with a generalized social phobia than of those with timidity (Millon, 1991a). However, we would also emphasize the fundamental definition of a personality trait when attempting to distinguish a generalized social phobia from AVD PD. To the extent that the social timidity, withdrawal, and insecurity involves a pattern of thinking, feeling, or relating to others that is characteristic of everyday functioning, has been evident since late childhood or early adolescence, and pervades most, if not all, social situations, it involves personality (whether or not the person meets the *DSM-IV* criteria for a generalized social phobia) (Widiger, 1992a).

DSM-III-R AVD PD consisted of seven items, any four of which were necessary for the diagnosis. Only one was not changed from *DSM-III-R*. Five of the seven were revised significantly, and one was replaced (the threshold for diagnosis remains at 4 of 7). The item replaced was "has no close friends or confidants (or only one)" (APA, 1987, p. 353). This item was also included in the *DSM-III-R* criteria for a schizoid PD (and a close variant is still included in the *DSM-IV* schizoid PD criteria set). Its inclusion within the criteria set for AVD clearly contributed to the confusion of these two personality disorders rather than to their differentiation. In addition, the absence of any close friends or confidants is more characteristic of schizoid PD than of avoidant PD (Millon, 1991a). Persons with avoidant PD intensely desire to obtain close relationships (a *DSM-III* criterion explicitly noted this desire; APA, 1980) and it is not surprising that they will, at times, be successful in obtaining a close relationship (to which they may then cling with considerable attachment and even dependency; Widiger & Frances, 1988). An initial proposal for *DSM-IV* was to revise this item to "few friends despite the desire to relate to others" (Millon, 1991a, p. 359), reverting back to some extent to a *DSM-III* item that indicated a "desire for affection and acceptance" (APA, 1980, p. 324). However, the proposal was eventually rejected because of its potential complexity (i.e., requiring that one assess both the number of and the desire for close friends, as well as that the presence of only a few friendships had occurred despite this desire). Table 5-1 presents the final *DSM-IV* criteria for the avoidant personality disorder diagnosis.

Table 5-1
DSM-IV Criteria for Avoidant Personality Disorder

A pervasive pattern of social inhibition, feelings of inadequacy, and hypersensitivity to negative evaluation, beginning by early adulthood and present in a variety of contexts, as indicated by four (or more) of the following:

(1) avoids occupational activities that involve significant interpersonal contact, because of fears of criticism, disapproval, or rejection
(2) is unwilling to get involved with people unless certain of being liked
(3) shows restraint within intimate relationships because of the fear of being shamed or ridiculed
(4) is preoccupied with being criticized or rejected in social situations
(5) is inhibited in new interpersonal situations because of feelings of inadequacy
(6) views self as socially inept, personally unappealing, or inferior to others
(7) is unusually reluctant to take personal risks or to engage in any new activities because they may prove embarrassing

Note. From *Diagnostic and Statistical Manual of Mental Disorders* (4th ed., pp. 164-165), by American Psychiatric Association, 1994, Washington, DC: Author. Copyright 1994 by American Psychiatric Association. Reprinted with permission.

Criterion AVD-1

Avoids occupational activities that involve significant interpersonal contact, because of fears of criticism, disapproval, or rejection.

Revisions and Rationale: The *DSM-III-R* version of this item included social as well as occupational activities. In *DSM-IV*, it is confined to occupational activities for simplification and to emphasize the occupational (as well as social) impairment that is often seen in persons with avoidant PD. This may be helpful in differentiating AVD PD from a social phobia that is confined to social dysfunction (Millon, 1991a)). However, given that the occupational activities are those that involve interpersonal contact, the overlap with social phobia may remain. The revision may still be helpful in differentiating among the avoidant PD items.

Equally important, *DSM-IV* adds that the avoidance is because of fears of criticism, disapproval, or rejection. This particular revision was made for compatibility with the respective criterion from the ICD-10 (Task Force, 1991; WHO, 1992). It will also be helpful in differentiating AVD from the schizoid PD. Schizoid persons will also avoid activities that involve significant interpersonal contact, but not because of fears of criticism, disapproval, or rejection. Persons with schizoid PD are generally indifferent to criticism or rejection (APA, 1987, 1994).

The *DSM-III-R* version of this item obtained the highest correlation with the diagnosis of AVD and the highest prototypicality rating in the *DSM-IV* MacArthur studies (Millon, 1991a). It was, therefore, placed at the top of the list in *DSM-IV*. This superiority in performance is not surprising, because the avoidance of social activities that involve significant interpersonal contact is obviously central to an avoidant personality disorder. However, it may no longer be the best item for diagnosing AVD PD, given the *DSM-IV* revision that now confines the item to an avoidance of occupational activities (Blashfield, Blum, & Pfohl, 1992). The avoidance of occupational activities that involve significant interpersonal contact is very diagnostic of AVD PD, but it may not be as diagnostic as some of the other items that emphasize or at least include relationships that exist outside of the realm of one's employment.

Rating:

0) Absent
1) Avoids occupational activities that involve significant interpersonal contact because of fears of criticism, disapproval, or rejection
2) Has received formal reprimands, poor evaluations, or left employment due to this avoidance

Questions:

a. Do jobs that require a lot of social contact make you uncomfortable or nervous?
b. Do you tend to avoid work that requires being closely involved with others? (*If "yes":*) Why?

Issues and Problems: The example provided in *DSM-III-R* for this item was refusing a promotion that would increase social demands (APA, 1987). This would represent a very avoidant act, but it is rarely seen in persons with avoidant PD (Millon, 1991a). Many avoidant persons will not have been offered a promotion that required a significant increase in interpersonal contact; they may not have been offered any promotions, or they may not even be employed in a setting wherein promotions are to be expected. More realistic or likely examples of this item include trying to avoid tasks, assignments, or responsibilities that require significant interpersonal contact (e.g., declining a request to lead or speak before a group, failing to attend meetings, avoiding informal lunch or happy hour "get-togethers," or declining invitations to social functions).

Some jobs may involve little or no interpersonal interactions within the immediate work responsibilities (e.g., assembly-line work, computer programming, and sorting mail). However, we do not confine this item to activities that are within the person's job description. We include informal social activities that occur with one's colleagues from work, such as happy hour gatherings, hallway discussions, softball games, and so forth. Occupationally related activities that involve significant interpersonal contact are often these more informal interactions, and the avoidance of such situations will often represent a major source of occupational impairment for persons with avoidant PD. It can be through these informal interactions that one obtains useful contacts, makes positive impressions on others, and resolves misunderstandings or problems. However, we would not include within this item activities that are primarily for the purpose of obtaining or developing a friendship outside of work (e.g., dates or a friendship with one particular person from work), as this would be more appropriately covered in subsequent items.

The *DSM-IV* revision may fail to distinguish AVD PD avoidance from Axis I social phobic avoidance. A common example of social phobia is a speech anxiety (APA, 1987, 1994) which is also a common occupational activity that would be avoided by persons with an avoidant PD. However, in order to consider the avoidant PD item to be present, there must be an avoidance of a variety of occupational activities that involve significant interpersonal contact, not just a phobia of public speaking. In addition, the avoidance of such situations in some persons may reflect specific difficulties or inadequacies that impair their interactions (e.g., poor fluency in the dominant language, or lack of familiarity or comfort with the social behavior and customs of a new culture).

Criterion AVD-2

Is unwilling to get involved with people unless certain of being liked.

Revisions and Rationale: This item was unchanged from *DSM-III-R*. The *DSM-III* version was "unwillingness to enter into relationships unless given unusually strong guarantees of uncritical acceptance" (APA, 1980, p. 324). Guarantees of uncritical acceptance was revised to a certainty of being liked in *DSM-III-R* because few avoidant persons would, in fact, require guarantees of uncritical acceptance. The *DSM-III* version could have suggested an assertive demand (or requirement) for no criticism when the intention was instead to convey a timid, insecure reluctance to assert oneself. Avoidant persons fail to approach others because they fear rejection, criticism, or embarrassment, so they will not approach someone until they are quite certain that they will be accepted. This item is particularly useful in distinguishing AVD PD from the schizoid and dependent PDs, as schizoid persons are largely indifferent to whether they are liked, and dependent persons will often throw themselves at persons who may have little or no interest in them.

Rating:

0) Absent
1) Is unwilling to get involved with people unless certain of being liked
2) Major or principal complaint of the person is the inability to develop close, personal relationships due to the expectation or presumption that he or she will not be liked

Questions:

a. Are you reluctant to let someone know you like them before you know how they feel about you?

b. Have you ever missed the chance to get involved with someone because you were too shy or too nervous to make the first move?

c. Is it especially difficult for you to make new friends?

Issues and Problems: A prototypic example of this item is failing to ever approach or indicate an interest in becoming romantically or sexually involved with someone because one is afraid of being rejected. Avoidant persons are so hypersensitive to rejection (a *DSM-III* criterion for AVD; APA, 1980) that they feel unable to take any risks or chances that will expose them to a possible rejection. They will often be able to describe many missed opportunities.

However, they may not say that they must be certain of being liked before they will approach someone. They are often so certain that they won't be liked that they would never require such a standard. Instead, they will often say that they are so convinced that they won't be liked that they won't even try. The end result, however, is largely the same.

An additional point concerning this item is that it can apply to friendships as well as to romantic or sexual relationships. Avoidant persons will be very slow to develop new friendships whenever they move to a new location, change jobs, or have old friends leave. They fear or expect others will find them boring or unappealing, with little to offer and are, therefore, very reluctant to approach others until they have enough reassurance and confidence that they won't be rejected or embarrassed. They may, indeed, eventually develop friendships, but these will typically develop quite slowly, and may be initiated and nurtured by the other person.

Criterion AVD-3

Shows restraint within intimate relationships because of the fear of being shamed or ridiculed.

Revisions and Rationale: The *DSM-III-R* version of this item was reticence in social situations "because of a fear of saying something inappropriate or foolish, or of being unable to answer a question" (APA, 1987, p. 353). The item was revised for *DSM-IV* to help differentiate AVD PD from generalized social phobia (Millon, 1991a). The fears listed within the *DSM-III-R* version involved public performance anxiety and were commonly seen in persons with even the more prototypic circumscribed social phobias (e.g., fear of public speaking or fear of performing in front of a group of people). The *DSM-IV* revision places less emphasis on public performance and more emphasis on inhibitions within personal, intimate relationships. Likewise, reticence was replaced with restraint to put less emphasis on speech inhibitions. And, finally, the threshold for its attribution was raised from simply a fear of saying something foolish to a fear of being shamed or ridiculed (Millon, 1991a).

Rating:

0) Absent
1) Shows restraint within intimate relationships because of the fear of being shamed or ridiculed
2) Relationships have failed to develop due to this restraint

Questions:

a. Is it difficult for you to talk about yourself within close, intimate relationships?

b. Have you often withheld intimate, personal feelings regarding someone close to you because of fears of appearing ridiculous or being rejected?

c. Do you generally feel inhibited in expressing or asserting yourself with people close to you?

Issues and Problems: The major difficulty in the assessment of this item concerns the fear of being shamed or ridiculed. The item might appear to suggest that the person expects to be admonished or ridiculed by others (i.e., fear of being shamed or ridiculed by others). Avoidant persons will, indeed, expect rejection or criticism, but their restraint will usually reflect their own severe self-criticism rather than an expectation of being criticized. Unrealistic or excessive expectations of criticism or ridicule from others is more paranoid than avoidant. Avoidant persons do not need the actual or expected ridicule of others to feel ashamed, embarrassed, humiliated, or foolish. They will be inhibited during an intimate or personal interaction even if they have no expectation of being ridiculed or admonished by that particular person. An example of this item is the failure to reveal one's feelings of warmth or affection for someone with whom one has been involved for some time because one is afraid that these feelings will not be reciprocated. Avoidant persons may not expect any ridicule or admonishment from this person. They may know the person well enough to realize that this is not likely to occur, but they may still feel ridiculous or foolish if the person does not reciprocate their feelings. As a result, they may refrain from expressing their real feelings for a long time and, even then, may give the misleading impression that they have little interest, feeling, or fondness for the person.

Avoidant persons will express their restraint in a variety of ways. They are generally very unassertive within intimate relationships. They will be very inhibited in expressing their opinions, concerns, or complaints; this is similar in many respects to persons with a dependent personality disorder. Dependent persons will also be very unassertive because they fear losing the relationship. It has been our experience that once persons with an avoidant PD finally obtain a relationship with someone, they will also be very passive, unassertive, and even submissive because they fear losing the relationship. They desired a relationship so badly, and it was so very difficult for them to obtain it, that they will cling to this person and may do just about anything to avoid being alone once again.

However, this item does not concern restraint (inhibition or unassertiveness) because of a fear of losing the relationship. The item concerns a fear of being shamed or ridiculed. Avoidant and dependent persons who are involved within an intimate relationship will share a fear of the loss of relationship, but dependent persons may not fear being embarrassed or ashamed by their feelings or expression of affection. Dependent persons will be much more willing and able to express such feelings than avoidant persons. Some persons with dependent PD will refrain from expressing such feelings to avoid losing the relationship (because they know that the other person would not want to hear them), but many dependent persons will be unable to restrain themselves. They will drive potential relationships away because of how quickly they develop and express their feelings for the other person. Another way to understand this difference is that dependent persons could become involved with avoidant persons because they would not restrain themselves, whereas avoidant persons would have difficulty becoming involved with dependent persons (or anyone else) because they might never cross the threshold of expressing their real feelings.

It is also important to recognize that there is substantial variation across cultures with respect to openness, restraint, and assertiveness within intimate relationships. What may appear to be excessive restraint to an interviewer may be, indeed, quite normative and adaptive for a particular subject. In addition, the requirement that the restraint is due to a fear of being shamed or ridiculed will not always be helpful in making the distinction, because persons may feel ashamed and may, in fact, be shamed or ridiculed by others for violating a social norm. The issues for a person with an avoidant personality disorder involve personal feelings of inadequacy and vulnerability rather than simply the failure to behave in the manner that is expected of one's social role or position.

Criterion AVD-4

Is preoccupied with being criticized or rejected in social situations.

Revisions and Rationale: The *DSM-III-R* version of this item was "easily hurt by criticism or disapproval" (APA, 1987, p. 353). Hypersensitivity to criticism and disapproval is very characteristic of persons with avoidant PD, but it is not particularly specific to avoidant persons. This item was, in fact, one of the *DSM-III-R* criteria for the diagnosis of dependent PD (APA, 1987) and a similar variant was part of the *DSM-III-R* criteria for narcissistic PD (i.e., reaction to criticism with shame or humiliation; APA, 1987). It was, therefore, replaced with a variant of an ICD-10 item, "excessive preoccupation with being criticized or rejected in social situations" (WHO, 1992, p. 206). The inclusion of rejection places more emphasis on concerns regarding social relationships rather than simply concerns regarding disapproval or criticism by an employer or someone else within a position of authority. Concerns regarding rejection are also more characteristic of avoidant persons than narcissistic persons (who may, in fact, deny any such concerns). The inclusion of a preoccupation raises the threshold for attribution because the person is now not only vulnerable or sensitive to criticism/rejection but is often thinking, ruminating, or worrying about being criticized or rejected.

Rating:

0) Absent
1) Is preoccupied with being criticized or rejected in social situations
2) Preoccupation with being criticized <u>and</u> rejected in social situations

Questions:

a. Do you often worry about what others may be thinking about you?
b. Do you often get the sense that people don't think well of you (e.g., they may think that you're not so bright, that you're unattractive, or that you're boring)?

Issues and Problems: It is also characteristic of dependent persons to be preoccupied with concerns about being rejected. They will ruminate excessively over whether their current relationships are failing. However, the intention of this item is not to characterize this particular preoccupation with rejection. In the assessment of this item, we emphasize ruminations or preoccupations with being criticized or rejected in everyday social situations. Avoidant persons worry about how almost everyone thinks about them. They will be inhibited, unassertive, and reticent in most social situations because they worry and fear that they will appear ridiculous, stupid, awkward, or unappealing. They will often feel embarrassed and apologetic, quickly taking the blame and responsibility for any error, misunderstanding, or confusion. They may even apologize when nothing has occurred. Most interactions seem to be a basis for a concern regarding whether they will be liked, respected, or accepted. Examples include worrying about whether a waiter thinks they don't know how to order correctly; whether persons in other cars think they are driving too slowly or too fast; whether strangers who might be overhearing a conversation think they are saying something stupid; and whether a salesperson was offended because they didn't buy something. They will be hypersensitive to cues of this expected or anticipated criticism or rejection, noting any real or imagined signs that might possibly suggest an impending rejection. Whenever they return from a date, a party, or any other social gathering, they will often describe how many times they "messed up," and why they felt that the other person(s) probably didn't like them.

Criterion AVD-5

Is inhibited in new interpersonal situations because of feelings of inadequacy.

Revisions and Rationale: The *DSM-III-R* version of this item was "fears being embarrassed by blushing, crying, or showing signs of anxiety in front of other people" (APA, 1987, p. 353). It was revised substantially for *DSM-IV* because the *DSM-III-R* version described a very common and even central symptom of an Axis I social phobia (APA, 1994). Many persons with AVD PD will have a social phobia. Avoidant persons will fear being embarrassed or showing signs of anxiety in front of other people. In such cases, both diagnoses should be given. However, generalized social phobia overlaps substantially with the avoidant personality disorder. One could provide both of these diagnoses to the same person, but it might be better in many of these cases to simply consider these two diagnoses as different ways of characterizing the same problem (Widiger, 1992a). Nevertheless, to facilitate the differentiation of AVD PD and generalized social phobia, "fears being embarrassed by blushing, crying, or showing signs of anxiety in front of other people" (APA, 1987, p. 353) was replaced with "is inhibited in new interpersonal situations because of feelings of inadequacy" (APA, 1994, p. 665). This version of the item describes a more general trait of social inhibition rather than simply a phobic performance anxiety, and it requires more fundamental feelings of inadequacy that may not be present in persons with social phobia (Millon, 1991a).

It is also of interest to note that an initial draft of this item for *DSM-III-R* had been "afraid of losing control or giving in to an unacceptable impulse, e.g., fear of crying or appearing anxious in public" (Work Group, 1985, p. 132). This version emphasized the dynamics that underly the analytic diagnosis of a phobic character (Fenichel, 1945; Frances & Widiger, 1987) that was influential in the development of the *DSM-III-R* version of the avoidant PD (Widiger et al., 1988). The *DSM-IV* version of this item represents, then, a substantial departure from the *DSM-III-R* version.

Rating:

0) Absent
1) Is inhibited in new interpersonal situations because of feelings of inadequacy
2) Often remains virtually speechless and silent in new interpersonal situations

Questions:

a. Do you often feel very nervous or inhibited when you meet new people? (*If "yes":*) Why?

b. Do you have trouble initiating conversations? (*If "yes":*) Why?

c. Do you worry a lot about making a bad first impression?

Issues and Problems: A difficulty in the assessment of this item is differentiating it from the other AVD items. We distinguish it in the following manner: (a) AVD-1 can involve new interpersonal situations at or related to work, but AVD-1 concerns the avoidance of these interpersonal situations whereas the current item concerns inhibition within these situations; (b) AVD-2 concerns inhibitions with respect to initiating new relationships (e.g., unable to call someone up for a date) whereas the current item concerns inhibitions during the interaction of a new relationship (e.g., unable to say anything on the date); (c) AVD-3 involves an existing or ongoing intimate relationship, whereas the current item involves a new relationship; (d) AVD-4 involves everyday (common) interpersonal situations, whereas the current item involves an interpersonal situation that is new to the person; (e) AVD-6 involves the belief that one is inadequate, whereas this item concerns inhibitions within new interpersonal situations that result from this belief; and (f) AVD-7 involves inhibitions related to potentially embarrassing new activities (discussed below), whereas the current item concerns inhibitions related to new interpersonal interactions.

Examples of this item include remaining virtually silent at parties or social functions that involve strangers; marked reticence on a first date despite reassurance and support by the date; or being unable to approach strangers to ask for advice, directions, or any other information. Interactions with strangers can be particularly stressful for persons with avoidant PD because of the many unknowns that come with strangers. Such persons feel they must make a good initial impression, but they have little confidence that this will be possible. They will feel frozen by how critical, impatient, disappointed, or annoyed the stranger will (presumably) be with their incompetence, clumsiness, inadequacy, and ineptitude.

An additional issue in the assessment of this item is the extent to which the feelings of inadequacy are realistic or accurate. Most persons who enter new social situations, particularly situations that involve very unfamiliar customs or norms, will feel inhibited. And, in some cases, the person may not, in fact, be adequately familiar with or adept at the new customs and norms. In order to consider this item to be present, the belief that one is inadequate should represent a distortion due to an inherent or fundamental low self-esteem (however, see also AVD-6).

Criterion AVD-6

Views self as socially inept, personally unappealing, or inferior to others.

Revisions and Rationale: This item was a new addition to *DSM-IV*. It replaces the *DSM-III-R* item of "no close friends or confidants" (APA, 1987, p. 353), the deletion of which was discussed above. This new item was obtained from the ICD-10 criteria for the anxious personality disorder (WHO, 1992), but it may also represent a return of the

DSM-III AVD PD criterion of low self-esteem (APA, 1980). This new item may be helpful in differentiating AVD PD from a social phobia. Persons with a social phobia may feel quite competent in most areas of functioning. It is only when they must give a speech (or some other particular area of public performance or display) that they become anxious and insecure. Persons with an avoidant PD believe that they are more fundamentally or consistently inept, inferior, or unappealing than other people.

Rating:

0) Absent
1) Views self as socially inept, personally unappealing, or inferior to others
2) Belief that one is socially inept, personally unappealing, <u>and</u> inferior to others

Questions:

a. Do you often feel inadequate or inferior to others?
b. Do you think of yourself as physically attractive or unattractive?
c. Do you think that you are good with others, or do you think that you are usually rather clumsy, awkward, and even inept in your interactions with other people?

Issues and Problems: Many persons with avoidant PD will have little difficulty in acknowledging their feelings of inferiority, inadequacy, and/or unattractiveness. Their low self-esteem may be a major reason they are seeking treatment. However, some will have difficulty acknowledging this problem. They may not want to draw any attention to a problem they find most painful. As noted above, persons with AVD PD feel quite inhibited within new interpersonal situations because of their feelings of inadequacy. Interviews with new clinicians or researchers regarding their problems (i.e., inadequacies) are often quite difficult. They may feel ashamed and embarrassed not only of their perceived inferiorities but also of their shame and embarrassment over their perceived inferiority (e.g., they are embarrassed by the degree of their embarrassment). For example, they may feel that they are very unattractive, perhaps even ugly, but any discussion of their appearance may be so difficult that they will avoid or deny such concerns, particularly with a new (strange) interviewer.

An additional issue is the extent to which there is any reality to the negative self-description. To understand this issue, it is helpful to consider a similar problem in the diagnoses of agoraphobia and social phobia (Schneier et al., in press). Persons who have suffered severe physical deformities (e.g., burn scars) may be inhibited and even fearful regarding their acceptance by others. They may be very reluctant to enter public places and thereby expose themselves to potential scrutiny or rejection. Complicating this inhibition is the fact that they may, indeed, be scrutinized and rejected by others. Such an occurrence would be clearly regrettable, but it is also important in their treatment not to convey a Pollyanna-like denial of the validity of their concerns. And, even if their concerns are exaggerated (i.e., they will receive much less negative attention and much more acceptance than they expect), their degree of concern may be quite common for persons with such an injury, scar, or deformity. Their inhibitions may be quite understandable and expected (although unrealistic and unnecessary), given their condition. In sum, it would not be appropriate to diagnose them with a mental disorder for having realistic inhibitions or inhibitions that are common to persons with their condition. The *DSM-IV* Anxiety Disorders Work Group, therefore, decided to emphasize that a mental disorder diagnosis should be given only when the fear is clearly in excess of that usually associated with the condition (APA, 1994).

A similar issue can also occur in the assessment of AVD PD. The avoidant PD item simply states that there is a belief that one is socially inept, unappealing, or inferior. It does not indicate whether the belief is inaccurate. We do not consider the item to be present unless the belief is inaccurate, excessive, or pervasive in its effects. Some avoidant persons will, in fact, be socially inept, unappealing, and inferior in one respect or another (Turner, Beidel, Dancu, & Keys, 1986). Their concerns regarding their acceptance by and appeal to others may not be entirely unrealistic. We would still consider the item to be present within such persons if these concerns and inhibitions pervade their self-evaluation and affect other activities, opinions, and expectations that have little or nothing to do with the realistic focus of their concern. This would then exclude persons whose feelings of inadequacy were confined to just one aspect of adjustment (e.g., adjusting to the norms or practices of a new culture).

Criterion AVD-7

Is unusually reluctant to take personal risks or to engage in any new activities because they may prove embarrassing.

Revisions and Rationale: The *DSM-III-R* version of this item involved exaggerating the potential difficulties, physical dangers, or risks involved in doing something ordinary but outside of one's usual routine (APA, 1987). It was included in *DSM-III-R* to represent the broader diagnosis of a phobic character that describes a person who is more generally inhibited with respect to a wide range of activities rather than simply socially inhibited (Frances & Widiger, 1987). However, the item obtained among the lowest sensitivity rates in the *DSM-IV* MacArthur studies (Millon, 1991a). Avoidant persons rarely exaggerate the physical dangers or risks of everyday activities (e.g., fears regarding potential traffic accidents or fires). The example provided in the *DSM-III-R* criterion, of cancelling social plans because one anticipated being exhausted by the effort of getting there (APA, 1987), is rarely seen. The new version places the emphasis on interpersonal issues, particularly with respect to feeling embarrassed.

Rating:

0) Absent
1) Is unusually reluctant to take personal risks or to engage in any new activities because they may prove embarrassing
2) Refuses to take personal risks or to engage in new activities because they may prove embarrassing

Questions:

a. Have you ever been real reluctant to join in on some group activity because you were likely to be embarrassed or to appear foolish? (*If "yes":*) Does this happen often?

b. Do you often just stay on the sidelines rather than join in the fun?

Issues and Problems: Examples of this item are fairly common. Avoidant persons may be too embarrassed by their physical appearance to go swimming when other people are around (e.g., embarrassed by pale skin, a wart, or being "fat"). They may fear appearing too clumsy, awkward, or incompetent to join colleagues in a friendly, informal game of softball or volleyball. They may fear appearing stupid if they play a board game or a card game, or appearing to be a rube or hick if they join a trip to a sophisticated event (e.g., museum or elegant restaurant).

Many persons who do not have an avoidant personality disorder will share these inhibitions and insecurities. It is quite common and natural to feel self-conscious when one is doing something new or different. It is important to determine whether the person often fails to do what is usually done by everybody else. Refusal to do the activity is not necessary for the item to be considered present (this is the requirement for the more severe rating), but rather, if the activity is done, then it is endured with considerable tension and dread. It is also important to determine if the inhibitions involve a wide range of activities (i.e., cross-situational) and are not confined to a particular type of activity (in which case the more appropriate diagnosis might be a phobia).

As noted above, persons with avoidant PD are often reluctant or embarrassed to acknowledge their flaws and fears, particularly when they could be said to be "absurd," "stupid," "crazy," or "neurotic." They may also fail to appreciate the extent of their inhibitions. Colleagues, friends, or a spouse may be particularly helpful in the assessment of this item, because they may recall many instances in which the person balked or refused to do something that was (or would have been) done by everybody else.

6

Borderline Personality Disorder

Overview: Borderline (BDL) personality disorder was a new addition to *DSM-III* (Frances, 1980). It was not recognized within the ICD-9, but ICD-10 now includes a borderline subtype to the emotionally unstable personality disorder (WHO, 1992). BDL PD has been the most frequently diagnosed *DSM-III-R* personality disorder (Widiger, 1991; Widiger & Frances, 1989b) and among the most heavily researched (Blashfield, 1993; Blashfield & McElroy, 1987). The major issues for *DSM-IV* were the inclusion of a new criterion concerned with psychotic-like experiences, its differentiation from other personality disorders, and its definition (Gunderson, Zanarini, et al., 1991).

The *DSM-III* criteria for BDL PD were developed by Spitzer, Endicott, and Gibbon (1979) on the basis of their survey of the literature and consultation with Drs. Gunderson, Sheehy, Stone, Rinsley, and Kernberg. They defined BDL PD as a "constellation of relatively enduring personality features of instability and vulnerability" (p. 17). This was revised somewhat in *DSM-III* to an "instability in a variety of areas, including interpersonal behavior, mood, and self-image" (APA, 1980, p. 321). BDL PD was defined in *DSM-III-R* as a pervasive pattern of "instability of mood, interpersonal relationships, and self-image" (APA, 1987, p. 347). This definition has been criticized for emphasizing two features that are among the most problematic with respect to reliability in assessment (self-image) and/or specificity (mood). A proposal considered for *DSM-IV* was to include within the definition of BDL PD a fear of and angry intolerance for being alone to emphasize the role of this dynamic in borderline psychopathology (Gunderson, Zanarini, et al., 1991), but this proposal was rejected for being too theoretically based. The definition was, therefore, revised only to add a marked impulsivity (APA, 1994). This addition was in response to the evidence that impulse dyscontrol is very common and perhaps central to the borderline personality disorder (Clarkin, Hull, & Hurt, 1993; Gunderson & Zanarini, 1987; Hilbrand & Hirt, 1987; Silverman et al., 1991; Zanarini, 1993).

The *DSM-III* criteria for BDL PD consisted of eight items, any five of which were necessary for its diagnosis. The only major revision for *DSM-III-R* was the replacement of "intolerance of being alone" (APA, 1980, p. 323) with "frantic efforts to avoid real or imagined abandonment" (APA, 1987, p. 347) (Widiger et al., 1988), the rationale for which will be discussed below. Three of the eight criteria were revised significantly for *DSM-IV*, two were unchanged, and three received minor revisions. In addition, a new item was added. The threshold for diagnosis remains at five. With the addition of the new item and no change in the threshold for diagnosis, the prevalence rate could increase somewhat (although this change may be offset by increased thresholds for the three items that were revised significantly). The complete *DSM-IV* criteria set is presented in Table 6-1.

Table 6-1
DSM-IV Criteria for Borderline Personality Disorder

A pervasive pattern of instability of interpersonal relationships, self-image, and affects, and marked impulsivity beginning by early adulthood and present in a variety of contexts, as indicated by five (or more) of the following:

(1) frantic efforts to avoid real or imagined abandonment. Note: do not include suicidal or self-mutilating behavior covered in criterion 5.

(2) a pattern of unstable and intense interpersonal relationships characterized by alternating between extremes of idealization and devaluation

(3) identity disturbance: markedly and persistently unstable self-image or sense of self

(4) impulsivity in at least two areas that are potentially self- damaging (e.g., spending, sex, substance abuse, reckless driving, binge eating). Note: do not include suicidal or self-mutilating behavior covered in criterion 5.

(5) recurrent suicidal behavior, gestures, or threats, or self-mutilating behavior

(6) affective instability due to a marked reactivity of mood (e.g., intense episodic dysphoria, irritability, or anxiety usually lasting a few hours and only rarely more than a few days)

(7) chronic feelings of emptiness

(8) inappropriate, intense anger or difficulty controlling anger (e.g., frequent displays of temper, constant anger, recurrent physical fights)

(9) transient, stress-related paranoid ideation or severe dissociative symptoms

Note. From *Diagnostic and Statistical Manual of Mental Disorders*, (4th ed., p. 654), by American Psychiatric Association, 1994, Washington, DC: Author. Copyright 1994 by American Psychiatric Association. Reprinted with permission.

Criterion BDL-1

Frantic efforts to avoid real or imagined abandonment. [*Note: Do not include suicidal or self-mutilating behavior, covered in criterion BDL-5.*]

Revisions and Rationale: This item was unchanged from *DSM-III-R*. As indicated above, it represented the only major revision of the *DSM-III* criteria for BDL PD. It was not, in fact, included in the first draft of the *DSM-III-R* BDL criteria set. Included instead was an interpersonal exploitativeness (Work Group, 1985). Frantic efforts to avoid abandonment, however, was included in the second draft of *DSM-III-R* (Work Group, 1986), and it replaced intolerance of being alone because of the poor performance of the former item within the published studies (Widiger et al., 1988). "Frantic efforts to avoid abandonment" provides a more accurate representation of the borderline's intense separation conflicts (Gunderson & Zanarini, 1987). It was moved to the top of the list in *DSM-IV* because it is considered to be central to the pathology of the borderline personality disorder (Gunderson, 1984; Gunderson, Zanarini, et al., 1991). However, it should be noted that other *DSM-III-R* criteria have been as, if not more, diagnostic of BDL PD, particularly impulsivity and unstable/intense relationships (Gunderson, Zanarini, et al., 1991; Nurnberg et al., 1991b; Widiger & Frances, 1989b; Zanarini, 1993).

Rating:

0) Absent
1) Frantic efforts to avoid real or imagined abandonment [*Note: Don't include suicidal or self-mutilating behavior, covered in criterion BDL-5.*]
2) Repeated history of desperate efforts to avoid loss of relationships with a variety of significant others, including therapists

Questions:

a. Has it usually been difficult for you when you learn that a relationship might end?
b. What are some of the things you have done to avoid losing your [*boyfriend/girlfriend/spouse*]?
c. Have you had similar difficulties with other persons, such as a therapist?
d. Has a [*former partner*] ever been real scared or angry at you because of things you did to try to stop the relationship from ending?

Issues and Problems: This item excludes suicidal or self-mutilating behavior used in the assessment of BDL-5. This exclusion is necessary to ensure that the diagnosis is not limited to a narrow range of behaviors (otherwise a series of suicidal acts might qualify for three of the five criteria), and to ensure that a pervasive pattern of behavior is being assessed. However, the exclusion is somewhat regrettable because suicidal threats and gestures provide a prototypic example of the extreme and volatile manner in which borderline patients will protest or fight a perceived abandonment. Additional examples include a history of pleading and begging for a relationship to continue through numerous phone calls, letters, and sudden, unexpected visits (e.g., repeated pleading to be seen "at least just this one more time"). Borderline persons will often refuse to accept or even acknowledge the ending of a relationship, at times acting as if it still continues. They may appear in places frequented by the person with whom they are (or were) involved, and they may even stalk the person. They will not only threaten their own lives but may also threaten the other person. These threats can include making scenes in public places, embarrassing the person somehow at work or in front of friends or colleagues, exposing secrets they might possess, or even inflicting physical harm or property damage.

A difficulty in the assessment of this item is differentiating it from the fears of abandonment that will be evident in persons with a dependent PD. One of the *DSM-III-R* criteria for dependent PD was a fear of being abandoned (APA, 1987). It was revised in *DSM-IV* to clarify that this fear is not necessarily of abandonment. Dependent persons will be preoccupied with fears concerning the end of a relationship even when they are reassured that they will not be abandoned. Fears of abandonment are more specific to persons with a borderline PD. Perceiving or characterizing the end of a relationship as involving "abandonment" does, itself, suggest the severe distortion that would be more indicative of a borderline than simply a dependent personality disorder (Kernberg, 1984b). However, persons with a dependent PD will often engage in frantic efforts to avoid losing a relationship (whether or not they expect to be abandoned may be irrelevant). Persons with borderline PD who exhibit frantic efforts to avoid abandonment will almost always exhibit the respective dependent criterion of an unrealistic preoccupation with fears of being left to take care of themselves; and dependent persons who have unrealistic preoccupations with fears about being left to take care of themselves will often engage in frantic efforts to avoid losing the relationship.

The observable distinction between the borderline and the simply dependent expression of this trait is that the effort to avoid (protest or fight) the end of a relationship tends to be more extreme, severe, and even dangerous, to the extent that the person has a borderline personality disorder. Persons with a dependent personality disorder who do not have a comorbid borderline PD will be unlikely to engage in the more severe behaviors, such as self-mutilation, threats of harm to the other person, or stalking. However, because it is not unusual for persons with a dependent PD, particularly those within an inpatient setting, to also meet the *DSM-III-R* (and *DSM-IV*) criteria for BDL PD, it will often be more informative with respect to this criterion to recognize that these personality disorders overlap and will often co-occur. Therefore, this item will often fail to differentiate these two personality disorders. Rather than conclude that a person has a borderline rather than a dependent personality disorder, it is often more informative to conclude that a person with a dependent personality disorder is at a borderline level of personality organization, using Kernberg's (1984b) terminology (although a *DSM-IV* diagnosis of BDL PD is not equivalent to Kernberg's diagnosis of a borderline level of personality organization). Or, using *DSM-IV* terminology, conclude that a person with a *DSM-IV* borderline personality disorder is characterized in particular by conflicts or issues concerning dependency.

Note as well the point made with respect to the dependent PD criterion, that some persons who are financially dependent upon another person may also become frantic and desperate to avoid losing the relationship. For example, an impoverished woman with many dependent children and little prospects for support or assistance may have many realistic fears and concerns about being abandoned by her husband, and her characterization of the end of the relationship as involving an abandonment may be quite accurate.

Criterion BDL-2

A pattern of unstable and intense interpersonal relationships characterized by alternating between extremes of idealization and devaluation.

Revisions and Rationale: This item was essentially unchanged from *DSM-III-R*. The only revision was to change overidealization to idealization; the meaning remains the same. Unstable and intense relationships has been cited as one of the most effective items for diagnosing BDL PD, particularly within inpatient settings (Widiger & Frances, 1989b). An early and often cited characterization of persons with borderline PD was that they were "stable in their instability" (Schmideberg, 1959, p. 398). The intensity and instability of their relationships is often a major reason such persons are so difficult to treat (Gunderson, 1984; Stone, 1990, 1992; Waldinger & Gunderson, 1987). Their relationships with their therapists can be as intense, unstable, and explosive as their relationships with their lovers.

It may be of some interest to note, however, that in the *DSM-III* version of this item, "manipulation (consistently using others for one's own ends)" (APA, 1980, p. 322) was included, along with idealization, devaluation, and marked shifts of attitude, as one of the examples of this item. Manipulation and exploitation are features of the borderline PD that have been considered for inclusion in various forms within the BDL criteria set (e.g., see earlier discussion of BDL-1). Manipulation was excluded in *DSM-III-R* due to the clear overlap with the antisocial and narcissistic PDs (Widiger et al., 1988).

This item does contain one of the more prototypic examples of the primitive defense mechanism of splitting emphasized by Kernberg (1984b), wherein one alternates between extreme, polarizing attitudes of idealization and devaluation. Many patients (and other persons) will have a history of unstable and intense relationships without clear periods of idealization. Persons with a dependent PD may have a history of unstable and intense relationships with little or no devaluation of their partner(s). They may continue to love, cherish, desire, and even honor the person, despite being neglected or abused. On the other hand, persons with an antisocial PD (particularly those with sadistic personality traits) may have a history of unstable and intense relationships with little or no idealization. They may continue to brutally exploit, viciously abuse, and denigrate their partner(s) without ever having any feelings of love, warmth, or affection, let alone idealization.

Rating:

0) Absent
1) A pattern of unstable and intense interpersonal relationships characterized by alternating between extremes of idealization and devaluation
2) This pattern characterizes most significant relationships, including those with therapists

Questions:

a. Have you had many fights with your [*lovers/spouses/partners*]?

b. Have you had many separations or break-ups?

c. Have you sometimes really hated the other person?

d. Has this anger or hatred occurred with your therapists as well, or with other persons?

Issues and Problems: A difficulty in assessing this item is determining what constitutes idealization and devaluation. An obvious example would be extreme feelings of love and hate toward the same person. Many persons become angry, bitter, and resentful when they feel mistreated, misled, or abandoned by a past or current love. They may even come to the point of truly hating this person, and they may certainly devalue and denigrate someone they once loved, cherished, and valued. We do not consider such changes of heart to reflect this item unless there is a pattern or history of occurrence. Assessing for this historical pattern is important because it is not unusual for persons in treatment to be currently ending a relationship or struggling with one that is very disappointing, bitter, depressing, and even volatile. The changes in attitude would not be characteristic of a borderline personality disorder unless there is a pattern of such relationships and changes.

Establishing this history will be difficult if the person has been involved primarily in just one relationship for an extended period of time. It is more characteristic of borderline persons to be involved in a series of volatile relationships. However, it is not unheard of for there to be one continuously unstable relationship. In such cases, we look for a history of volatile fights/separations and idealized reconciliations. The borderline person will alternate between feelings of passionate love and bitter hatred toward the same person, with little apparent reason or justification for each fluctuation. Most persons who have experienced such degrees of disappointment, resentment, bitterness, or anger toward a particular person would not so readily forget and quickly return to the relationship. Their perceptions of this other person will be modified or modulated by their experiences. Borderline persons, however, seem just to fluctuate from one extreme to another, never appearing to learn much from their past experience.

It will also be difficult to observe this history in young adults who have not yet had the opportunity or time to establish such a pattern (Stone, 1993). One may often observe this pattern during adolescence, but it is important to appreciate that the turmoil of adolescence may not continue into adulthood. What will be characteristic of adulthood may not be apparent from what is characteristic of adolescence (Costa & McCrae, 1993). Many adolescents who might appear to have a borderline personality disorder (i.e., unstable, intense relationships, impulsivity, intense anger, and identity disturbance) are better thought of as having an adjustment disorder, identity problem, or phase of life problem (APA, 1994). It is indicative of a borderline personality disorder that this turmoil, instability, and volatility does not begin to dissipate until well into middle age.

In these circumstances, it is often useful to consider other relationships in the person's life, particularly persons who have been especially meaningful or significant to the subject. It is unusual for a person with a borderline personality disorder to develop a significant or meaningful relationship that does not eventually (and often quickly) become volatile and explosive. They tend not to have relationships that remain dispassionate, calm, or controlled. Inquiries with respect to their relationships with their significant friends, parents, teachers, caseworkers, or therapists are often informative. However, it is also important not to presume that some current (or prior) relationship should be (or should have been) intense. It is very unusual for a person with borderline PD not to develop an intense relationship with someone who is significant and meaningful to them; however, if he or she did not find the relationship to be personally significant or meaningful, then no intensity of feelings will likely develop.

A common experience within new therapeutic relationships is for borderline persons to devalue prior therapist(s) and indicate how pleased, gratified, and/or optimistic they are with their current therapist (Gunderson, 1984). Idealization and devaluation of different members of the same treatment team are also common (Gunderson, 1984; Stone, 1993). However, we do not consider this idealization and devaluation to necessarily qualify for this item unless there is a concomitant intensity of affect. Narcissistic persons will also idealize and devalue various members of a treatment team, but often without the intensity in the relationship that is characteristic of BDL PD.

Criterion BDL-3

Identity disturbance: markedly and persistently unstable self-image or sense of self.

Revisions and Rationale: Identity disturbance has been included in the *DSM-III*, *DSM-III-R*, and *DSM-IV* criteria for BDL PD, but it has also been one of the most problematic criteria. It is one of the few *DSM* borderline items that is not also explicitly included within the DIB (Gunderson et al., 1981) or the DIB-R (Zanarini, Gunderson, et al., 1989). It represents instead one of the three fundamental features of Kernberg's (1984b) borderline personality organization (i.e., identity diffusion, primitive defenses, and poor reality testing in object/interpersonal relations). The major problem with the item is that it has been very difficult to assess reliably. It was the one *DSM-III-R* BDL item that was considered for deletion (Gunderson, Zanarini, et al., 1991).

The *DSM-III* version was "identity disturbance manifested by uncertainty about several issues relating to identity, such as self-image, gender identity, long-term goals or career choice, friendship patterns, values, and loyalties (e.g., 'Who am I?', 'I feel like I am my sister when I am good')" (APA, 1980, p. 323). A major difficulty with this version was that it could easily be interpreted as describing normative adolescent or young adult questions regarding identity and future. It is not unusual for young adults to be unclear as to their long-term goals, career goals, values, and even their self-image. The illustrative quotations provided in *DSM-III*, in fact, seemed to encourage this association with normal issues of adolescence. *DSM-III* provided an exclusion criterion for the borderline PD that a person under age 18 could not meet the criteria for an Identity Disorder (APA, 1980, p. 323). However, normative concerns regarding identity will continue past the age of 18 (e.g., college students who have delayed decisions regarding their future) and the identity concerns of childhood and adolescence are often below the threshold for a borderline identity disturbance (Kernberg, 1984b). The *DSM-III-R* identity disorder of adolescence has, in fact, been moved out of the mental disorders section and into the (V-code) section for conditions that may be a focus of clinical attention, and the name has been appropriately shifted from an identity disorder to simply an identity problem.

DSM-III-R attempted to address this problem with the BDL criterion by indicating that there was a "marked and persistent" identity disturbance (APA, 1987, p. 347), but the examples that were provided still conveyed the impression of simply the normative issues that are present within many young adults. *DSM-III-R* also required that at least two of these concerns must be present, but that did not really address the problem because normative issues concerning identity will rarely be confined to just one area.

A proposal considered for *DSM-IV* was to replace the examples of career choice, long-term goals, and preferred values with "they may feel like they don't exist or that they embody evil" (Gunderson, Zanarini, et al., 1991, p. 346). However, it was decided that this would be swinging the pendulum too far in the other direction. These examples are at the level of a psychotic or a psychotic-like break with reality. Psychotic-like experiences are not unusual in borderline persons (Zanarini, Gunderson, & Frankenburg, 1990), but the identity disturbances of borderline persons are not typically at this level of pathology (Kernberg, 1984b). A subsequent proposal was to redefine the item as involving "persistent and markedly disturbed, distorted, or unstable self-image" (Task Force, 1993, p. T:5), but it was then suggested that disturbed and distorted self-images are common within most personality disorders (e.g., the low self-esteem of the dependent person and the grandiosity of the narcissistic). The final decision was to emphasize the persistent instability of the sense of self and to move the examples out of the criteria set and into the text so there would be room for further discussion and clarification.

Rating:

0) Absent
1) Identity disturbance: markedly and persistently unstable self-image or sense of self
2) Significant social or occupational decisions have been made on the basis of distortions in identity

Questions:

a. How would you describe your personality? What is distinct or unique about you?

b. Do you ever feel that you don't know who you are or what you believe in?

c. Has your sense of who you are, what you value, what you want from life, or what you want to be, been fairly consistent, or has this often change significantly?

Issues and Problems: The major issue in assessing this item remains its reliability, particularly with respect to the distinction between normative versus pathologic questioning of one's identity and future. One approach we take with this item is to consider the age of the respondent. Uncertainty regarding long-term goals, values, career, and types of friends are more indicative of identity disturbance in persons who are well past adolescence (and college). However, even in adults, one must be careful not to confuse a preferred absence of direction with borderline identity disturbance. For example, many antisocial persons who do not have borderline personality traits may lack clear plans or direction because they are pursuing a hedonistic, irresponsible, aimless, and/or impulsive lifestyle. The distinction in such cases may be that these nonborderline antisocial persons may be able to describe themselves as being rebellious, criminal, or hedonistic. That is, they will have a clear self-identity as someone who lacks a definite life plan.

It is also important to carefully consider cultural variations in the sense of identity and self (Landrine, 1992). Statements regarding individualized values, career plans, or goals can vary substantially across cultures. What may appear to be vague or noncommittal to the Western culture may be normative within other cultures.

Major shifts in one's goals, values, or vocations can be indicative of an identity disturbance (APA, 1994). Some borderline persons will express clear and strong values, plans, or aspirations, but have a history of whimsical shifts. Histrionic persons will also display sudden and dramatic changes in beliefs and commitments, reflecting their suggestibility. However, the shifts in histrionic persons are often in response to the influence of others; they are less likely to make these changes on their own. The major changes in the goals and values of the borderline person may also lack the theatrical or dramatic nature seen in histrionic persons, as they will reflect simply the inability to sustain a clear sense of themselves (i.e., what they want, need, value, or desire).

Kernberg (1984b) has emphasized the inability of borderline persons to describe themselves or others in such a way that one can obtain a clear sense of the person being described, either because the description was unclear and shallow, or because it was contradictory and inconsistent. We do find it helpful in the assessment of identity disturbance to ask persons to describe themselves and also to describe other persons, in order to determine whether their descriptions are shallow, vague, or contradictory. However, we also find that many persons have considerable difficulty with such open-ended questions regarding descriptions of oneself and others. Vague, unclear, shallow, and even contradictory descriptions will often reflect one's level of verbal skills, intelligence, or familiarity with the language, as well as one's motivation and interest in the question. In addition, an individual's response may be affected substantially by current life circumstances. One's sense of one's goals, values, and aspirations in life can be understandably disrupted and confused by an inpatient hospitalization for a mood disorder, psychosis, substance dependence, or other Axis I disorder.

Unstructured psychological tests may also be useful in assessing for the absence of a clear sense of identity or for the presence of a severely distorted or disturbed identity, such as the feeling of not existing or embodying evil (Gunderson & Singer, 1975; Kernberg, 1984b). Borderline persons do tend to lean heavily on structure to maintain their grip on reason, clarity, and reality, and projective tests can be quite useful in assessing self-image in the absence of such structure (Kwawer, Lerner, Lerner, & Sugarman, 1980; Lerner, 1991). However, we also encourage subsequent discussions of any aberrant psychological test responses to obtain whatever clarification or meaning can (or cannot) be provided by the persons themselves.

Criterion BDL-4

Impulsivity in at least two areas that are potentially self-damaging (e.g., spending, sex, substance abuse, reckless driving, binge eating). [*Note: Do not include suicidal or self-mutilating behavior, covered in criterion BDL-5.*]

Revisions and Rationale: The only real change to this item was the deletion of shoplifting from the list of examples. This deletion reflects the clinical experience that shoplifting is not particularly common or characteristic of persons with borderline personality disorder. Binge eating, sexual promiscuity, and substance abuse are much more common than shoplifting.

Self-damaging impulsivity is a central and common feature of borderline PD. This item has been the most consistent in obtaining among the highest correlations with a borderline diagnosis (see Gunderson, Zanarini, et al., 1991). Borderline persons often live, as the name can imply, chaotic and dangerous lives, engaging in a variety of impulsive acts that usually result in some eventual harmful and even disastrous consequences.

Rating:

0) Absent
1) Impulsivity in at least two areas that are potentially self-damaging (e.g., spending, sex, substance abuse, reckless driving, binge eating) [*Note: Do not include suicidal or self-mutilating behavior, covered in criterion BDL-5.*]
2) Impulsivity in at least three areas, at least one of which has been physically self-damaging

Questions:

a. Did you ever spend so much money that you had trouble paying it off?

b. Did you ever go on a drinking or eating binge?

c. Have you ever taken any major chances or risks with drugs?

d. Did you ever do anything impulsive that was risky or dangerous?

e. Have you ever become sexually involved with someone in a risky or dangerous way?

Issues and Problems: Two of five areas of impulse dyscontrol are necessary, but it is important to note that one can consider areas of dyscontrol beyond the five presented within the list. The list of five provides a set of examples or possibilities. One is not confined to these particular five. Obvious additional possibilities would be two behavioral patterns that were included in *DSM-III-R*: shoplifting and recurrent physical accidents. The requirement is that the behavior pattern reflects an area of impulse dyscontrol that is potentially self-damaging. Shoplifting was removed from the list not to ensure that it would not be used but because the remaining five occur more frequently. Impulsive, reckless shoplifting can (and should) still be considered (although careful, calculated shoplifting may not reflect borderline impulsivity).

One could also rank-order the remaining five with respect to their diagnostic value. It has been our experience that the three most common are substance abuse, sex, and binge eating, followed by spending and reckless driving (we would be reluctant to rank-order the behaviors within these two groups). Overspending that simply reflects financial impoverishment (e.g., due to lack of employment or income) should not be included, unless the spending is, indeed, quite impulsive, reckless, and irresponsible given the current financial condition.

One also finds examples of borderline impulsivity that are confined to just one area. For example, we have been tempted to consider this item to be present when there was substantial dyscontrol only of sexual behavior (e.g., sex with many strangers with no protection, including bizarre and/or abusive sex acts). We would consider this to be more suggestive of a borderline PD than a history of defaulting on debts and speeding tickets (i.e., mild dyscontrol in two different areas). Nevertheless, it is important to follow the *DSM-IV* criteria to ensure consistent, replicable assessments. Impulse dyscontrol must be present in at least two different areas.

The impulse dyscontrol must also be severe enough that it is potentially self-damaging. One way of operationalizing this threshold is meeting the *DSM-IV* criteria for a respective Axis I disorder (e.g., gambling, substance abuse, paraphilia, or bulimia). However, there are no respective disorders for some of the impulse dyscontrol that one often observes in borderline persons (e.g., sex, spending, and reckless driving). Our threshold for attribution is when the person has suffered (or will likely suffer) substantial social, occupational, or physical consequences if the behavior continues (e.g., loss of marriage, job, or savings; or severe danger to physical health). We would not consider a history of speeding tickets or nicotine dependence to be sufficient (multiple traffic accidents or cocaine abuse are more characteristic).

The requirement that one must document the presence of impulsivity in at least two different areas ensures that one does to confuse an Axis I disorder with BDL impulsivity (Stone, 1993). If only one such behavior was required, then almost any person with a long history of an Axis I substance-related, paraphilic, gambling, or bulimic disorder might be said to have a borderline personality trait. The presence of such behaviors in at least two areas is helpful in determining whether the behavior pattern is, indeed, pervasive (Axis II) rather than being confined to a circumscribed domain (Axis I). However, the 2+ algorithm does not really ensure that one will not confuse an Axis I disorder with a borderline personality disorder because many persons can, indeed, have impulse dyscontrol in two or more areas without having a borderline personality disorder. On the other hand, many borderline persons will develop a substance-related, eating, or other Axis I disorder as a result of their borderline psychopathology. Meeting the *DSM-IV* criteria for an Axis I disorder does not (in our opinion) negate or rule out the possibility that the Axis I behavior is due to a borderline personality disorder (Widiger & Shea, 1991).

This issue has been particularly problematic with respect to bulimia. Many borderline persons will develop bulimia, but the impulsivity and affective dyscontrol of persons with bulimia contribute to an overdiagnosis of BDL PD within eating-disordered populations (Pope & Hudson, 1989; Widiger & Shea, 1991). If the person does meet the *DSM-IV* criteria for an Axis I paraphilic, substance-related, gambling, or eating disorder that has been present since late adolescence or early adulthood, we then prefer to rely on the other eight criteria for a diagnosis of BDL PD (using the same threshold). This is admittedly a more restrictive threshold than is required for *DSM-IV*, but it is not terribly restrictive because a BDL diagnosis would require four additional criteria anyway. We are simply requiring that the fifth criterion be one other than the item that involves explicitly the Axis I symptomatology. This more restrictive threshold would affect a diagnosis only in a case that was literally on the boundary of the diagnosis. In such cases, it is perhaps best to provide both diagnoses so that the issues that concern each disorder (Axes I and II) are not neglected in the treatment program.

Criterion BDL-5

Recurrent suicidal behavior, gestures, or threats, or self-mutilating behavior.

Revisions and Rationale: This item was unchanged from *DSM-III-R*. The *DSM-III* version was more broadly defined as physically self-damaging acts, including recurrent accidents and physical fights (APA, 1980). Physical fights, however, are more appropriately covered within the item concerned with dyscontrol of anger (BDL-8). In any case, recurrent physical accidents that do not explicitly reflect suicidal behaviors are not particularly common in borderline persons and are readily covered within the item concerned with self-damaging impulsivity (BDL-4).

Recurrent suicidal and self-mutilative behavior is commonly seen in borderline inpatients (often providing the impetus for hospitalization) but may not be as common among borderline persons who are rarely hospitalized (Widiger & Frances, 1989b). Self-mutilative behavior (e.g., slashing or burning oneself) is a prototypic borderline act that is relatively specific to persons (particularly adults) with borderline personality disorder. Persons with a mood disorder who do not have a comorbid borderline PD will be suicidal but are much less likely to display impulsive self-mutilation. Self-mutilation is often precipitated by threats of separation, rejection, or loss, but may also occur during episodes of depersonalization or derealization (APA, 1994; Gunderson, 1984).

Rating:

0) Absent
1) Recurrent suicidal behavior, gestures, or threats, or self-mutilating behavior
2) Recurrent suicidal behavior, gestures, or threats, and self-mutilating behavior

Questions:

a. Ever threaten suicide or try to kill yourself?

b. Ever hurt yourself physically? (e.g., by cutting, slashing, or burning yourself)?

Issues and Problems: Recurrent self-mutilation in an adult (without schizophrenia, mental retardation, or other relevant Axis I disorder) has high positive predictive power but low negative predictive power for the diagnosis of BDL PD. That is, when it does occur, it is very diagnostic of BDL PD (positive predictive power) but its absence is not as helpful in ruling out the presence of a borderline personality disorder (negative predictive power) (Widiger, Hurt, Frances, Clarkin, & Gilmore, 1984) because many borderline persons will fail to engage in self-mutilative behavior, but few nonborderlines engage in this behavior (although one might observe acts of self-mutilation within certain religious or spiritual rituals).

An issue that is problematic for assessment even when suicidal or self-mutilative behaviors occur is that they can be quite infrequent in their occurrence. It would be unusual for a year to pass without a borderline person exhibiting affective instability, intense/unstable relationships, impulsivity, feelings of emptiness, or dyscontrol of anger (although the occurrence of these behavior patterns will depend, in part, on the life circumstances of the person; Gunderson, 1987). However, this would not be unusual in the case of suicidal behavior and self-mutilation. Some researchers approach this problem by allowing just one suicidal act within a 5-year period to be sufficient to consider the item to be present. However, this would readily confuse suicidal behavior that is resulting from an Axis I disorder (e.g., major depression) with suicidal behavior resulting from borderline personality disorder (Widiger & Sanderson, in press-a), a differentiation that is already very problematic (Gunderson & Phillips, 1991; Widiger, 1989). In addition, the item specifies that the suicidal behavior is recurrent. One act during the past 5 years, or perhaps two during the past 10 years, is not really recurrent. However, the item does include suicidal gestures and threats, along with suicidal acts and self-mutilation. One might observe suicidal gestures or threats during the years that precede or follow an explicit suicidal act by someone with a borderline personality disorder. To the extent that such an act reflects recurrent suicidal behavior in someone with a borderline personality disorder, one would expect to observe further indicators of this trait over the next few years. An exception, however, would be when the person's life has been stabilized through treatment or other intervention (e.g., by a nurturant, patient, and tolerant spouse) (Gunderson, 1987).

Criterion BDL-6

Affective instability due to a marked reactivity of mood (e.g., intense episodic dysphoria, irritability, or anxiety usually lasting a few hours and only rarely more than a few days).

Revisions and Rationale: Affective instability was one of the three BDL items to receive substantial revision for *DSM-IV*. In *DSM-III-R*, affective instability was defined as marked shifts in mood (APA, 1987). The differentiation of BDL PD from a mood disorder is one of the more difficult issues (Gunderson & Elliott, 1985; Gunderson & Phillips, 1991; Stone, 1993; Widiger, 1989). The affective instability item has not only been unhelpful in differentiating BDL from a mood disorder, it has contributed to the confusion.

One of the revisions for *DSM-IV* was to replace depression with dysphoria. As noted in the *DSM-IV* text discussion, the predominant mood of persons with borderline PD is dysphoria, which is often disrupted by periods of anger, panic, or despair and is rarely relieved by periods of well-being (APA, 1994). This is quite different from the descriptions provided in *DSM-III* and *DSM-III-R*, which referred to a baseline mood that would shift to either depression, irritability, or anxiety. The baseline mood was, in fact, characterized as a normal mood in *DSM-III* (APA, 1980). A predominant mood of dysphoria will be helpful in distinguishing BDL affective instability from cyclothymic affective instability, as the latter will have a euthymic (normal) baseline mood (Gunderson, Zanarini, et al., 1991).

It is also noted in *DSM-IV* that the moods involve intense dysphoria, irritability, or anxiety. *DSM-III-R* indicated that the affective instability involved marked shifts in mood, placing more emphasis on the change in the mood state than on the severity or intensity of the mood state. The *DSM-IV* revision will be helpful in increasing the threshold for the attribution of the item.

Finally, there is the indication that the affective instability involves a marked reactivity of mood, rather than simply momentary and fleeting shifts in mood states that could occur without any precipitating event. The mood of the borderline person is very sensitive. It takes little to cause a severe eruption of anger, panic, or dysphoria. A passing, innocent remark, an apparently innocuous suggestion, or a seemingly minor slight can have an explosive effect. Most importantly, this revision reflects an effort to link the mood states to interpersonal crises and to diminish the suggestion of autonomous mood shifts (Gunderson & Phillips, 1991). Although quite sensitive and easily exploded, the mood of the borderline person is, nevertheless, reactive rather than endogenous.

Rating:

0) Absent
1) Affective instability due to a marked reactivity of mood (e.g., intense episodic dysphoria, irritability, or anxiety usually lasting a few hours and only rarely more than a few days)
2) Intense mood shifts are also apparent during interview and are described as a daily problem

Questions:

a. Does your mood tend to shift from one feeling to another, even during the same day?

b. Does it seem to take very little to get you upset, anxious, or angry?

Issues and Problems: Many persons currently in treatment, particularly those within inpatient settings, will feel dysphoric, depressed, or anxious, and it is not unusual for them to complain of affective instability. This will be particularly evident in persons with a mood disorder. It is then important to document the presence of this item since late childhood or adolescence and prior to the onset of any current mood disorder. Requests for examples for this item are also particularly important (but, as indicated in chapter 1, this should be asked for all items) to assess whether the mood shifts are, indeed, very intense and reactive. Interviews with persons who have known the subject for many years can also be very helpful in the assessment of this item.

The histrionic PD also involves affective instability. In this case, it is characterized as a rapidly shifting and shallow expression of emotions (APA, 1994). It will often be very difficult to distinguish intense episodic dysphoria, irritability, and anxiety that usually lasts only a few hours from a rapidly shifting and shallow expression of emotions. A distinction that may, at times, be helpful is that the borderline mood shifts are typically reactive to an interpersonal event (and are characteristically more intense) whereas the histrionic mood shifts can be more autonomous and may even be inexplicable to the observer. This distinction, however, may not always be evident.

Criterion BDL–7

Chronic feelings of emptiness.

Revisions and Rationale: Chronic feelings of emptiness or boredom was included in both the *DSM-III* and *DSM-III-R* criteria for BDL PD (APA, 1980, 1987). It was obtained from an early version of the Diagnostic Interview for Borderlines (Gunderson & Kolb, 1978; Gunderson, Kolb, & Austin, 1981), but it has since become evident that it has been emptiness and not boredom that is discriminative (Gunderson, Zanarini, et al., 1991). Chronic feelings of boredom will be more characteristic of the antisocial, narcissistic, and schizoid personality disorders than of the borderline PD. Chronic feelings of emptiness are also more indicative of the identity diffusion of borderline persons than simply boredom (Kernberg, 1984b). Boredom can trivialize the severity of the pathology, perhaps implying that what is wrong is simply that one has nothing to do (a common complaint within some inpatient settings), rather than that one is feeling without substance, purpose, or meaning.

Rating:

0) Absent
1) Chronic feelings of emptiness
2) Chronic feelings of emptiness are a spontaneous and central complaint of the person

Questions:

a. Do you sometimes feel like you have no meaning or purpose in life?

b. Do you feel rather empty much of the time?

Issues and Problems: At times, we have found that some persons will not know what is meant by feeling "empty," or feeling "without meaning, purpose, or substance." We might, then, revert to using the term "boredom" only to initiate a discussion, and then ask the person for a more precise description in his or her own words of how he or she feels. The person may say, for example, "I don't know who I am," "I'm not really here," or "Nothing seems to really matter." Probing and clarification are almost always necessary in the assessment of this item.

It is also important to document that these feelings of emptiness are chronic. We interpret chronic to mean that such feelings have been with the person throughout adult life, but they may come and go during this time. However, this would not include fleeting thoughts or occasional existential reflections late at night. This item concerns, instead, sustained periods of emptiness that are typically very disturbing to the person and are often difficult to escape. They may, in fact, be evident during periods when the person is within a relatively stable relationship, as it is during such times that the borderline person may experience an inability of other persons to resolve, fulfill, or cure their inherent loneliness and emptiness (Gunderson, 1987).

Some of these periods of emptiness may qualify as dissociative episodes of depersonalization or derealization. If so, we would still consider them to reflect the current item, and we would then exclude them from consideration for BDL-9 (which can involve other dissociative symptoms, as well as paranoid ideation). On the other hand, the simple presence of statements that the person has often felt a lack of meaning or purpose may be more appropriately considered for BDL-3 (identity disturbance). Chronic feelings of emptiness involve the more visceral feeling that might accompany the experience of an identity disturbance (Kernberg, 1984b) rather than simply the belief or cognition.

Criterion BDL-8

Inappropriate, intense anger or difficulty controlling anger (e.g., frequent displays of temper, constant anger, recurrent physical fights).

Revisions and Rationale: This item was essentially unchanged from *DSM-III-R*. The only revision from *DSM-III* to *DSM-III-R* was the addition of recurrent physical fights to the list of examples (moved from the examples of physically self-damaging acts). The physical fights of borderline persons are more reflective of their dyscontrolled anger than of their propensity to engage in suicidal or self-mutilative behavior. Persons with a borderline personality disorder are prone to explosive outbursts of rage, which will often have a devaluative or manipulative effect (APA, 1994). Borderline anger may also be more chronic and sustained, expressed through extreme sarcasm or enduring bitterness (APA, 1994). Anger can, in fact, appear to be the prominent trait of this disorder, as it is a symptom that will often require the most patience of the clinician and staff to accept and to tolerate.

Rating:

0) Absent
1) Inappropriate intense anger or difficulty controlling anger (e.g., frequent displays of temper, constant anger, recurrent physical fights)
2) Episodes of severe rage

Questions:

a. Do you often feel bitter or angry?

b. What usually happens when you get angry?

c. Did you ever get into a real screaming and yelling fight?

d. Did you ever throw or break things?

e. Did you ever get into any physical fights?

Issues and Problems: The angry hostility of borderline persons is one of the easier items to assess, as it is readily evident to those around them, including therapists and any clinic or hospital staff. However, it is also important not to exaggerate its importance and overdiagnose BDL PD on the basis of having an angry, hostile patient. In clinical lore, a euphemism for borderline personality disorder is that it applies to any patient that one dislikes. This symptom may be the major culprit for therapeutic countertransference, impatience, and/or annoyance. Contributing to a potential overdiagnosis is the fact that the item appears to include the full range of anger, from a low-level constant anger (examples provided in the text of *DSM-IV* are sarcasm and bitterness; APA, 1994) to rage and physical fights. We emphasize that the anger must be inappropriate and intense. Sarcasm and bitterness are characteristic of borderline persons, but we would not consider this item to be present unless the antagonism was particularly extreme and/or punctuated by occasional episodes of explosive rage.

Recurrent physical fights are not as common as constant bitterness and resentment with episodes of rage. Repeated physical fights can be more characteristic of persons with an antisocial PD. The fights of the antisocial person, however, will often be more calculated, controlled, and even premeditated. They will often reflect an explicit effort to subjugate, control, humiliate, or harm someone (e.g., an assault), whereas the fights of a person with borderline PD will tend to be more impulsive, explosive, and dyscontrolled. It is more indicative of a borderline person than the antisocial or psychopathic person to initiate a fight that he or she clearly cannot win ("physical fights" was, in fact, included within the borderline criterion of physically self-damaging acts in *DSM-III*; APA, 1980, p. 323). However, antisocial and psychopathic persons can be very impulsive and hotheaded (Hare, 1992). Many of their fights will reflect dyscontrolled outbursts of anger, particularly when they are under the influence of a drug (Widiger & Trull, 1993).

Criterion BDL-9

Transient, stress-related paranoid ideation or severe dissociative symptoms.

Revisions and Rationale: This item is a new addition to *DSM-IV*. The question of whether such an item should be included within the criteria set for BDL PD has been controversial since the development of the original criteria set for *DSM-III* (Frances, 1980; Gunderson, Zanarini, et al., 1991; Spitzer et al., 1979; Widiger, Miele, & Tilly, 1992). It was noted within the associated features section of *DSM-III* that "during periods of extreme stress transient psychotic symptoms of insufficient severity or duration to warrant an additional diagnosis may occur" (APA, 1980, p. 322).

Psychotic and psychotic-like symptoms were a major part of the original formulation of borderline PD developed by Gunderson and his colleagues (Gunderson & Kolb, 1978; Gunderson & Singer, 1975), and they have been included within the original (DIB) and revised (DIB-R) Diagnostic Interview for Borderlines (Gunderson, Kolb, & Austin, 1981; Zanarini, Gunderson, Frankenburg, & Chauncey, 1989). However, the odd thinking, aberrant perceptual experiences, and paranoid ideation assessed by the DIB and DIB-R are also characteristic of schizotypal persons. Many are included within the *DSM-III-R* and *DSM-IV* schizotypal criteria set (e.g., suspicious-paranoid ideation, unusual perceptual experiences, ideas of reference, and odd, magical thinking; APA, 1987, 1994) and "occasional transient quasi-psychotic episodes with intense illusions" is included within the ICD-10 criteria for schizotypal disorder (WHO, 1992, p. 96). The co-occurrence of the BDL and schizotypal PD diagnoses is already substantial, and the inclusion of this criterion may only diminish rather than improve their differentiation. The distinction between the BDL and schizotypal PDs has been of less concern to Gunderson and his colleagues, in part because their original formulation of borderline personality disorder included the schizotypal traits. They did not, at first, recognize the existence of this different variant of (literally) borderline psychopathology that was eventually developed by Spitzer et al. (1979) for *DSM-III* (Gunderson & Kolb, 1978; Gunderson & Singer, 1975; Siever & Gunderson, 1979; Widiger, Miele, et al., 1992).

The new *DSM-IV* item was developed, in part, through pilot tests with analogue cases (Sternbach, Judd, Sabo, McGlashan, & Gunderson, 1992). It emphasizes that the paranoid ideation and dissociative symptoms are transient and stress-related. This is to help distinguish them from the cognitive and perceptual aberrations that are seen in persons with schizotypal PD. Schizotypal cognitive and perceptual aberrations are likely to be more stable and enduring and are less likely to be clearly related to stress (Gunderson, Zanarini, et al., 1991). An additional proposal considered for *DSM-IV* was to require that the schizotypal cognitive and perceptual aberrations not be associated with mood states of depression, anxiety, or anger (Siever, Bernstein, & Silverman, 1991; Task Force, 1991), whereas this would often be the case for the borderline symptoms.

In sum, there is no doubt that borderline persons will, at times, experience brief episodes of psychotic and psychotic-like symptomatology, and that such symptoms will be of considerable importance in treatment (Gunderson, Zanarini, et al., 1991). To the extent that transient, stress-related paranoid ideation and severe dissociative symptoms are not characteristic of persons with schizotypal personality disorder, the inclusion of this item would contribute to the differentiation of the borderline and schizotypal PDs.

Rating:

0) Absent
1) Transient, stress-related paranoid ideation or severe dissociative symptoms
2) Transient, stress-related paranoid ideation <u>and</u> severe dissociative symptoms

Questions:

a. Have you had any odd or unusual perceptual experiences?
b. Have you at times felt that things were unreal, that you weren't really here, or that you were detached or separate from life?
c. Did you ever find that time had passed and you didn't know what you had been doing?
d. Have you ever become very suspicious of other people, or felt sure they were plotting against you or out to get you?
e. Do these experiences occur only when you are under stress?
f. Do these experiences tend to be persistent, or are they fleeting or transient?

Issues and Problems: It is important in the assessment of this item to confirm that the symptoms are, indeed, transient and stress-related. To the extent that any cognitive or perceptual aberrations precede, endure, or occur independent of severe stress, this item would not be considered as present. The aberrations should be evident only when the person is under severe stress (particularly with respect to an interpersonal stressor) and be clearly related to an intensely dysphoric mood state (Gunderson, Zanarini, et al., 1991). The most characteristic example would be fleeting paranoid or dissociative experiences that rapidly remit with the provision of structure (e.g., hospitalization) or relief from stress.

The *DSM-IV* criterion describes these cognitive-perceptual aberrations as involving paranoid ideation or severe dissociative symptoms. However, in an initial draft of the *DSM-IV* text discussion of this criterion, they were described as psychotic-like symptoms, notably hallucinations, body-image distortions, ideas of reference, and hypnagogic phenomena (this description was shifted to the associated descriptive features in the final version; APA, 1994). It has been difficult to confine the description of these experiences (Gunderson, Zanarini, et al., 1991; Widiger, Miele, et al., 1992; Zanarini et al., 1990). The particular form or content of these symptoms is, perhaps, less important than the extent to which they are transient and stress-related.

The inclusion of severe dissociative symptoms will also highlight the association and differentiation of BDL PD from post-traumatic stress disorder (PTSD) (Gunderson & Sabo, 1993). Borderline persons have often suffered from very severe stress, and they tend to continue to live chaotic and even dangerous lives. They may contribute to the eventual experience of additional stress, and they are certainly poor at avoiding or coping with stress. Thus, it is to be expected that many persons with borderline PD will also suffer from PTSD. Given the importance of being aware of the presence (vs. absence) of borderline personality traits in persons with PTSD, we would not consider the presence of PTSD to exclude the relevance of the dissociative symptoms for the diagnosis of BDL PD. That is, we would encourage that both diagnoses be given if the person meets the criteria for both disorders; and we would still consider the dissociative symptoms to be diagnostic of BDL PD, even if the person also meets the *DSM-IV* criteria for PTSD.

The dissociative symptoms seen in borderline persons may not have been evident since late childhood, and many borderline persons will develop PTSD later in life. If there is little indication of borderline personality traits prior to the onset of a severe stressor that occurred since adolescence, then the more appropriate diagnosis would be simply PTSD. However, the ICD-10 does include a diagnosis of enduring personality change after catastrophic experience (WHO, 1992, p. 209). This diagnosis was considered for *DSM-IV* (Task Force, 1991) but was not included because of insufficient documentation that it could be distinguished reliably from Axis I disorders, such as PTSD.

One final note concerns the occurrence of unusual or dissociative experiences that are consistent with cultural, spiritual, or religious practices. One should be careful not to consider an experience as aberrant or pathological simply because it is deviant or unusual from the perspective of one's own cultural background. On the other hand, membership within a particular cultural group does not negate a diagnosis of borderline PD. One should consider whether the experience is excessive within that person's particular cultural or religious heritage.

7

Dependent Personality Disorder

Overview: The dependent (DEP) personality disorder was included as a subtype to the passive-aggressive personality in *DSM-I*, "characterized by helplessness, indecisiveness, and a tendency to cling to others as a dependent child to a supporting parent" (APA, 1952, p. 37). It was not included in *DSM-II* (APA, 1968) but was returned in *DSM-III* (APA, 1980). It was defined in *DSM-III-R* as a "pervasive pattern of dependent and submissive behavior" (APA, 1987, p. 354). This definition is rather circular, and was, therefore, revised in *DSM-IV* to emphasize that the disorder involves "a pervasive and excessive need to be taken care of that leads to submissive and clinging behavior and fears of separation" (APA, 1994, p. 665). The purpose of this revision was to provide a more specific definition that emphasizes the attachment component of dependency and emotional reliance upon others rather than simply a low self-confidence (Benjamin, 1993; Hirschfeld, Shea, & Weise, 1991; Livesley, Schroeder, & Jackson, 1990; Pilkonis, 1988). This emphasis has also been made in many of the individual item revisions.

There has been some question regarding the validity of the dependent personality disorder (e.g., Kaplan, 1983; Perry, 1990). The *DSM-IV* revisions to the criteria set emphasized the differentiation of dependent PD from the borderline and avoidant PDs and concerns regarding potential sex bias (Hirschfeld et al., 1991). *DSM-III-R* provided nine items, any five of which were necessary for the diagnosis. In *DSM-IV*, one of these items was deleted, and the threshold for diagnosis remains at five (of eight). All of the remaining eight items have been revised significantly. Being "easily hurt by criticism or disapproval" (APA, 1987, p. 354) was deleted because it is nonspecific to dependency. It was, in fact, one of the *DSM-III-R* criteria for the avoidant PD (APA, 1987). Many persons who have feelings of inadequacy or conflicts regarding their self-esteem (e.g., persons with a narcissistic PD) will be easily hurt by criticism or disapproval. The complete *DSM-IV* criteria set is presented in Table 7-1.

Criterion DEP-1

Has difficulty making everyday decisions without an excessive amount of advice and reassurance from others.

Revisions and Rationale: This item was not among the *DSM-III* criteria for DEP PD (APA, 1980). It was added to *DSM-III-R* to emphasize that the dependent person has difficulties with everyday, as well as major life decisions. *DSM-III* had confined its attention to the major areas of life, but many persons who are not dependent have considerable difficulty with the major decisions of life (e.g., marriage, job changes, or moving). The dependent person needs advice and reassurance even for the most simple, everyday decisions.

Table 7-1
DSM-IV Dependent Personality Disorder Criteria

A pervasive and excessive need to be taken care of that leads to submissive and clinging behavior and fears of separation, beginning by early adulthood and present in a variety of contexts, as indicated by five (or more) of the following:

(1) has difficulty making everyday decisions without an excessive amount of advice and reassurance from others.

(2) needs others to assume responsibility for most major areas of his or her life.

(3) has difficulty expressing disagreement with others because of fear of loss of support or approval. Note: Do not include realistic fears of retribution.

(4) has difficulty initiating projects or doing things on his or her own (because of a lack of self-confidence in judgment or abilities rather than a lack of motivation or energy).

(5) goes to excessive lengths to obtain nurturance and support from others, to the point of volunteering to do things that are unpleasant.

(6) feels uncomfortable or helpless when alone, because of exaggerated fears of being unable to care for himself or herself.

(7) urgently seeks another relationship as a source of care and support when a close relationship ends.

(8) is unrealistically preoccupied with fears of being left to take care of himself or herself.

Note. From *Diagnostic and Statistical Manual of Mental Disorders* (4th ed., pp. 668-669), by American Psychiatric Association, 1994, Washington, DC: Author.

A proposal considered for *DSM-IV* was to italicize the word "everyday" to emphasize this point (Hirschfeld et al., 1991).

The *DSM-III-R* version of this item was being "unable to make everyday decisions" (APA, 1987, p. 354). It was among the least frequently observed in dependent persons (i.e., low sensitivity) in the *DSM-IV* MacArthur studies (Hirschfeld et al., 1991). It has, at times, been among the most diagnostic (e.g., Pfohl & Blum, 1990). It may not be particularly common, but when it does occur, it is often diagnostic of the dependent PD (i.e., good positive predictive power; Widiger et al., 1984). It was retained at the top of the list in *DSM-IV* largely for the purpose of historical continuity. The results of the MacArthur studies may not have provided a clear ordering of the diagnostic value of each DEP PD criterion.

The revision may also improve its diagnostic value by lowering the threshold for its attribution. Few persons may be truly unable to make everyday decisions. Difficulty with such decisions provides a more realistic and accurate description of the difficulties of the dependent person, and lowering the threshold for its attribution may improve its sensitivity.

Rating:

0) Absent
1) Has difficulty making everyday decisions without an excessive amount of advice and reassurance from others
2) Is unable to make everyday decisions without an excessive amount of advice or reassurance from others

Questions:

a. Do you like to make your own decisions?

b. Do you like to get the advice and suggestions of others, even for everyday decisions?

c. Do you tend to feel nervous or insecure if you have to get by without some advice or reassurance?

Issues and Problems: A common difficulty in the assessment of this item is the meaning of "everyday." Some may interpret the item to mean that the dependent person asks for excessive advice and reassurance every day and throughout each day. This very stringent threshold is consistent with a literal interpretation of the *DSM-III-R* and *DSM-IV* wording. A person who truly has difficulty making everyday decisions without excessive advice and reassurance should be displaying this incapacity every day and throughout the day because each day will be filled with such decisions. This stringent interpretation may help to explain its low prevalence and low sensitivity in the *DSM-IV* MacArthur studies. We rarely find a dependent person who is that disabled. Our interpretation of this item is that the person frequently or often has difficulty making decisions that are of the nature of an everyday decision. These are people who will require excessive advice and reassurance for many "everyday decisions." In other words, everyday does not necessarily mean every day, but simply that the decisions for which they seek excessive advice and reassurance are largely trivial, inconsequential, or commonplace. These are decisions for which reassurance and advice should not be that necessary.

Examples provided in *DSM-IV* include decisions about what color shirt (or blouse) to wear to work and whether to take an umbrella (APA, 1994). These are, indeed, everyday decisions. However, it is perhaps common to ask in the morning for advice regarding what clothes to wear or whether one should bother with an umbrella. It is important to emphasize that the dependent request for advice and reassurance is excessive or beyond the range of what is normal or common. We would not score this item as present simply because the person usually or almost always asks for advice regarding what to wear that day. It is a reflection of dependency when the request conveys feelings of insecurity and inadequacy. Dependent people are not simply asking for one's advice or an opinion, they feel unable to make the everyday decision without this advice or reassurance.

An additional problem concerns the distinction from obsessive-compulsive PD doubts and ruminations. Indecisiveness is characteristic of both dependent and the obsessive-compulsive PDs (indecisiveness was a *DSM-III-R* criterion for the obsessive-compulsive PD; APA, 1987). Obsessive-compulsive indecisiveness, however, results from ongoing rumination and doubt rather than from a need to be taken care of by others. The obsessive-compulsive person will often gain little solace or reassurance from the advice of others because opinions of others are equally flawed, inadequate, and subject to critical review. The dependent person desires, seeks, and is often reassured by such advice.

In some cultures, wives are expected to seek the advice of their husbands regarding matters that might be considered trivial in our culture (Alarcon & Foulks, in press; Brown, 1986). This criterion should also be applied with great caution to women who are being physically or sexually abused or otherwise dominated by their partners (Walker, 1984). Abusive husbands frequently intrude on even trivial matters in their partners' lives. For example, an excessively domineering husband might carefully monitor a spouse's appearance, reacting angrily or even violently to styles which he views as seductive. The husband may likewise attach great importance to other details of household life, such as meals, cleaning, and spending, again reacting abusively or violently to violations of his strict standards. Thus, women in these circumstances may always be seeking the advice of their husbands simply for self-protection.

Criterion DEP-2

Needs others to assume responsibility for most major areas of his or her life.

Revisions and Rationale: *DSM-III-R* stated only that the person allows others to make most of the important decisions (APA, 1987). This was problematic because it could result simply from a friendly agreeableness rather than (as intended) a maladaptive submissiveness. The agreeableness could also reflect a social-cultural role, wherein one member of the family is given the authority to make most, if not all, of the important decisions. An initial draft of the *DSM-III-R* version was "prefers others to make most or all of his or her life decisions" (Work Group, 1985, p. 132). This draft version was, perhaps, preferable to the final version because it emphasized that the motivation is intrinsic to the person. The *DSM-III-R* Work Group, however, was concerned with the difficulty in assessing an inferred motivation, and, therefore, preferred the overt behavior of allowing others to make the decisions (Widiger et al., 1988). The ICD-10 uses the wording of "encouraging or allowing others to make most of one's important life decisions" (WHO, 1992, p. 206). The 1978 draft for *DSM-III* was similar to this ICD-10 version, as it used the wording, "gets" others to assume responsibility for major areas of one's life (Task Force, 1978, p. K:25).

The ICD-10 version was considered for *DSM-IV* (Task Force, 1991). Encouraging others to make one's decisions implies more than simply a passive or friendly acquiescence. The final decision for *DSM-IV* was to state that there is a need within the person to have others assume the responsibility for major areas of his or her life. The presence of an inferred need may be difficult to assess, but it does emphasize that there is a personal, internal motivation for the abdication of authority and responsibility.

Rating:

0) Absent
1) Needs others to assume responsibility for most major areas of his or her life
2) As a result of this need, most major life decisions are in fact made by someone else

Questions:

a. Have you ever let someone else make important decisions for you, such as where you'll live or what job you'll take?

b. Is there someone you rely on to make important decisions in your life?

c. Do you want this person to make these decisions?

d. Would you feel uncomfortable or unable to make these decisions yourself?

Issues and Problems: The *DSM-IV* text discussion indicates that this item is present if the person allows others to make most, if not all, major life decisions, such as where to live, whether to change jobs, whether to get married, or whether to have children (APA, 1994). However, a person who is simply agreeable, tolerant, or acquiescent may also allow others to make many important life decisions. A passive agreeableness is not sufficient for the item to be present. *DSM-III* addressed this problem by requiring that the acquiescence result from an inability to function independently (APA, 1980). This solution was problematic because an inability to function independently could result from mental retardation or any other severe disability or handicap. *DSM-IV* specifies that there be a need within the person but does not indicate how to assess for this need beyond simply observing that "the difficulty in taking responsibility must go beyond what would normally be associated with [a particular] condition or disability" (APA, 1994, p. 665). We ask if the person wants someone else to make respective decisions or would feel uncomfortable or unable to make the decisions alone when it is necessary (being sure to rule out any actual, realistic disability). The agreeable but potentially independent person would be willing and comfortable to make the decisions when others are not present. An additional approach would be to ask directly whether the person needs someone to make important decisions, but we have found that dependent persons are rarely that insightful or willing to acknowledge the need for someone to make their decisions.

It is also stated in the *DSM-IV* text discussion that "adolescents with this disorder may allow their parent(s) to decide what they should wear, with whom they should associate, how they should spend their free time, and what school or college they should attend" (APA, 1994, p. 665). However, passive deference to culturally sanctioned authorities is normative in some cultures. In fact, modern Western culture may be exceptional or excessive in its endorsement of assertive independence (Alarcon & Foulks, in press). In some cultures, one is encouraged (if not required) to seek and follow the advice of elders, clergy, or other community leaders for major life decisions. Likewise, in some cultures, young adults are expected to follow the dictates of parents or grandparents in such life decisions as whom to marry or what occupation to pursue. In addition, some young adults (in any culture) may remain financially dependent on their parents well into adulthood and after marriage. Some young adults in these circumstances feel compelled to defer to parents' wishes because of this financial dependence. For example, a male college student may feel obliged to select the major that his father prefers because the father is paying his tuition, or a young woman may defer to her parents' wishes that she not move, because she is financially dependent upon her parents for their continued support.

In addition, it is normative in some cultures for wives to defer to husbands in major life decisions (Alarcon & Foulks, in press; Brown, 1986). Some religious groups emphasize the submission of wives to husbands, giving the husband decision-making power in major life areas. Or, husbands have assumed or demanded this authority, and wives have not had adequate support, encouragement, or ability to object. Deference in major life areas might be expected in unusually hierarchical marriages.

In sum, all of these potential situations should be considered when assessing this item. One should not confuse one's own personal values, culture, or preferences for what is ideal, normative, or healthy independence with what is valued or preferred by the person being assessed. On the other hand, maladaptively dependent submissiveness can occur within the context of a culture or society that encourages this behavior (e.g., a person raised within a family that has exaggerated normative sex roles to such an excessive degree that the person is clearly impaired in his or her ability to function within a marital or occupational relationship).

Criterion DEP-3

Has difficulty expressing disagreement with others because of fear of loss of support or approval [*Note: Do not include realistic fears of retribution*].

Revisions and Rationale: *DSM-III-R* had specified that the agreeableness reflected a fear of being rejected (APA, 1987). In *DSM-IV*, the emphasis is placed on a fear of loss of care or support. "It is not the rejection per se that motivates the compliance, but rather the consequences of rejection, that is, the loss of care and support" (Hirschfeld et al., 1991, p. 145). Fear of rejection is seen in many personality disorders, including the histrionic, avoidant, narcissistic, and borderline. The dependent person is concerned not only with being rejected but also with losing the care and support that a relationship provides.

The initial draft of this item included a fear of anger along with a fear of losing support (Hirschfeld et al., 1991). However, this was revised to a fear of losing support or approval. Victims of actual or threatened abuse will have considerable difficulty expressing disagreement as a result of their realistic fear of anger (Walker, 1984, 1987, 1994). The final version of the item, in fact, emphasizes that realistic fears of retribution do not qualify in order to encourage clinicians to assess whether the submissiveness is due to threats of verbal or physical abuse.

Rating:

0) Absent
1) Difficulty expressing disagreement with others because of fear of loss of support or approval [*Note: Do not include realistic fears of retribution.*]
2) Fails to express disagreement with others because of fear of loss of support or approval

Questions:

a. Is it difficult for you to openly disagree with others? Do you tend to avoid an argument at all costs?

b. Do you tend to keep your opinions to yourself to avoid an argument?

c. Did you ever pretend to agree with your spouse [boyfriend/girlfriend] in order to get along? How often?

Issues and Problems: This item can be scored as present if the fear concerns a loss of support or approval. The dependent person need not fear loss of support. He or she need only fear a loss of approval, and a fear of loss of approval can result in a much lower threshold for attribution than a fear of loss of support. For example, a college student can have considerable difficulty expressing disagreement with a professor because of a fear of a loss of approval but may have no issues concerning dependency upon this professor (some may be expressing issues of narcissism rather than dependency). However, in such cases, it is useful to assess for cross-situational difficulties in expressing disagreement (e.g., difficulties with subordinates, friends, and lovers, as well as with persons in authority). We do not consider the item to be present if the fear only concerns a loss of approval from persons within positions of authority.

A more common example of this trait is the patient who is very reluctant to disagree with his or her therapist. Patients with issues of dependency upon their therapist will often be very agreeable, fearing that the expression of disagreement will result in a loss of the therapist's approval. However, these patients are not seeking simply a formal permission for or a confirmation of a belief or opinion (i.e., the more denotative meaning of the word approval). They are seeking an implied expression of continued concern and care. Disapproval by the therapist may suggest a discouragement, disappointment, or annoyance that could contribute to an eventual loss of interest by the therapist. The dependent patient wants approval as an affirmation of care, interest, and concern. In sum, we place more emphasis on a fear of loss of support than on a fear of loss of approval.

Again, it is important to examine this criterion in the context of explicit or implicit hierarchies of authority that may be inherent to the person's culture. For example, open disagreements with elders are discouraged, if not forbidden, in some cultures. Continued emotional support and approval may be contingent upon continued acquiescence and submission. Assertiveness in women may also be discouraged in some cultures.

This item also specifies that one should not consider realistic fears of retribution as constituting a difficulty in expressing disagreement. People who are being threatened with physical or sexual abuse, divorce or separation, or some other actual injury, danger, or loss of support, will be understandably reluctant to express disagreements. Their reluctance is realistic. Many victims of abuse and threat will appear dependent within the context of the abusive relationship (Koss, 1990; Walker, 1984, 1987). It is very important to assess the extent to which fears are, in fact, realistic.

However, the presence of an actual threat does not necessarily mean that a dependent personality disorder is not present. A person with a dependent PD can become involved with an abusive person and will be more easily exploited or abused than persons who lack a dependent personality disorder (Strube, 1988). It is particularly helpful in these cases to assess for difficulties in expressing disagreements across time (e.g., within prior relationships) and across situations (e.g., at work, with friends, or with subordinates). An additional caution is that people are often quite reluctant to reveal the presence or a history of abuse. One may not become aware of this abuse until well into a psychotherapeutic relationship. It is readily missed within a single clinical interview (Jacobson & Richardson, 1987).

Criterion DEP-4

Has difficulty initiating projects or doing things on his or her own (because of a lack of self-confidence in judgment or abilities rather than a lack of motivation or energy).

Revisions and Rationale: The revision to this item was the addition of the parenthetical clause. Its addition emphasizes that the difficulty reflects an impairment in self-confidence rather than any actual impairment in ability, motivation, or energy (e.g., secondary to low intelligence, physical impairment, or indifference). The dependent person would be fully capable of initiating or completing projects if not for the lack of self-confidence.

Rating:

0) Absent
1) Has difficulty initiating projects or doing things on his or her own due to lack of self-confidence in judgment or lack of self-confidence in abilities rather than a lack of motivation or energy
2) Fails to initiate or finish many tasks due to lack of self-confidence in own judgment

Questions:

a. Are you confident regarding your abilities?

b. Is it hard for you to get started on things and to do them well? (*If "yes":*) What do you suppose is the problem?

c. Do you often need advice or help?

Issues and Problems: The corresponding *DSM-III* criterion was low self-confidence (APA, 1980). This earlier version was, in one respect, preferable to *DSM-III-R* because it is the presence versus absence of self-confidence that is the key issue, and simply inquiring as to a difficulty initiating projects or doing things on one's own can often miss this issue entirely.

Patients and research subjects also vary widely in what they understand is meant by "projects" or "doing things." Do they have difficulty in completing college, finishing a term paper, washing the dishes, painting a house, getting off drugs, finding employment, or holding a job? One can't really specify the task because it will depend on the person's baseline level of ability and competence, that is, whether their impaired self-confidence inhibits, restrains, or prevents them from doing (whatever) things that are readily within their range of ability or expertise.

One qualification is that we would not include such difficulties as asking someone out, giving public speeches, or going to a party. These social behaviors can involve a difficulty in doing things on one's own, and dependent persons may lean heavily on others for help in social assertiveness and public performance. However, these social phobic behaviors are more indicative of the avoidant PD.

It is also noted in the *DSM-IV* text discussion of DEP that the low self-confidence may not impair performance if the person is given the assurance that someone is supervising or approving (APA, 1994). This point is important. Dependent persons may perform quite well with close support, encouragement, and/or reassurance. In fact, an expression or demonstration of ineptness, helplessness, or incompetence may be to elicit this expression of support and concern. As long as it is provided, the person may perform quite well.

Criterion DEP-5

Goes to excessive lengths to obtain nurturance and support from others, to the point of volunteering to do things that are unpleasant.

Revisions and Rationale: In *DSM-III-R*, it was stated that dependent persons volunteered to do unpleasant or demeaning things in order to get people to like them (APA, 1987). This was changed to obtaining nurturance and support because the issue is not simply wanting to be liked; the dependent person wants to be cared for, supported, and nurtured (Hirschfeld et al., 1991). Volunteering to do something unpleasant in order to be liked could be said to be present in most persons (e.g., attending an unpleasant dinner, function, or event as a favor to a friend).

The reference to demeaning activities was also deleted to minimize a potential overlap and confusion with the self-defeating personality disorder (that was in the appendix to *DSM-III-R* and deleted entirely from *DSM-IV*) and to discourage an overdiagnosis of dependency in victims of abuse. Persons with a dependent PD will often be victimized (in one way or another). The 1978 draft of this criterion for *DSM-III* had cited the tolerance of an abusive spouse as an example (Task Force, 1978), and it was noted in the *DSM-III* text that "a wife with this disorder may tolerate a physically abusive husband for fear that he will leave her" (APA, 1980, p. 325). A criterion proposed for *DSM-III-R* was "remains in relationships with people who mistreat him or her, because of fear of being alone" (Work Group, 1985, p. 132). However, there may also be a tendency to overdiagnose dependency in persons who remain within abusive relationships (Walker, 1987; Widiger & Frances, 1989a). Given the controversy and cost of blaming a victim for abuse, the Work Group recommended deleting the reference to doing something demeaning.

Rating:

0) Absent
1) Goes to excessive lengths to obtain nurturance and support from others, to the point of volunteering to do things that are unpleasant
2) Does or accepts things that are demeaning or abusive in order to gain nurturance and support

Questions:

a. Have you ever felt used by someone because you wanted them so badly or were afraid to lose them?

b. Have you ever been willing to do things for someone that you now regret, or that were in any way unpleasant, demeaning, or exploitive? (*If "yes":*) Has this happened often?

Issues and Problems: A difficulty in the assessment of this item is the apparent contradiction in going to excessive lengths to do simply unpleasant things. The item states that one goes to excessive lengths to do things to the point of volunteering to do things that are unpleasant. We have found that many patients and subjects will consider taking out the garbage, cleaning the bathroom, and changing the diapers to be unpleasant. If one takes this item literally, then anyone who volunteers to do these unpleasant things for his or her spouse has gone to excessive lengths.

The type of acts and behaviors that should actually qualify for this item are not simply unpleasant. Unpleasant is best understood as a euphemism for being exploited, used, abused, humiliated, degraded, or demeaned (e.g., sexual acts that are experienced as demeaning, prostitution for a lover, tolerance of physical abuse, or loss of substantial property or funds). It is, in fact, stated in the *DSM-IV* text discussion of this item that dependent persons "may make extraordinary self-sacrifices or tolerate verbal, physical, or sexual abuse" (APA, 1994, p. 666). Our minimal threshold for this item is anything that the person experiences as (very) unpleasant in order to be consistent with the *DSM-IV* revision, but we also emphasize the extent to which the person is being exploited, abused, demeaned, or humiliated. One must be careful not to overdiagnose dependent PD in persons who are or have been victimized, but one should also not minimize the extent of being mistreated, used, exploited, or victimized by equating these experiences with things that are simply unpleasant.

The distinction with (the deleted) self-defeating PD is that dependent people do these things in order to obtain or to avoid losing a relationship (i.e., care, nurturance, and support), whereas self-defeating people would do these things because they feel they do not deserve any better or because they have accepted the role and life of a victim (Hirschfield et al., 1991; Widiger & Frances, 1989a). The motivations for these behaviors can be quite different. However, it is again important to emphasize that one must determine if the person is currently being victimized or abused. If so, then the person is quite possibly being compelled or forced rather than a "willing victim." This is a very sensitive and important distinction because one does not want to blame the victim for being victimized (Koss, 1990; Walker, 1987). One should determine whether the behavior is evident across time (e.g., with prior lovers) and across situations (e.g., with friends). And, again, be advised that people who are being humiliated, degraded, demeaned, or simply embarrassed will be understandably reluctant to talk about this openly (Jacobson & Richardson, 1987). Open discussion of the victimization can be quite humiliating and embarrassing (particularly with a member of the opposite sex or a person who fails to convey sufficient empathy).

In addition, some persons are compelled to remain within undesirable relationships because of financial need, and they may be compelled to perform humiliating or dangerous acts (e.g., transportation of drugs, prostitution) as a desperate effort to pay for debts (Belle, 1990). In such a case, the person is compelled to perform the humiliating or dangerous act by a financial rather than an emotional dependency.

Criterion DEP-6

Feels uncomfortable or helpless when alone because of exaggerated fears of being unable to care for oneself.

Revisions and Rationale: In order to try to help distinguish DEP PD from borderline PD, *DSM-IV* added the clause that the discomfort or helplessness is because of fears of being unable to care for oneself (Hirschfeld et al., 1991). Borderline persons may also feel uncomfortable or helpless when alone, but it has often been observed that borderlines do not seek others to take care of them; they seek others to overcome feelings of emptiness and to help them obtain a sense of identity. *DSM-III-R* had also included the option of going to great lengths to avoid being alone (APA, 1987). This behavior is characteristic of dependent persons who feel helpless when alone and are unable to care for themselves but, when the motivation for the behavior is not considered, it will also be characteristic of many borderline persons.

Rating:

0) Absent
1) Feels uncomfortable or helpless when alone because of exaggerated fears of being unable to care for himself or herself
2) Feels uncomfortable and helpless when alone because of exaggerated fears of being unable to care for himself or herself

Questions:

a. Do you like being alone, or do you hate being by yourself?

b. Do you like to go on trips by yourself or spend a lot of time by yourself?

c. Do you ever feel uncomfortable when you're alone? (*If "yes":*) What have you done to avoid this?

d. Have you ever felt really terrible or lonely when you were by yourself for a period of time?

Issues and Problems: A difficulty in the assessment of this item concerns what is meant by "alone." It is not difficult to characterize a fear of living by oneself for the rest of one's life. However, this fear is covered by item 8 (preoccupation with fear of being left to care for oneself). The current item involves more brief or limited periods of time, including (or especially) when the person is within a relationship. "Alone" in this context means being physically alone for any particular period of time. Dependent persons may go to great lengths to avoid taking a trip or spending even an evening by themselves. They may dread having their spouse leave them for even an evening. Dependent persons could very well enjoy some evenings alone and may have some peaceful, pleasurable activities that they often do by themselves (e.g., reading, gardening, or drugs), but, at other times, dependent persons may also dread these moments. The item would be considered to be present if there was a history of desperately trying to avoid inconsequential, everyday times by oneself (e.g., pleading, staying on the phone), other than times that would be of special significance to most persons, such as holidays or anniversaries.

The requirement in *DSM-IV* that the dread of being alone involve a fear of being unable to care for oneself will complicate this assessment if the person is currently involved with someone. The dread of being alone for any particular period of time rarely involves a fear of being unable to care for oneself during that limited period of time, or, at least, it is rarely articulated by the person in this manner. Persons may dread being alone and will go to great lengths to avoid these experiences, but they may have (an understandable) difficulty in describing it as a fear of being unable to care for themselves for one particular evening or during a business or social trip. Therefore, in persons who are currently involved (and living) with someone, we do not require an explicit description of the dread of being alone as a fear of being unable to care for oneself.

Persons who live within dangerous neighborhoods may have a realistic fear of being left alone. In addition, immigrants and other persons who have recently moved to a new, strange community or environment may be very reluctant, and even fearful, of being left alone. One should be cautious in attributing this trait to such persons.

Criterion DEP-7

Urgently seeks another relationship as a source of care and support when a close relationship ends.

Revisions and Rationale: This item replaces the *DSM-III-R* item of "feels devastated or helpless when close relationships end" (APA, 1987, p. 354). Dependent persons do feel devastated and helpless when a close relationship ends, but, then, so will many other people. To the extent that a relationship was significant and meaningful (with a realistic expectation of longevity), it may not be unusual to feel devastated and helpless when it ends. One should be cautious in inferring that a person has a disorder if he or she feels devastated or helpless about losing something that is of considerable importance and significance. What is more specific to, and pathologic of, dependent persons is that they will quickly and indiscriminately find someone else to fill the void.

In this respect, the *DSM-IV* revision is also helpful in distinguishing DEP PD from the avoidant PD. Avoidant persons will become dependent and clinging when they finally do get involved with someone, but they will revert to their isolation when it ends (Trull, Widiger, & Frances, 1987). Persons with dependent PD, on the other hand, will often waste little time in finding a new partner. Avoidant and dependent persons may act quite similarly when they have someone, but not when they are alone. In dependent persons, the history of negligent, abusive, unreliable, or exploitative partners is due, in large part, to their failure to be careful, selective, or discriminating.

An earlier version of this item was "indiscriminately seeks another relationship to provide nurturance and support" (Task Force, 1991, p. R:13). It was thought that this revision would be helpful in addressing concerns regarding potential sex bias (Kaplan, 1983; Widiger & Spitzer, 1991) because the "immediate seeking of another relationship may be a common expression of dependency in males" (Hirschfeld et al., 1991, p. 147). However, being indiscriminate can be as indicative of an indifference towards others as it is of a dependency upon others. Some persons may be quite indiscriminant in their selection, because the presence of the person actually means very little to them. The item was revised to "urgently seeks another relationship" (APA, 1994, p. 669) to emphasize the desperate need to find a replacement, not simply the indiscriminate nature of the selection.

Rating:

0) Absent
1) Urgently seeks new relationship as a source of care and support when a close relationship ends
2) History of obtaining negligent, unreliable, exploitative, or abusive partners due to urgent need to be involved with someone

Questions:

a. Do you tend to desperately look for a new relationship as soon as one ends?
b. Do you tend to fall in love quickly?
c. Have you often found that your feelings have led you astray?
d. How well have you known the people with whom you have become sexually or romantically involved?

Issues and Problems: A difficulty in assessing this item is the potential implication that there should be a particular period of time between the ending of one relationship and the beginning of another. It is not simply a matter of the amount of time, but the sense of urgency and need. If one relies solely on how quickly a new partner is found, then one may also confuse indifference with dependency. Persons who are entirely indifferent may quickly obtain a new relationship because they simply don't care one way or the other. They do not actively seek a new relationship; they simply accept whoever expresses an interest. What makes it an issue of dependency is the urgency or the intense need to become attached and cared for once again (APA, 1994). People with a dependent PD will quickly fall in love, and these feelings will often lead them astray.

This urgency is often suggested by the indiscriminate nature of the selection of a new partner. Dependent persons may be unaware of or deny serious flaws in their selection. They may know very little about the other person before they become emotionally attached. Even if they are aware of the other person's history, the anticipated consequences and problems may be dismissed initially as trivial and insignificant. It is only some time into the relationship that they begin to appreciate what a serious mistake they might have made. However, as noted above, a history of indiscriminate selections are not, by themselves, sufficient to consider the item to be present. One must also document that the indiscriminate selection reflected a sense of urgent, desperate need or a fear of being all alone and left to care for themselves.

Again, some persons may be compelled to move indiscriminately into relationships because of financial rather than emotional needs (Belle, 1990). They will urgently seek another relationship as a source of care and support because they will become financially impoverished and destitute without a partner to provide financial support. This will be particularly evident in persons who are unemployed or who have many dependent children.

We emphasize that the concern for care and support involve a concern for emotional care and support, not financial.

Criterion DEP-8

Is unrealistically preoccupied with fears of being left to take care of himself or herself.

Revisions and Rationale: The *DSM-III-R* wording of this item concerned a fear of being abandoned (APA, 1987). Some dependent persons who are currently involved with someone may, indeed, fear being abandoned, but it is not so much how the relationship might end (e.g., through an unforeseen and abrupt abandonment) as the fact that it might end at all. Receiving plenty of forewarning and more than adequate alimony will not ease the fear and sorrow for the dependent person. Concerns regarding abandonment may also be more specific to persons with a borderline PD (Hirschfeld et al., 1991).

Rating:

0) Absent
1) Is unrealistically preoccupied with fears of being left to care for self
2) Unrealistic preoccupation with fears of being alone even when the person is closely involved with someone

Questions:

a. Are you often afraid that you will be alone, without someone to love and care for you?
b. Do you worry about this a lot even when you are involved with someone?
c. Does it worry you that you would be left to care for yourself?

Issues and Problems: The emphasis throughout the *DSM-IV* criteria on the need to be taken care of can, at times, be problematic, and particularly for this item. Dependent persons with adequate-to-good employment may not describe themselves as being afraid of being left to care for themselves; and, on the other hand, nondependent persons with tremendous financial burdens can be quite afraid of the prospect of being left to care for themselves. One should not confuse financial dependency with emotional dependency. A woman with six children, no savings, no house or apartment, and few job skills, may be quite preoccupied with a fear of being left to care for herself (and her children) (Belle, 1990). As a result, she may even tolerate a neglectful, abusive, and selfish husband. It would not be appropriate to characterize her financial dependency as an emotional dependency. Therefore, we find it helpful to describe a fear of being emotionally alone, or without the love and care of another person, rather than simply a fear of being left to care for oneself.

It is also important to distinguish a realistic versus an unrealistic preoccupation. Dependent persons are preoccupied with a fear of being alone, even when they are involved with someone. Their constant demands for reassurance and their clinging needfulness may be a principal factor in driving a spouse away. However, some people will be preoccupied for a very good reason. If the spouse is, indeed, unavailable, ungiving, and self-centered, then it would be understandable for the person to feel needy and emotionally alone. If the spouse is unfaithful and threatens abandonment, it is quite understandable for the person to fear being left emotionally alone.

8

Histrionic Personality Disorder

Overview: Histrionic (HST) personality disorder is defined in *DSM-III-R* and *DSM-IV* as a pervasive pattern of excessive emotionality and attention-seeking (APA, 1987, 1994). A proposal considered for *DSM-IV* was to emphasize that the purpose of the attention-seeking behavior and exaggerated emotionality was to evoke and maintain the interest and appreciation of others (Pfohl, 1991). The inclusion of the apparent motivation was to distinguish HST PD from a mood disorder that is characterized by simply emotional dyscontrol.

Much of the focus in the revision of the *DSM-III* HST criteria concerned the extent to which the *DSM-III* criteria set was too heavily influenced by the relatively low-functioning hysteroid dysphoria diagnosis developed by Liebowitz and Klein (1981) rather than the more traditional concept of an hysterical character (Cooper, 1987; Gunderson, 1983; Kernberg, 1984a; Widiger et al., 1988). The emphasis in *DSM-III* on the diagnosis of hysteroid dysphoria may have also contributed to the substantial overlap with the borderline and dependent PDs. Therefore, deleted from the *DSM-III* criteria set were manipulative, suicidal behaviors and angry outbursts or tantrums (seen in borderline persons) and dependency or helplessness (seen in dependent persons); "inappropriately sexually seductive" (APA, 1987, p. 349) was added to provide a better representation of the more traditional formulation of HST PD (Widiger et al., 1988).

The issues that were emphasized for *DSM-IV* were again (a) the extent to which the criteria set adequately recognized the clinical concept of histrionic personality disorder (Pfohl, 1991) and (b) the differentiation of HST PD from the other personality disorders, particularly the borderline, dependent, and narcissistic PDs and, to some extent, the antisocial (Pfohl, 1991; Task Force, 1991). Also of substantial concern was the question of a potential sex bias (Blashfield, Sprock, & Fuller, 1990; Kaplan, 1983; Widiger & Spitzer, 1991).

The *DSM-III-R* criteria for HST PD consisted of eight items (four of which were necessary for the diagnosis). Three received significant revision for *DSM-IV*, one received only a minor revision, two were unchanged, two were deleted, and two were added. In addition, the threshold for the diagnosis was raised to 5 of 8 to make it more restrictive and distinct (Pfohl, 1991). One of the items deleted was "constantly seeks or demands reassurance, approval, or praise" (APA, 1987, p. 349). This item had the lowest specificity of the HST criteria (Pfohl, 1991). It was quite common in other PDs, particularly borderline and dependent. Histrionic persons will often seek reassurance, approval, or praise, but this is also characteristic of dependent persons (a criterion for dependent PD is the need for advice and reassurance) and narcissistic persons (a criterion for narcissistic PD is a need for admiration).

The other item that was deleted was "self-centered, actions being directed toward obtaining immediate satisfaction; has no tolerance for the frustration of delayed gratification" (APA, 1987, p. 349). This item also obtained among the lowest specificity values of the HST criteria (Pfohl, 1991). Self-centeredness is also characteristic of narcissistic persons and no tolerance for frustration is characteristic of antisocial persons. In addition, this *DSM-III-R* item actually involved two criteria (self-centeredness and low frustration tolerance) that could, at times, involve quite different behaviors. An initial proposal was to replace the item with being "intolerant of, or frustrated by, situations involving delayed gratification" (Pfohl, 1991, p. 162) but it was decided that it was unlikely that this revision would actually resolve (or even decrease) the problem of low specificity. The complete *DSM-IV* criteria set is presented in Table 8-1.

Table 8-1
DSM-IV Criteria for Histrionic Personality Disorder

A pervasive pattern of excessive emotionality and attention seeking, beginning by early adulthood and present in a variety of contexts, as indicated by five (or more) of the following:

(1) is uncomfortable in situations in which he or she is not the center of attention
(2) interaction with others is often characterized by inappropriate sexually seductive or provocative behavior
(3) displays rapidly shifting and shallow expression of emotions
(4) consistently uses physical appearance to draw attention to self
(5) has a style of speech that is excessively impressionistic and lacking in detail
(6) shows self-dramatization, theatricality, and exaggerated expression of emotion
(7) is suggestible, i.e., easily influenced by others or circumstances
(8) considers relationships to be more intimate than they actually are

Note. From *Diagnostic and Statistical Manual of Mental Disorders* (4th ed., pp. 657-658), by American Psychiatric Association, 1994, Washington, DC: Author. Copyright 1994 by American Psychiatric Association. Reprinted with permission.

Criterion HST-1

Is uncomfortable in situations in which he or she is not the center of attention.

Revisions and Rationale: This item was unchanged from *DSM-III-R*. It was moved to the top of the list in *DSM-IV* because the *DSM-IV* MacArthur studies had indicated that it was the most diagnostic symptom of HST PD (i.e., relatively more sensitive and specific to this disorder than the other items; Pfohl, 1991). Attention-seeking (along with excessive emotionality) is one of the defining features of HST PD. Histrionic persons need to be the center of attention and may become quite uncomfortable, distressed, or despondent when they are not adequately noticed. This need can be a source of substantial strain and annoyance to their friends and colleagues (APA, 1994).

Rating:

0) Absent
1) Uncomfortable in situations in which he or she is not the center of attention
2) Humiliated or dismayed when not noticed by others

Questions:

a. Do people tend to notice you a lot; do you easily catch people's attention?

b. Do you like being the wallflower, outside of attention, or does it bother you when nobody notices you?

c. Have you ever done anything to be noticed, to set yourself apart from the crowd?

d. Have you ever felt upstaged at a social gathering?

Issues and Problems: A difficulty in assessing this item is that it is usually denied by histrionic persons. Such an admission may occur during the course of treatment, but we have found that histrionic persons are often reluctant to acknowledge, and may not be particularly aware of, the extent of this need. Histrionic persons may acknowledge an intense desire to be noticed, flattered, or appreciated, and may feel terribly slighted, humiliated, or dismayed when they are not noticed, but they rarely go so far as to say that they need to be the center of attention. On the other hand, a need to be the center of attention is, at times, evident in their difficulty in "sharing the spotlight" with someone else or in feeling "upstaged" by someone else.

The histrionic person enjoys intensely being the "belle of the ball" or the "life of the party." Anything less might be experienced as being simply a humiliated "wallflower." Histrionic and narcissistic persons share the intense need or desire to stand out from the pack; they cannot accept being simply one of the crowd. Both may obtain attention and admiration through dramatic and flamboyant appearance or behavior. However, the histrionic person will, at times, seek attention through melodramatic helplessness and emotional outbursts that could be experienced as denigrating and humiliating to the narcissistic person. The narcissistic person ultimately desires admiration, whereas the histrionic person desires whatever attention, interest, or concern can be obtained. What would constitute a "belle of the ball" can vary substantially across different situations. The prototype, of course, involves ebullient, dramatic, and sexually provocative displays at a social gathering (that are excessive and extreme even within the person's particular cultural or ethnic group). However, equally successful for the histrionic person are dramatic stories of suffering and abuse during group therapy; tearful explosions or angry diatribes at family gatherings, patient meetings, or social functions; bizarre, dramatic or provocative symptomatology for the interest of a therapist; and bold criminal acts for the attention of a gang. Interviews with people who would have an opportunity to observe such behaviors can then be very informative and helpful.

An additional issue in the assessment of this item is its differentiation from other HST PD items. Histrionic persons will draw attention to themselves by being sexually provocative, emotional, or melodramatic, but these behaviors are also central to HST-2 (sexually seductive or provocative behavior), HST-3 (rapidly shifting and shallow emotions), HST-4 (use of physical appearance to draw attention), and HST-6 (self-dramatization, theatricality, and exaggerated expression of emotions). However, it is useful to emphasize that the current item involves not simply the drawing of attention to oneself but being uncomfortable when this attention is not provided. This discomfort may, at times, have to be inferred on the basis of blatant and repeated attention-seeking behavior, but the criterion is the presence of this discomfort and not just the attention-seeking behavior.

The reader may notice the use of a female metaphor to illustrate this criterion (i.e., belle of the ball). This is not to imply that the histrionic person is necessarily female. A variety of studies have indicated that clinicians often overdiagnose HST PD in females (e.g., Ford & Widiger, 1989; Hamilton, Rothbart, & Dawes, 1986). A common error is to diagnose an antisocial female with histrionic PD. Nevertheless, the prototypic histrionic patient is female, as the prototypic antisocial patient is male. A comparable male variant of the belle of the ball metaphor would be "cock of the walk," which suggests narcissistic traits (needs for admiration) that tend to occur more often in males than in females (APA, 1987, 1994).

Criterion HST-2

Interaction with others is often characterized by inappropriate sexually seductive or provocative behavior.

Revisions and Rationale: The *DSM-III-R* version of this item was inappropriately sexually seductive in appearance or behavior (APA, 1987). This item was revised in *DSM-IV* to minimize the occurrence of a potential sex bias. HST appears to occur more often in females than in males, but it is important for the diagnostic criteria not to require or impel this to occur by including items that are confined to one sex or gender, particularly items that are readily confused with normal functioning (Widiger & Spitzer, 1991). The concern in this case involved the assessment of inappropriate sexually seductive appearance. Normal sexual attractiveness can be readily confused with sexual seductiveness. Males will be as sexually seductive in behavior as females, but females may be perceived as more sexually seductive in appearance, given the social pressure for physical attractiveness. For example, social stereotyping can contribute to the perception that beautiful women who dress attractively are being sexually seductive but handsome men who dress attractively are not. The item was, therefore, revised to place emphasis on sexually seductive or provocative behavior, rather than simply on appearance.

Rating:

0) Absent
1) Interaction with others is often characterized by inappropriate sexually seductive or provocative behavior
2) Interaction with others is usually characterized by inappropriate sexually seductive <u>and</u> provocative behavior

Questions:

a. Do people find you sexually attractive?
b. Would you say that you are somewhat flirtatious?
c. Has anyone ever said that you were "a flirt"?
d. Have you ever flirted with someone at a company, church, or family gathering?
e. Have you ever flirted with a therapist or with clinical staff?

Issues and Problems: An issue in the assessment of this item is the appropriate meaning of being "sexually provocative." Sexual harassment is inappropriate sexually provocative behavior. However, we would not typically include sexual harassment here because such behavior will usually reflect sadistic, antisocial, or narcissistic traits (i.e., interpersonal exploitation, dominance, or humiliation) rather than histrionic traits. The distinction can, at times, be subtle. Sexually lewd remarks (at conferences, restaurants, or any other public gathering) can have the purpose of trying to draw attention to oneself. However, to the extent that they are antagonistic, they would be more appropriately considered to be indicative of sadistic, antisocial, or psychopathic traits (Widiger, Trull, et al., 1994). This form of sexually provocative behavior often reflects a lack of empathy (i.e., no consideration or respect for those who might be offended by the behavior) and antagonism (i.e., an implicit, if not explicit, intention to offend) rather than an intention to attract interest or involvement with oneself. In other words, we would emphasize the seductive, rather than the provocative, nature of the behavior.

This item concerns the general tendency of histrionic persons to use their sexuality to draw attention to themselves and to infuse most situations with sexuality even when inappropriate. However, it can be difficult to determine when such behavior is inappropriate and even whether sexuality is, in fact, present. Sexuality is often more implicit than explicit. The most obvious examples are overt sexual flirtations with a variety of persons that are not appropriate to the situation (e.g., allusions to a sexual liaison or provocative caresses during a church function, treatment setting, or professional meeting). However, we have, at times, found considerable disagreement among raters regarding whether a person was, in fact, being flirtatious or seductive. Judgments during clinical interviews will, at times, depend upon the sex of the interviewer and/or interviewee (e.g., heterosexual male interviewers may not perceive male interviewees as sexually seductive), the cultural and ethnic background of the interviewer and interviewee (e.g., normative physical contact or display within one culture may be perceived as inappropriate within another), and the perception of the physical attractiveness of the interviewer and/or interviewee. The optimal assessment would be to view the person interacting with others, preferably across a series of social functions. Interviews with close friends or colleagues can be informative in this respect. However, it is important to note that the perceptions of close friends and colleagues can also be clouded by whatever issues or biases they may have with respect to sexuality (e.g., they may have an excessively high or low threshold for a judgment regarding what is inappropriate sexuality) or with respect to the person in question (e.g., anger, bitterness, or jealousy toward the person).

Criterion HST-3

Displays rapidly shifting and shallow expression of emotions.

Revisions and Rationale: This item was unchanged from *DSM-III-R*. Histrionic persons display rapidly shifting and apparently shallow emotions. Their moods may change throughout a single day, contributing to intense dysphoria; confusion regarding what one really feels; readily changing opinions, plans, and goals; and interpersonal conflicts. The *DSM-III-R* version was derived from the *DSM-III* criterion of being perceived by others as shallow and lacking genuineness (APA, 1980). As noted in the *DSM-IV* text, the emotions of the histrionic person seem to come and go too quickly to be deeply felt, at times leading others to accuse the person of being phony or superficial (APA, 1994). *DSM-III-R* and

DSM-IV, however, emphasize not how others might think or feel toward the person (which is filtered through the other person's own issues, biases, and conflicts) but how the person actually behaves.

Rating:

0) Absent
1) Displays rapid shifting and shallow expression of emotions
2) Episodes of intense rage, tears, fright, and/or elation have had substantial effects on his or her relationships

Questions:

a. Does your mood tend to have a life of its own, shifting from one time to another?

b. Do you tend to get upset easily, and then later feel quite differently about it?

c. Have shifts in your mood caused you any troubles with others, or resulted in impulsive decisions?

Issues and Problems: This item is more straightforward to assess than many of the other HST items because histrionic persons are usually quite aware of the rapid shifts in their feelings, and they will have little difficulty in acknowledging them. The rapid shifting of mood may, in fact, be a major factor in the seeking of treatment.

However, it can be difficult to distinguish histrionic shifts in mood from a mood disorder. One should always assess whether these mood shifts are of a recent origin or have been present since childhood. Chronicity, however, may not rule out some mood disorders, such as cyclothymia. Persons with cyclothymia may also be characterized by rapidly shifting and shallow expressions of emotion since late childhood (cyclothymia was diagnosed as a personality disorder in *DSM-II*; APA, 1968). Prototypic cases of cyclothymia will involve shifts between clear and sustained episodes of hypomania and dysthymia but some cases will also be characterized by more rapid, transient, and complex shifts (Akiskal & Akiskal, 1992). An additional basis of distinction is that the rapidly shifting and shallow emotions of the histrionic person are often provocative or manipulative. The purpose of the emotionality of the histrionic person will often be to evoke or maintain the interest and involvement of others, whereas no such motivation drives cyclothymia.

The manipulative nature of histrionic emotions, however, can also be difficult to assess. A histrionic person may be quite aware of and willing to acknowledge the mood shifts, but quite unaware of or unwilling to acknowledge manipulative intentions or effects. A useful analogy here would be hysterical conversion reactions. Conversion symptoms are also typically reactive and may also be manipulative but they will lack conscious intent, willful control, and even subjective awareness. Histrionic persons are typically quite manipulative, but they may have little conscious awareness or control of this manipulativeness, particularly with respect to their rapid shifts in mood. They may use their emotionality and mood shifts to gain attention and involvement, but they will also bemoan the existence of this apparent emotional dyscontrol.

One final note with respect to this item is to be careful to avoid gender or cultural biases in its assessment. Some cultural and ethnic groups may be less inhibited and more expressive in their emotions than the interviewer, and females will tend to be more expressive and open with their feelings than males. What may appear to be excessive, rapidly shifting, or shallow to one person may not appear so to another. The subjective experience of the interviewee of feeling dyscontrolled or experiencing the feelings as excessive or problematic is important to consider in the assessment of this item.

Criterion HST-4

Consistently uses physical appearance to draw attention to self.

Revisions and Rationale: The *DSM-III* version of this item was vanity (APA, 1980), which *DSM-III-R* attempted to define more specifically as being "overly concerned with physical attractiveness" (APA, 1987, p. 349). However, the *DSM-III-R* revision was problematic because it was difficult to assess, may have contributed to sex biased assessments, and has contributed to an overlap with the narcissistic PD (i.e., narcissistic persons will also be characterized by vanity and an overconcern with appearance).

It is unclear, for example, what constitutes an overconcern. Histrionic persons rarely characterize the attention they give to their physical appearance as representing excessive overconcern. They might even suggest (appropriately perhaps) that the interviewer should be more concerned with his or her own physical appearance. Overconcern would occur when it was, in some respects, maladaptive, but it is difficult to specify when a concern with one's physical appearance becomes maladaptive (i.e., the social and/or, occupational impairments that result from this apparently excessive concern). Efforts to assess the *DSM-III-R* version readily degenerated into questions such as, "how much make-up should one wear," "how long should it take to get ready to go out on a date," "how often should one wear perfume or cologne," "how often should one check one's hair, tie, or makeup," and "should one obtain cosmetic surgery, wear a wig or toupee, or lose weight." Everyone probably has had the experience of noticing someone who appeared to be excessively or overly concerned with his or her physical appearance, but this is often a matter of taste, value, or personal preference, rather than a consideration of maladaptivity.

In the absence of a clear threshold for when concern becomes overconcern, and the presence of differential sex-role expectations and normative behavior with respect to concerns regarding one's physical attractiveness, the item has the potential to be applied in a sex-biased manner (Kaplan, 1983; Widiger & Spitzer, 1991). To the extent that a woman extends more effort and attention to her physical appearance, there is the potential for considering what is normal for a woman as representing an overconcern.

The item was, therefore, revised in *DSM-IV* to emphasize that the concern with physical appearance is to draw attention to oneself. The item no longer requires an assessment of when a concern becomes excessive. The issue is now tied directly to the excessive seeking of attention, a trait that is central to histrionic PD. The use of physical attractiveness to obtain and hold attention is comparable to the use of emotionality, sexual seduction, self-destructive behavior, and dramatic theatricality to draw and hold attention to oneself. The revision may also be helpful in distinguishing histrionic PD from narcissistic PD by placing less emphasis on vanity and more on attention-seeking.

Rating:

0) Absent
1) Consistently uses physical appearance to draw attention to oneself
2) Dress and/or appearance is usually inappropriately sexually provocative

Questions:

a. Do people ever notice you because of the way you appear or dress?

b. Do you enjoy dressing in a sexually attractive, perhaps even provocative manner?

c. Do you tend to emphasize your sexuality in the way you dress or appear?

d. Has anyone ever told you to tone down how you dress or appear?

Issues and Problems: A difficulty with this item is that, taken literally, it does not necessarily suggest a maladaptive behavior pattern. Wearing makeup every day might constitute a consistent use of physical appearance to draw attention to oneself. The term "consistent" does not convey sufficient implication of dysfunction. Our approach to this item is to interpret consistent to mean an inappropriate or excessive use of physical appearance to draw attention to oneself.

A prototypic example would be a sexually provocative appearance in inappropriate situations. Histrionic persons are not sufficiently responsive to cues that indicate when sexuality is inappropriate to the situation. They may wear sexually revealing clothing at professional meetings, church functions, family reunions, or within clinic or hospital settings. Both male and female variants are readily evident (e.g., low-cut dress in a woman and open shirt in a man).

This item now captures the inappropriate sexually seductive appearance that was deleted from HST-2 (discussed above). Sexually provocative behavior is considered for HST-2; sexually provocative appearance is covered by the current item. However, it is important to note that this item does not require that the appearance involve sexuality. Any flamboyant use of physical appearance could be considered, included tattoos, hair coloring, or excessive muscle development. Extending the item into these domains, however, brings additional problems. Members of a counter-culture group may consistently dress and appear in a provocative manner, perhaps even to draw attention to themselves. However, very few (if any) will have a histrionic personality disorder. We would recommend considering whether the dress or appearance is excessive even within (or relative to) the particular cultural group to which the person belongs, including accepted as well as counter-culture groups. Styles of dress and hairstyles are obviously strongly culturally determined. What appears to be provocative or inappropriate to the interviewer may be entirely acceptable and common within the interviewee's cultural group. It would also be helpful to consider the motivation for drawing attention to oneself. For example, a histrionic person's motivation for attention may reflect an insecurity with respect to other domains of relating to others (e.g., avoiding a more meaningful or personal relatedness by sexualizing the relationship), rather than the rebellious (and perhaps angry) provocation of a member of a counter-culture group.

Criterion HST-5

Has a style of speech that is excessively impressionistic and lacking in detail.

Revisions and Rationale: This item was new to *DSM-III-R* (APA, 1987), and it received only a minor revision for *DSM-IV* (APA, 1994). The revision involved moving the specific example of describing one's mother in no more detail than "she was a beautiful person" out of the criteria set and into the text discussion (consistent with the general policy discussed in chapter 3). The purpose of this item is to consider the style of speech along with behavioral and interpersonal indicators of HST PD. It has traditionally been suggested that the thinking and speech of the histrionic person is impressionistic, complementary to the overly precise and intellectualized speech of the person with obsessive-compulsive PD (Shapiro, 1965).

Rating:

0) Absent
1) Style of speech that is excessively impressionistic and lacking in detail
2) History of dramatic, Pollyanna-like, or extreme impressions that are unsupported by facts or details and contribute to poor (maladaptive) decisions

Questions:

a. Do you tend to form a quick impression of people? (*If "yes:*) Has this impression ever proved to be horribly wrong, such that you have been very disappointed?
b. Why do you say that [*insert person*] is [*insert extreme, dramatic, or pollyanna-like impression of someone or something expressed during interview*]?

Issues and Problems: Assessment of this item may be based entirely on statements made during the interview, with no need for specific questions. However, this item obtained among the worst sensitivity rates in the *DSM-IV* MacArthur studies (Pfohl, 1991). Many researchers either do not observe this style of speech in persons with HST PD, or they are reluctant to assess it as present. However, some do find that it is highly diagnostic of HST PD when it is clearly present (Pfohl, 1991). We find it to be the most difficult HST item to assess. One difficulty is that many people will provide quite vague, brief, general, and/or perfunctory responses that lack detail because they are depressed, mildly retarded, guarded, medicated, tired, disinterested, annoyed, inexperienced with the language of the interviewer, or lack verbal skills. In addition, we have found many histrionic persons to have no difficulty in providing sufficiently detailed examples for why they consider their mother to be "wonderful," "beautiful," or "horrible."

We do find it useful to ask persons to explain why they have a particular belief, preferably one that is held strongly or appears to be impressionistic (e.g., a strong impression of a person that was expressed during the interview). Histrionic persons will come to quick judgments without much reasoning or rationale. It may also be helpful to indicate contradictions or inconsistencies to assess whether these lapses in reasoning are thoughtfully addressed or simply dismissed with another "gut-reaction." Clear examples of this item include "Pollyanna-like" or naive impressions of others that are quite likely to lead to an eventual disappointment. Pollyanna-like optimism is particularly useful because it also documents the maladaptive nature of the cognitive style.

Criterion HST-6

Shows self-dramatization, theatricality, and exaggerated expression of emotion.

Revisions and Rationale: The *DSM-III-R* version of this item was "expresses emotion with inappropriate exaggeration" (APA, 1987, p. 349). The primary reason for the revision was to obtain compatibility with the respective item from the ICD-10 criteria set, which is "self-dramatization, theatricality, exaggerated expression of emotions" (WHO, 1992, p. 205). This conversion to the ICD-10 for international congruency is somewhat ironic, as the ICD-10 version was probably based, in large part, on the *DSM-III* version, which was "self-dramatization, e.g., exaggerated expression of emotions" (APA, 1980, p. 315). *DSM-IV* has, thus, returned to *DSM-III* to be congruent with the international community. However, there is also a conceptual rationale for this revision to emphasize the histrionic (attention-seeking) nature of the emotional exaggeration. Emotional exaggeration by the histrionic person has a melodramatic or theatrical flair, as its purpose is, in part, to obtain or maintain the attention, interest, or concern of others. The histrionic person experiences life as a series of major crises that require all of the resources, time, and help that others could possibly provide (or, more accurately perhaps, that are beyond the time, energy, or capacity of others to provide).

Rating:

0) Absent
1) Shows self-dramatization, theatricality, and exaggerated expression of emotion
2) Describes history of many melodramatic crises, largely of his or her own making

Questions:

a. Tell me about some of the more dramatic crises you have experienced.
b. How do you handle it when you get really upset? Do things ever really get out-of-control?

Issues and Problems: The examples given in *DSM-III-R* for this item included embracing casual acquaintances with excessive ardor, uncontrollable sobbing on minor sentimental occasions, and temper tantrums (APA, 1987). *DSM-III* also noted an overreaction to minor events (APA, 1980). The more typical clinical example, however, would be a melodramatic, tearful pleading for help. Threats of suicide, of being unable to continue, and resignation to complete helplessness are common.

A difficulty in the assessment of this item is that persons who are in the midst of a severe depression or panic attack will also experience and describe themselves as being within a major crisis. They may also describe their life in a grossly exaggerated fashion as a direct result of their mood or anxiety disorder (e.g., seeing no alternative other than death). It is always important to verify that the dramatic nature of their experiences has been characteristic throughout their adult life. Interviews with close friends, colleagues, or relatives may be particularly useful for this item.

This item can also be difficult to assess because the threshold for what is exaggerated or excessive is unclear. The example of uncontrollable sobbing is helpful because it conveys the sense of maladaptivity (i.e., uncontrollable). However, it is also important to recognize that the perception of another person's excessive emotionality may reflect one's own emotional inhibition or constriction. The more extreme examples of histrionic emotionality are unlikely to contribute to culture- or gender-biased assessments (e.g., threats of suicide or resignation to complete helplessness), but less extreme variants (e.g., embracing casual acquaintances with excessive ardor) are prone to culture, ethnic, or gender bias. As we noted in our discussion of HST-3 (shifting and shallow expressions of emotions), the common or accepted emotionality of one culture or gender may appear to be excessive and inappropriate to another. The emotionality should be excessive and inappropriate within the person's own cultural group. We also emphasize the melodramatic and theatrical nature of the emotional display (e.g., self-control becomes more evident when other persons are not present, or there is a distortion of events for the purpose of increasing the sense of tragedy).

Criterion HST-7

Is suggestible (i.e., easily influenced by others or circumstances).

Revisions and Rationale: This item was a new addition to the HST PD criteria set. It was not among the original proposals for *DSM-IV* (Pfohl, 1991; Task Force, 1991). It was included to contribute to the congruence between *DSM-IV* and ICD-10 (Frances et al., 1991), as the research criteria for ICD-10 HST PD contain the criterion "suggestibility, easily influenced by others or by circumstances" (WHO, 1992, p. 205). Suggestibility, however, was also included within the earlier Lazare, Klerman, & Armor (1966) description of the hysterical personality. A prototypic, yet extreme, example of this suggestibility would be the development of memories, symptoms, or disorders suggested by a clinician (or some other source). Histrionic patients might develop memories of childhood abuse, alternate personalities, and other symptoms that would generate substantial attention, interest, and involvement on the part of their clinicians. They are prone to becoming converts to faddish therapeutic movements, adopting whatever rationale or theory is offered by a charismatic therapist to explain their distress and dysphoria.

Rating:

0) Absent
1) Is suggestible (i.e., easily influenced by others or circumstances)
2) Suggestibility has resulted in the development of significant beliefs, memories, or symptoms that are later abandoned

Questions:

a. Do you think that you are easily influenced by others or by the circumstances you are in?

b. What have been some of the more unusual treatment programs you have tried?

c. Did you ever believe in something with all your heart that you now realize wasn't true?

Issues and Problems: A potential difficulty in assessing this item is determining the credibility of a belief. This assessment may not be problematic if there is a history of abandoning or rejecting beliefs that were once held with substantial commitment (e.g., the person now acknowledges the absence of a childhood history of abuse, or now acknowledges the misrepresentation of multiple personalities, or has repeatedly joined and left various groups). However, a histrionic person may currently be devoted to a particular group or treatment program that a clinician considers to be faddish or "cultish," or the interviewer may be skeptical regarding a current belief in having been sexually abused or having multiple personalities. The assessment of the credibility of such beliefs is, indeed, very difficult and controversial (Briere & Conte, 1993; Fahy, 1988; Frankel, 1990; Loftus, 1993, 1994; Singer, 1991) (see also the letters in response to Loftus, 1993, that are published along with Loftus, 1994). It is important to emphasize that there has not yet been any systematic research to document that persons with a histrionic PD are prone to false or induced memories or alternate personalities. One must be careful not to let one's own biases and presumptions against a particular treatment program, group, retrospective memory, or diagnostic construct interfere with or impair one's ability to provide an objective, valid assessment. However, it is no accident that histrionic persons will be involved in areas that are controversial, as such controversy provides the drama and theatrics they are seeking. For example, some persons diagnosed with borderline PD may, in fact, be histrionic persons who desire the borderline diagnosis because of its melodramatic reputation. The differentiation of an actual borderline personality disorder from a histrionic borderline personality disorder would, indeed, be quite difficult (and perhaps illusory).

An additional difficulty in assessing this item involves differentiating histrionic suggestibility from dependent agreeableness. Dependent persons will also be easily influenced by others to the point of accepting beliefs they know to be wrong or doing things that they find demeaning or humiliating (APA, 1987, 1994). However, one distinction is that the dependent person would be more aware that the belief is, in fact, untrue. Dependent persons express beliefs they know to be wrong in order to maintain a relationship, whereas histrionic persons readily adopt new beliefs as their own. In addition, the motivation for the dependent person is a fear of losing a relationship, whereas for the histrionic person, it is to obtain attention. We would emphasize the melodramatic, theatrical nature of the histrionic person's suggestibility (i.e., beliefs that will bring notoriety or attention) as opposed to the submissiveness of the dependent person's agreeableness (i.e., beliefs that will sustain a particular relationship).

Criterion HST-8

Considers relationships to be more intimate than they actually are.

Revisions and Rationale: This item is a new addition to the *DSM-IV*. It was developed as a result of a survey of eight experts on the histrionic PD diagnosis (Pfohl, 1991). Four experts rated this item as having a high likelihood of usefully discriminating patients with HST PD, and four rated it as having a medium likelihood of discriminative value (Pfohl, 1991). These results were as good as those obtained for many of the existing HST items and were better than any of the other new items that were considered. The examples provided in *DSM-IV* for this item include romantic fantasies regarding persons one has met, describing almost every acquaintance as "my dear friend," or referring to physicians met only once or twice under professional circumstances by their first name (APA, 1994). It is also of interest to note that a 1978 draft criterion for the *DSM-III* HST PD included "indulgence in frequent flights of romantic fantasy" (Task Force, 1978, p. K:13) as one of the four features of the poor sexual adjustment of persons with HST PD.

Rating:

0) Absent
1) Considers relationships to be more intimate than they actually are
2) History of romantic fantasies regarding various persons

Questions:

a. Do you tend to become friends with people you have worked with?
b. Have you ever fallen in love with any of these people?
c. Have you ever become personally involved with clinical staff? [*Also consider other professional relationships.*] (*If "yes":*) Does this tend to happen often?

Issues and Problems: The example provided in *DSM-IV* of referring to physicians by their first names helps illustrate difficulties in the assessment of this item. Narcissistic persons will also presume a "first-name basis" with persons of authority, power, or status. However, this will reflect a need to place themselves on equal footing with these persons (i.e., to elevate their own status) or to avoid acknowledging any status, authority, or superiority in the other person (i.e., to deflate the status of the other person). They may also refer to casual acquaintances as "dear friends," but, again, this may reflect the desire to obtain a vicarious status (consistent with name-dropping during a conversation to display one's importance to an audience, indicating that one personally knows or is a personal friend of someone who is very important). The motivation for the histrionic person, on the other hand, is not to deflate or inflate status; instead, it may reflect a desire for the relationship to be more personally significant to the other individual than is actually the case. Histrionic persons will quickly develop romantic involvements that do not last. This is similar to the quick and unreflective attachments developed by persons with a dependent personality disorder; however, dependent persons tend to remain attached, whereas histrionic persons may just as quickly lose interest and fall out of love.

An additional difficulty in the assessment of this item is a presumption that certain relationships should not be intimate or personal. Friendly, informal, or casual persons may also refer to physicians (clinicians, lawyers, professors, or other persons who have a professional relationship to the subject) by their first names without implications of narcissistic or histrionic issues. Cultural groups can also vary substantially in the extent to which they accept and encourage informality. In addition, persons in positions of authority may also expect or impose a degree of deference that is unrealistic or excessive. The issue is not so much that histrionic persons use first names without adequate permission, or even that they desire a degree of informality or involvement that is not desired by a clinician, but that they act as if they have a personal relationship that does not actually exist. One indication of this presumed intimacy is using the clinician's first name. Other indications include phone calls at home, inquiries about the clinician's personal life, and giving presents to the clinician. None of these behaviors, alone, is necessarily inappropriate, but taken together and in the context of no encouragement on the part of the clinician, they do suggest a presumption or experience of an intimate, personal relationship that does not actually exist.

9

Narcissistic Personality Disorder

Overview: The narcissistic (NAR) personality disorder was a new addition to the *DSM-III* (Frances, 1980; Spitzer et al., 1980). It was not recognized within the ICD-9, but it is noted among the residual set of other personality disorders in ICD-10 (along with the eccentric, haltlose type, immature, passive-aggressive, and psychoneurotic PDs; WHO, 1992). It is described in *DSM-IV* as a pervasive pattern of grandiosity, need for admiration, and lack of empathy (APA, 1994). This description represents only a minor change from *DSM-III-R*, wherein NAR PD was described as involving a hypersensitivity to the evaluation of others (APA, 1987). Hypersensitivity to the evaluation of others is not actually specific to NAR PD, as it is also quite evident in paranoid, avoidant, and dependent PDs. The hypersensitivity of the narcissistic person involves the need for admiration (i.e., fragile self-esteem). Narcissistic persons may, at times, convey substantial disinterest in the opinions of others (i.e., as if they were not at all sensitive), but this apparent indifference is a bravado display of denial rather than a true security in their sense of self-worth.

The *DSM-III-R* criteria for NAR PD included nine items (any five of which were necessary for the diagnosis). Two received only minor revision for *DSM-IV*, five received significant revision, and one was replaced. Only one item was left unchanged. The revisions focused, in particular, on the differentiation of narcissistic PDs from antisocial and histrionic PDs (Task Force, 1991). The item concerned with a hypersensitivity to criticism was deleted because of its lack of specificity and difficulties with its assessment (Gunderson, Ronningstam, & Smith, 1991). The *DSM-III* version of this item was quite broad and nonspecific: "cool indifference or marked feelings of rage, inferiority, shame, humiliation, or emptiness in response to criticism, indifference of others, or defeat" (APA, 1980, p. 317). This version covered the full array of possible reactions to criticism, rebuke, or defeat. *DSM-III-R* attempted to clarify the item by specifying a reaction "feelings of rage, shame, or humiliation (even if not expressed)" (APA, 1987, p. 351). However, this version might have been even more problematic because it encouraged an interviewer to attribute the presence of hypersensitivity when there were no overt signs whatsoever (at least *DSM-III* had required a "cool" indifference). The complete *DSM-IV* criteria set is presented in Table 9-1.

Criterion NAR-1

Has a grandiose sense of self-importance (e.g., exaggerates achievements and talents, expects to be recognized as superior without commensurate achievements).

Revisions and Rationale: The revision to this item consisted of changing the parenthetical example from expecting to be noticed as special to expecting to be recognized as

Table 9-1
DSM-IV Criteria for Narcissistic Personality Disorder

A pervasive pattern of grandiosity (in fantasy or behavior), need for admiration, and lack of empathy, beginning by early adulthood and present in a variety of contexts, as indicated by five (or more) of the following:

(1) has a grandiose sense of self-importance (e.g., exaggerates achievements and talents, expects to be recognized as superior without commensurate achievements)

(2) is preoccupied with fantasies of unlimited success, power, brilliance, beauty, or ideal love

(3) believes that he or she is "special" and unique and can only be understood by, or should associate with, other special or high-status people (or institutions)

(4) requires excessive admiration

(5) has a sense of entitlement, i.e., unreasonable expectations of especially favorable treatment or automatic compliance with his or her expectations

(6) is interpersonally exploitative, i.e., takes advantage of others to achieve his or her own ends

(7) lacks empathy: is unwilling to recognize or identify with the feelings and needs of others

(8) is often envious of others or believes that others are envious of him or her

(9) shows arrogant, haughty behaviors or attitudes

Note. From *Diagnostic and Statistical Manual of Mental Disorders* (4th ed., p. 661), by American Psychiatric Association, 1994, Washington, DC: Author. Copyright 1994 by American Psychiatric Association. Reprinted with permission.

superior (APA, 1987, 1994). A grandiose sense of self-importance will, at times, be evidenced by an unrealistic or exaggerated expectation of being noticed or treated as special, but a sense of being superior is a more obvious example of grandiosity (Ronningstam & Gunderson, 1990). The *DSM-III-R* use of the term "special" was, to some extent, a concrete carry-over from the *DSM-III* version of this item, which indicated a focus on the special nature of one's problems (APA, 1980). The *DSM-III* version was useful in indicating a particular manifestation of narcissism within the treatment relationship. However, the belief that one's problems have a special or unique nature became a separate item in *DSM-III-R* (APA, 1987). The term "special" then remained in the grandiosity criterion, which was referring now to a more general expression of grandiosity.

One might consider this revision to represent only minor clarification, but, given that being superior represents a change in content from being special, we do consider this to represent a significant revision. Perhaps the most substantial revision, though, is its placement at the top of the list, indicating that grandiosity is considered to be the most diagnostic or central feature of narcissism (e.g., Ronningstam & Gunderson, 1991).

Rating:

0) Absent
1) Grandiose sense of self-importance (e.g., exaggerates achievements and talents, expects to be recognized as superior without commensurate achievements)
2) Loss of relationships or job have been direct result of grandiosity

Questions:

a. Do you have any special talents or abilities?

b. What are your future goals or ambitions?

c. How would you evaluate your achievements?

Issues and Problems: Most, if not all, of the NAR items are difficult to assess through direct questions. Some narcissistic persons will have so much "chutzpa" that they will have no qualms acknowledging that they are grandiose and conceited. Some may also be quite aware of their narcissistic conflicts and needs. However, to the extent that they believe that they are, indeed, superior, they may not characterize this belief as being grandiose or exaggerated. One approach to this problem is to provide a stimulus probe to solicit expressions of grandiosity (Widiger, 1993b). Therefore, we ask persons to describe any special talents, abilities, or achievements they might have, and we then assess whether the resulting description is exaggerated, pompous, pretentious, or grossly unrealistic. Reference to a likelihood that one will someday become a great writer, athlete, star, or tycoon are the most obvious examples, but narcissistic persons will often have enough reality-testing not to provide such extreme responses. This assessment will, of course, presume sufficient knowledge of the person's actual talents and abilities. However, it has been our experience that narcissistic persons will often need little encouragement to discuss their talents and abilities (e.g., brag, boast, posture, or display themselves in some manner).

This item, however, is, at times, scored on the basis of subsequent or prior comments. Narcissistic persons may avoid the bait of a direct inquiry but will eventually be unable to resist the need to describe their achievements, talents, or other special qualities. Narcissistic persons wear their achievements and talents "on their sleeves" so that they will be admired and praised by others. It is not unusual for the conversation to eventually divert to some special accomplishments, qualities, or talents they wish to be noticed. It is also difficult for narcissistic persons to remain quiet while others are talking about their accomplishments. Rather than offer any sincere praise or compliment to another person, they will remind the "audience" of their own accomplishments or talents. Such fishing for compliments will usually be considered to reflect NAR-4 (excessive need for admiration). However, even when discussing trivial or inconsequential matters, narcissistic persons will divert the conversation to their own lives, as if what is most interesting is how they have experienced any issue or event (such as injuries, bills, vacations, or even the weather).

Another approach to the problem that narcissistic persons may deny their grandiosity is to ask if they have ever been described as or accused of being somewhat conceited, pompous, or grandiose. This is an approach emphasized in other instruments (Widiger & Sanderson, in press-a). At times, it may be useful, particularly when the problem is simply a lack of awareness. Other people are often more aware of the narcissist's traits than the narcissist. However, we would not suggest relying upon this approach. It will not be useful when nobody has, in fact, provided this feedback (such a confrontation is often avoided), when the person fails to remember that such feedback has occurred, or when the person is unwilling to acknowledge its occurrence. This approach can be as transparent in its intention as a direct inquiry. To the extent that persons have difficulty acknowledging to themselves or to the interviewer that they are conceited, immodest, or grandiose, they will likely have difficulty acknowledging to the interviewer that other people have described them in this manner.

A related approach is to interview a close friend, colleague, or relative. Indeed, friends and colleagues may be much more aware of the grandiosity within the narcissistic person. To the extent that a significant other is more aware, it would be preferable to simply interview this other person directly. However, it is also important to note that significant others do not necessarily provide objective assessments. They can have their own "axe to grind" and may overestimate the subject's tendency to exaggerate his or her achievements.

Criterion NAR-2

Is preoccupied with fantasies of unlimited success, power, brilliance, beauty, or ideal love.

Revisions and Rationale: This item is unchanged from *DSM-III-R* and essentially unchanged from *DSM-III*. It concerns the tendency of narcissistic persons to be preoccupied with fantasies that would provide, nurture, support, or confirm their sense of being special, chosen, unique, or superior (APA, 1994).

Rating:

0) Absent
1) Preoccupation with fantasies of unlimited success, power, brilliance, beauty, or ideal love
2) Preoccupations have resulted in significant disappointments within career or relationships

Questions:

a. Do you know much about successful or famous people? Do you follow their lives?
b. What are your expectations regarding yourself? Do you think or dream a lot about what you might accomplish?
c. Have you ever been severely disappointed when your hopes or expectations weren't realized?

Issues and Problems: At times, this item is taken too literally, as if it refers to the tendency of a person to spend an inordinate amount of time daydreaming about being rich, famous, powerful, brilliant, or romantically involved. Some narcissistic persons will, indeed, spend a considerable amount of time in excessive daydreaming, but the preoccupation within a fantasy world can also be less transparent. We include within this item being absorbed, obsessed, or preoccupied with the world of fame, status, power, and brilliance. This might be evident in such behaviors as "always buying the best" (particularly when it is irrelevant or unnecessary), excessive displays of status symbols, or any other absorption in the lifestyles of the rich and famous. Our consideration of such behavior is analogous to the *DSM-III-R* item for sadistic PD of being fascinated by violence, weapons, martial arts, injury, or torture (APA, 1987). Just as the sadistic person was said to be absorbed in the artifacts, tools, and symbols of sadism, the narcissistic person is absorbed in the artifacts, tools, and symbols of status.

There are qualifications to this approach. Absorption in the fantasy world of ideal love (e.g., romance novels) tends to be more indicative of a dependent PD than a narcissistic PD. Likewise, a preoccupation with beauty may be more indicative of histrionic PD, and a preoccupation with becoming rich may be more indicative of antisocial PD. The confusion in these latter two cases reflects, in part, the inherent overlap of the narcissistic PD with the histrionic (Gunderson, Ronningstam, et al., 1991) and the antisocial (Hare et al., 1991; Perry & Cooper, 1989) PDs. We are more confident in our assessment of narcissism when the preoccupation concerns matters of success, brilliance, fame, power, or status, rather than beauty, love, or money. Note, as well, that the symbols of each will vary (i.e., the symbols of success and status in one profession will be different from those in another).

Another issue is the fact that what is excessive, showy, flamboyant, or pretentious to one person may not be so to another. Some people will always buy the best simply because they can readily afford the expense. There may also be cultural variation in the extent to which such behavior is considered to be acceptable, common, and perhaps even encouraged. On the other hand, some wealthy persons may be revealing their narcissism through an excessive display of their wealth. Being wealthy does not exclude the possibility of being narcissistic.

A useful analogy for the assessment is provided by the sexual, substance, gambling, and other disorders of dyscontrol (or behavioral dependence), wherein a person becomes obsessed or absorbed within an activity that eventually dominates his or her life (e.g., increasing amounts of time spent within the activity; sacrificing of other important social, occupational, or recreational activities; continuation despite significant opposition or criticism by others; and inability to avoid or resist the activity) (Goodman, 1990; Orford, 1985). In this case, one would assess whether the person's life appears to be dominated by or to revolve around symbols of status, fame, power, or brilliance, and whether the person appears to be driven to continually seek and obtain such symbols.

Criterion NAR-3

Believes that he or she is "special" and unique and can only be understood by, or should associate with, other special or high-status people (or institutions).

Revisions and Rationale: The *DSM-III-R* version of this item was confined largely to a manifestation within treatment: a belief that one's problems are unique and could be understood only by other special people (APA, 1987). The item was broadened considerably in *DSM-IV* because it is best not to require that the person be in treatment in order to assess the item. The *DSM-III-R* version of this item also presumed that the person had acknowledged the presence of problems, which may not be the case for many narcissistic persons. The belief that one's problems are unique or special would still apply to this item, but beliefs in a special uniqueness outside of therapy will now also apply.

Rating:

0) Absent
1) Believes that he or she is special, unique, and can only be understood by or should only associate with other persons of comparable status
2) Requires therapist of substantial status, or makes similar demands outside of treatment setting

Questions:

a. Do you know any important people?

b. Are you affiliated with any important institutions, organizations, or groups?

c. What do you think should be the qualifications of your therapist?

d. Have your prior therapists been able to understand your problems? Were they sufficiently qualified?

Issues and Problems: The belief that one's problems are unique or special, and can be understood only by the more brilliant, talented, or gifted therapist, remains one of the best examples of this item. However, this presumption might become evident only within the eventual course of treatment (Kohut, 1971, 1984). It can be suggested within an initial evaluation interview through inquiries by the subject regarding the experience, education, or success of the therapist. Such inquiries can, of course, be entirely appropriate. Narcissism might be revealed by asking the person to describe the special qualities and/or failings of the person's prior therapists (e.g., assessing for signs of devaluation or idealization of prior therapists). When narcissistic persons do not, in fact, get the very best therapist, they may elevate the therapist they got to the very best. Such idealization will also occur in persons with borderline PD, but narcissistic persons are less likely to eventually devalue these same persons (unless they feel rejected or snubbed by them).

The belief that one should be associated with or treated by only the very best may also result in an idealization of colleagues and associates, as well as therapists. Indications of narcissism outside of therapy include references to well-known institutions or persons with whom the person claims some form of special relationship or significance. An analytic term for this is "mirroring" (Cooper & Ronningstam, 1992; Kohut, 1971). A simple example would be name-dropping, as when the name of a prestigious university (with which the person is somehow affiliated) keeps being mentioned, perhaps with the implication that this affiliation provides the person with some sort of special authority or credibility. It is particularly revealing when no actual affiliation exists. It is, of course, true that a "Harvard physicist" will have more credibility than a "Muskogee physicist" (no offense, please, to those from Muskogee), but even in such instances where there is some reality to the implication, it will remain a reflection of narcissism to the extent that others are continually reminded of a title, affiliation, or status to buttress a fragile self-esteem. Institutions and organizations that can provide this credibility may, in fact, attract narcissistic persons who will sacrifice a great deal for the affiliation.

Criterion NAR-4

Requires excessive admiration.

Revisions and Rationale: The *DSM-III-R* version of this item included a need for both attention and admiration. It is confined to admiration in *DSM-IV* to help differentiate NAR PD from HST PD (Gunderson, Ronningstam, et al., 1991). This is somewhat ironic because the 1978 draft version of the respective histrionic criterion for *DSM-III* was "drawing attention to oneself to obtain admiration" (Task Force, 1978, p. K:13). Both histrionic and narcissistic persons will crave attention, obtained, in part, through flamboyant, provocative, dramatic, and/or seductive appearances and behaviors. Histrionic attention-seeking, however, will also include dramatic suicidal gestures, displays of helplessness, and emotional outbursts that are not characteristic of the narcissistic PD (APA, 1994). The attention sought by the narcissistic person is usually confined to admiration (rather than pity or concern).

An additional revision was to replace the adjective "constant" with "excessive." The adjective "constant" was used in *DSM-III-R* to ensure that the criterion would not contribute to false negative assessments (i.e., a diagnosis of a personality disorder in someone who was not, in fact, narcissistic). Most persons desire and value some degree of admiration from others; there may be nothing pathological in this desire. Requiring constant admiration is clearly pathological. However, this threshold for diagnosis was also unrealistic. Nobody requires constant admiration (i.e., every minute of every day). The threshold for clinical significance is when the need is excessive.

Rating:

0) Absent
1) Requires excessive admiration
2) Requires excessive admiration and becomes outraged if he or she experiences a rebuke, slight, or criticism

Questions:

a. Do people often come to you for advice?

b. Do you tend to get the admiration of others?

c. Do you feel that you haven't gotten the attention or admiration you deserve?

d. Have you ever felt slighted, insulted, or rebuked?

Issues and Problems: A difficulty in assessing this item is determining when a desire or need for admiration is excessive. Interviewers will often have different thresholds for this attribution. An example provided in *DSM-IV* is fishing for compliments (APA, 1994). As noted earlier (NAR-1), narcissistic persons wear their achievements on their sleeves, providing not so subtle cues for praise and admiration. Fishing for compliments, however, may not always be evident within a clinical interview. A narcissistic person may feel little need or value in being admired by the interviewer. The situation may lack enough meaning, importance, or personal significance to potentiate the need for admiration. A need for admiration, however, will certainly become evident at some point within a psychotherapeutic relationship (Kohut, 1971). The requirement for excessive admiration is also evident in social gatherings, where the narcissistic person will desire to be recognized. Narcissistic persons will remind other guests or participants of special status, talents, or abilities that raise them above the rest of the crowd.

We also include here expressions of outrage and anger in response to criticism or rebuke (e.g., "how dare he criticize me"). To the extent that one needs to be "constantly" admired, one will protest, deny, or dismiss suggestions of flaws and failings. Nobody is without flaws, but narcissistic persons have substantial difficulty in acknowledging their inadequacies, failings, and errors (e.g., it was not their mistake; it was the fault of somebody or something else). As noted in the above overview for NAR PD, expression of anger in response to criticism was included within the *DSM-III* and *DSM-III-R* criteria for NAR PD (APA, 1980, 1987). Anger in response to criticism is also evident within passive-aggressive persons. However, the rebuke of passive-aggressive persons will reflect their disdain and criticism of authority in general rather than a counterattack to a threat to their self-esteem.

Prior versions of this criterion have also included reactions of shame and humiliation (*DSM-III*). Narcissistic persons may react to criticism with shame, embarrassment, or humiliation. However, such reactions can also suggest a characteristically low self-esteem evident in persons with depressive, avoidant, or dependent PD. Reacting to criticism with humiliation could suggest an excessive need for admiration, but we recommend being quite cautious in making this inference. Inferring the presence of a need for excessive admiration from anger or rage in response to criticism may also represent an incautious leap, but some degree of inference is, at times, necessary as many narcissistic persons will not be aware of or will not acknowledge their need for excessive admiration.

Criterion NAR-5

Has a sense of entitlement (i.e., unreasonable expectations of especially favorable treatment or automatic compliance with his or her expectations).

Revisions and Rationale: A sense of entitlement was included in the *DSM-III* and *DSM-III-R* criteria for NAR PD (APA, 1980, 1987). The revisions have concerned how this criterion was defined. In *DSM-III*, it was defined as an expectation of special favors without assuming reciprocal responsibilities (APA, 1980); in *DSM-III-R*, it was defined as an unreasonable expectation of especially favorable treatment (APA, 1987); and in *DSM-IV*, it is defined as an unreasonable expectation of especially favorable treatment or automatic compliance with one's expectations (APA, 1994). However, each revision was intended to provide a clarification in meaning rather than an actual change in content. We, therefore, consider this to represent only a minor revision in wording.

An expectation of automatic compliance is a very common expression of narcissistic entitlement (i.e., that one won't or should not have to experience any delays or impediments). The narcissistic person is someone who acts as if he or she lives with a special "gold card," such that the rules, demands, obligations, or delays do not apply to them. They should not have to suffer the petty annoyances that are suffered by everybody else. The truly rich, beautiful, famous, and powerful are treated with special favors and attention; the narcissistic person expects equal treatment.

Rating:

0) Absent
1) A sense of entitlement (i.e., unreasonable expectations of especially favorable treatment or automatic compliance with his or her expectations)
2) Outrage or humiliation when special treatment is not provided

Questions:

a. Have you ever failed to get what you deserved? That is, have you ever felt slighted, insulted, or mistreated?

b. Do you ever break the rules or pull strings to get what you need?

Issues and Problems: There are a variety of ways in which a narcissistic sense of entitlement may be expressed. One example was provided in *DSM-III-R*: the assumption that one does not have to wait in line while others must wait. However, there are a multitude of other possible ways to express a sense of entitlement, such as a refusal of accommodations that are beneath one's level of importance or status, continually interrupting others under the implicit assumption that one's own opinions are more worthwhile or informative, failing to express any gratitude or appreciation for favors, and failing to complete tasks because they were too petty for one's level of importance.

This item, along with most of the other NAR items, is difficult to assess, in part because of its social undesirability. At times, one will interview narcissistic persons who will boldly claim that they do deserve special treatment or that they can't be bothered with petty demands and annoyances that are meant "only for the little people." However, an overt acknowledgment of entitlement can also be transparently rude. Many narcissistic persons believe they have the right and expect to be treated like royalty, but have enough understanding of social etiquette to keep this expectation to themselves. They will act as if the special treatment will occur; and will be appalled, humiliated, or enraged if it does not occur, but they may deny that they have any such expectation. Therefore, we ask for examples of having been slighted, insulted, or mistreated to assess whether a sense of entitlement does become evident.

An additional difficulty with this item is that a sense of entitlement may, at times, be realistic or within cultural norms and expectations. The extent to which persons of authority, status, or power are provided special treatment, consideration, and attention can vary substantially across cultures. Truly rich, famous, beautiful, talented, or handsome persons may be given special consideration and treatment, and it is natural to expect to receive what one has been receiving. For example, it might be narcissistic for the average student to expect special treatment at a university, but not for a star athlete. It may not be right, just, or good that this athlete receives special treatment, but it would not be narcissistic for the athlete to expect to receive what is received by other such athletes. It would be modest and humble for the athlete to refuse this treatment, but, again, it is not narcissistic for the athlete to expect to receive what is typically provided. The same reasoning applies to the beautiful, handsome, brilliant, or rich person who is given (and therefore expects) special attention (e.g., at restaurants, stores, or social functions). Those who are envious of this special treatment must be careful not to attribute narcissism to those who expect to receive what has typically been provided.

On the other hand, a history of special treatment can contribute to the development of a narcissistic sense of entitlement. Truly rich, famous, beautiful, talented, bright, or handsome people are certainly not immune to narcissism, and their experiences can contribute to or exacerbate their narcissism. It is specified in *DSM-IV* that the expectation is "unreasonable," or beyond the normal level of expectation for a person of comparable merit (e.g., the talented athlete who expects much more than is commonly provided to talented athletes, or the beautiful person who expects special treatment in situations in which beauty is not of relevance or interest to the other persons involved).

Criterion NAR-6

Is interpersonally exploitative (i.e., takes advantage of others to achieve his or her own ends).

Revisions and Rationale: This item was essentially unchanged from *DSM-III-R*, receiving only minor revisions to sentence structure (APA, 1987). Narcissistic persons will exploit, use, and take advantage of other persons. Antisocial persons will also be exploitative, but their exploitation is often for direct material gain (e.g., theft for money or rape for sex). Narcissistic exploitation will reflect a self-centered indifference, as if other people are simply tools or objects to be used. The benefits obtained by this exploitation will typically concern matters of status or power.

Rating:

0) Absent
1) Is interpersonally exploitative (i.e., takes advantage of others to achieve his or her own ends)
2) Has been repeatedly exploitative without any regret or concern for other persons

Questions:

a. Are you able to get other people to do the little, petty, annoying, or unpleasant things for you?

b. Has it ever been necessary for you to go through someone or over someone in order to get ahead?

c. Have you ever seduced or manipulated someone into doing something?

Issues and Problems: The distinction between narcissistic PD and antisocial PD with respect to this trait will often be difficult and may, at times, be illusory (Hare et al., 1991; Widiger, 1993a). A criminal act is inherently exploitative (i.e., any theft, rape, assault, extortion, or deception involves some form of exploitation). It would be quite unusual to find an antisocial or psychopathic person who was not interpersonally exploitative. The *DSM-III* version defined interpersonal exploitation, in part, as a "disregard for the personal integrity and rights of others" (APA, 1980, p. 317) which is almost synonymous with the *DSM-IV* definition of antisocial PD as a pervasive pattern of "disregard for and violation of the rights of others" (APA, 1994, p. 649).

On the other hand, the exploitation by narcissistic persons will often be more subtle than an overt criminal act (Kernberg, 1989; Stone, 1993). The narcissistic person may never steal or extort, but may instead "walk over people" to gain success, status, or power. Narcissistic persons will be colleagues or friends as long as it is to their advantage or benefit. Once their friends become useless or a burden to further success or advancement, they may be abandoned.

To the extent that one wishes to differentiate the narcissistic PD from the antisocial PD, we would not include here overt criminal acts of robbery, rape, or extortion. Instead, we would emphasize the more subtle acts of exploitation, such as seduction for the sake of sexual conquests or demanding substantial sacrifice on the part of subordinates or friends for one's own personal gain. Exploitation of others for the purpose of gaining status, glory, or fame should be emphasized.

Criterion NAR-7

Lacks empathy: is unwilling to recognize or identify with the feelings and needs of others.

Revisions and Rationale: Lack of empathy was included in *DSM-III* and *DSM-III-R*, but it was described in *DSM-III-R* as an inability to recognize and experience how others feel (APA, 1987). It has been revised in *DSM-IV* to an unwillingness to recognize or identify with the feelings and needs of others (APA, 1994). The purpose of this revision was to clarify that narcissistic persons may have an ability to recognize, but may not be at all concerned with, how others feel (Gunderson, Ronningstam, et al., 1991). This revision is, in fact, comparable to an initial, earlier draft of the *DSM-III-R* version of the item, which stated that the person "is aware of but indifferent to the feelings of others" (Work Group, 1985, p. 128). Narcissistic persons will, at times, be quite knowledgeable of how others feel, but these feelings will be of little concern to them.

Rating:

0) Absent
1) Lacks empathy: is unwilling to recognize or identify with the feelings and needs of others
2) Overtly acknowledges absence of concern regarding the feelings of others

Questions:

[*Present the conflict, loss, or illness of significant other, provided earlier by person, and then ask the following:*]

a. Can you tell me how it has been for [insert name of significant other]?

b. How is he or she feeling?

Issues and Problems: *DSM-IV* specifies that the narcissistic person is "unwilling" to recognize or identify with the feelings and needs of others. The word "unwilling," however, can be misunderstood to imply a passive-aggressive or hostile refusal. Thus, the word "unwilling" can suggest that the person consciously (willfully) decides not to be concerned about how others feel. However, narcissistic persons can be entirely unaware of their lack of empathy. They may be fully aware of how others feel and express no concern for these feelings but have little awareness that this behavior suggests a lack of empathy. It is not so much that narcissistic persons choose or decide to ignore the feelings of others, but rather that they appear to be capable of appreciating the feelings of others and fail to do so.

A distinction is at times made between a cognitive and an emotional empathy. The former refers to a knowledge of how others feel; the latter to an emotional appreciation or concern for how others feel. Empathy is also not synonymous with sympathy. The failure to express any sympathy for an illness or loss experienced by another person is indicative of a lack of empathy, whereas simply being aware that such a loss or illness is likely to be painful or difficult for another person is not an expression of much sympathy. Therapists are, at times, instructed to avoid expressions of any sympathy while, at the same time, they are instructed to express empathy. This admonition can be important to minimize a personal involvement. But, empathy for some therapists can be more cognitive than personal (e.g., the way a scientist understands the behavior of an experimental subject or rat, rather than the way a friend understands the sorrow and loss of another friend).

An example given in *DSM-III-R* was annoyance or surprise when a friend who is seriously ill cancels a date (APA, 1987). This would, indeed, be a good example of a lack of empathy (i.e., no appreciation for the suffering of this friend), but, in our experience, we have not yet found a person who has been this narcissistic. A more common and useful example is provided in *DSM-IV*, whereby the narcissistic person boasts of good health to an ill person, or makes similar exclamations of pride or joy to someone who has recently experienced a loss or suffering in the same area (APA, 1994). A comparable example is complaining about a minor ailment when a friend reveals a quite serious illness (e.g., in response to a friend indicating that she might have cancer, the narcissistic person may say, "I know how you feel, I am afraid I may have arthritis").

As noted under NAR-1, narcissistic persons continually refer all matters and issues to their own lives, opinions, or experiences. It is difficult for them to appreciate the suffering of others, and they would rather talk about themselves than about someone else. When this self-reference demonstrates a lack of empathy for the suffering, pain, or loss of the other person, we consider it as an example of the current item. When the self-reference is only to emphasize their own importance (i.e., does not involve ignoring pain or suffering in the other person), then we would consider it reflective of NAR-1. When it involves a fishing for compliments, we consider it to reflect NAR-4 (need for admiration).

Another common example is the inability to understand or appreciate the concerns or problems that others might have with them. Narcissistic lack of empathy will be particularly evident within marital conflicts. Spouses will complain that narcissistic persons don't seem to understand or care, and they would be correct. Narcissistic persons may even be disdainful of the spouse's emotional needs, perceiving the spouse as overly dependent, childish, or weak. They will have considerable difficulty "walking in the spouse's shoes," understanding the conflict from the viewpoint and perspective of the other person.

Our approach to this item is to ask the person to discuss or describe a conflict with or a loss experienced by another person. We then assess whether the person expresses any feelings of empathy or sympathy. This item is one of the least reliably assessed, which is not surprising given the considerable degree of judgment involved. Another approach is to ask directly whether the person has difficulty recognizing or appreciating how others feel, but, as noted earlier, narcissistic persons have considerable difficulty acknowledging their inadequacies and limitations. Admitting to being unempathic is, to some extent, inconsistent with being narcissistic. They may also confuse a cognitive understanding ("I do appreciate the infantile and dependent needs of my spouse") with an emotional understanding. Another approach is to ask if others have ever accused them of being unempathic. However, if they can't or won't acknowledge their lack of empathy to the interviewer, it may be just as difficult for them to acknowledge that others have accused them of being unempathic.

Lack of empathy will also be observed in persons with antisocial PD (Cooper & Ronningstam, 1992; Kernberg, 1989) and is, in fact, one of the criteria used by Hare (1992) to diagnose psychopathy (lack of empathy is now noted in the *DSM-IV* text discussion of associated features of antisocial PD; APA, 1994). Narcissistic and psychopathic persons will tend to be callous, cynical, and cruelly tough-minded. They may consider both feelings of sympathy and emotional empathy as signs of weakness. In response to the losses experienced by their victims, psychopathic persons will indicate that "I can't be bothered," "I haven't thought about it," "Life is tough," or "It's not my problem." Narcissistic persons will describe the people they have used, exploited, or taken advantage of in a similar manner. There may not be any meaningful distinction between the lack of empathy in narcissism and the lack of empathy in psychopathy.

Criterion NAR-8

Is often envious of others or believes that others are envious of him or her.

Revisions and Rationale: The *DSM-III-R* version of this item was a preoccupation with feelings of envy (APA, 1987). Preoccupation was clarified to mean being often envious of others. More importantly, *DSM-IV* now includes the belief that others are envious of them. Narcissistic persons are often envious of others, particularly those who have the status, recognition, or fame for which they yearn. However, consistent with their grandiosity, they may (falsely) believe that others are envious of them.

Rating:

0) Absent
1) Is often envious of others or believes that others are envious of him or her
2) Preoccupied with feelings of envy and the belief that others are envious of him or her

Questions:

a. Have some of your colleagues and friends been more successful than you?

b. Has their success been justified or deserving?

c. Are any of your colleagues or friends envious of you?

Issues and Problems: The inclusion of the belief that others are envious of them was a helpful revision because we have found that narcissistic persons will often be reluctant to acknowledge their envy of others. Such an admission may only occur later in therapy as the person becomes more willing and able to acknowledge needs for admiration and esteem. Their envy of others, however, may, at times, be expressed indirectly, through disdainful criticism, gratuitous derogatory remarks, and devaluations of successful or famous persons (e.g., "they were just lucky," "they don't deserve it," "they aren't that good," or "did you know that they are, in fact, in serious trouble?") (APA, 1994). We will, at times, consider such statements to reflect envy, but this inference can also confuse narcissistic envy with passive-aggressive (negativistic) scorn and disdain. Passive-aggressive disdain and scorn, however, are typically aimed at persons in positions of authority or power, whereas narcissistic persons aim their arrows at anyone with the status, fame, or recognition that they desire.

The inclusion of polar opposite expressions of envy provides a very accurate description of narcissistic behavior (Ronningstam & Gunderson, 1988, 1989, 1990). Narcissistic persons will, at one time, be very envious of others but, at other times, believe that others are very envious of them. The presence of both extremes is consistent with the severe conflicts or issues concerning self-esteem (Cooper & Ronningstam, 1992; Kohut, 1971). However, it is also of some interest to note that the prior attempt to represent polar opposite expressions was not particularly successful. The *DSM-III* criteria for NAR PD included both cool indifference or marked feelings of rage in response to criticism; cool indifference was deleted in *DSM-III-R* (Widiger et al., 1988). The difficulty in the assessment of such items is that either behavior alone is sufficient for the item to be considered present, but the presence of both behaviors is particularly characteristic of and unique to narcissistic persons. It is for this reason that we give the presence of both behaviors a higher rating. However, at any one point in time, only one pole may be evident, and during such times the narcissistic person may have little memory or willingness to acknowledge the opposite pole.

A belief that others are envious of them is more readily acknowledged by narcissistic persons because this belief will support rather than question their own self-esteem. Being envious of others is an admission of an injury to one's self-esteem; believing that others are envious of them is a means to boost one's self-esteem. A belief that others are envious of them may also be expressed indirectly through expressions of suspiciousness or anger that others are working against them (APA, 1994). The narcissistic person will believe that there are foes or opponents to their success who wish to topple them from their pedestal. Both assumptions may be wrong (i.e., that they are on a pedestal or that anyone really cares enough to want them removed). That is, the narcissistic person believes he or she is much more important in the eyes or minds of others than is actually the case. Inferring envy from suspicion, however, can readily confuse narcissistic with paranoid traits. To be considered a reflection of narcissism, the suspicion should involve issues of status, success, or fame (i.e., that others wish to undermine their fame, authority, or success, not just that others are working against them).

Criterion NAR-9

Shows arrogant, haughty behaviors or attitudes.

Revisions and Rationale: This item is a new addition to the criteria for NAR PD. It concerns more general expressions of arrogance, such as snobbish, disdainful, haughty, contemptuous, or patronizing attitudes or behaviors (APA, 1994). Arrogance is central to NAR PD, and research has indicated that it is more useful in diagnosing NAR PD than many of the *DSM-III-R* items (Ronningstam & Gunderson, 1988, 1989, 1990). Gunderson, Ronningstam, et al. (1991) suggested that "it helpfully differentiates narcissists from histrionics, antisocials, and borderlines who are, respectively, self-centered but coquettish, distant but callous, and entitled but needy" (p. 174).

Rating:

0) Absent
1) Shows arrogant, haughty behaviors or attitudes
2) Openly disdainful and disparaging of friends, colleagues, and subordinates

Questions:

a. How talented [bright, attractive, successful] are your friends or colleagues?

b. Do you ever become impatient when you have to explain something to someone?

c. Do you often get annoyed with the incompetence one finds every day?

Issues and Problems: A difficulty with this item is that it overlaps substantially with many of the other NAR PD items. Conceit or grandiosity (NAR-1), a belief that one is a special person who can be understood or helped only by the very best analyst (NAR-3), a sense of entitlement such that one demands the very best treatment or an automatic compliance with one's wishes (NAR-5), and the belief that everybody is envious of oneself (NAR-8), are all expressions of arrogance. To avoid redundant assessments, we recommend waiting until all prior items have been considered before assessing this item, and then confining its assessment to expressions of arrogance that were not previously considered.

Examples of arrogance provided in *DSM-IV* include complaints of a clumsy waiter's "rudeness" or "stupidity," or concluding a clinical assessment with a condescending evaluation of the clinician (APA, 1994). Another example would be patronizing advice (e.g., an unsolicited explanation of the operation or functioning of some device that is provided in a patronizing manner so that it could be understood by the apparently ignorant audience). A further example would be disdainful or derogatory descriptions of one's friends or subordinates. Disdain of famous, successful, or other high-status persons will usually be considered as expressions of NAR-8 (envy), but narcissistic persons will also be excessively critical, disdainful, and derogatory of both their equals (e.g., colleagues and friends) and their subordinates (e.g., students and staff). Such disdain bolsters their own esteem (i.e., magnifying their own worth by devaluing the worth of others). Additional examples of arrogance include highfalutin, pompous, or pretentious speech and mannerisms (e.g., an oratorical, bombastic, or flamboyant manner of presenting what could have been said in a simple and straightforward manner).

This item, along with lack of empathy, the requirement for excessive admiration, a sense of entitlement, and interpersonal exploitation, may also be best assessed through an interview with a close friend, relative, or colleague of the person. As indicated above, narcissistic persons may deny or be unaware of narcissistic traits that are clearly evident to those who interact with them (Benjamin, 1993; Cooper & Ronningstam, 1992). Narcissistic persons, for example, may describe themselves as having few problems with self-consciousness or vulnerability, whereas their friends and colleagues will describe them as being very self-conscious and vulnerable (Costa & McCrae, 1990). Once again, however, one must be careful not to take at face-value a critical assessment by a close friend or colleague, who may perceive arrogance where there is only a natural or realistic level of self-confidence.

10
Obsessive–Compulsive Personality Disorder

Overview: The obsessive-compulsive (OBC) personality disorder has been included in all prior editions of the *DSM*. The *DSM-IV* PD Work Group was concerned about the name because it contributes to a confusion and misinterpretation of the extent of relationship with the Axis I obsessive-compulsive anxiety disorder (Pfohl & Blum, 1991). OBC PD does not appear to be closely related to OBC anxiety disorder, nor is it even the most common PD among persons with OBC anxiety disorder. The ICD-10 uses the term anankastic (WHO, 1992), but this name lacks any apparent meaning or familiarity within America. Consideration was given to reverting back to *DSM-III* compulsive PD because this name does have historical precedent, familiarity, succinctness, and at least fails to be equivalent to the name for the anxiety disorder. However, this reversion could itself be viewed as simply obsessive indecisiveness on the part of the authors of the *DSM*, as the name has alternated between compulsive PD and obsessive-compulsive PD across the history of the *DSM* (compulsive in *DSM-I*, obsessive-compulsive in *DSM-II*, compulsive in *DSM-III*, and obsessive-compulsive in *DSM-III-R*; APA, 1952, 1968, 1980, 1987). Reverting back to compulsive PD might fail to represent any real advancement.

OBC PD was defined in *DSM-III-R* as a "pervasive pattern of perfectionism and inflexibility" (APA, 1987, p. 356). Perfectionism and inflexibility, however, do not provide a particularly vivid or clear description. Perfectionism is only one of the nine criteria, and inflexibility is relatively nonspecific. Inflexibility could imply stubbornness (which is characteristic of both the passive-aggressive and paranoid PDs) or a general inflexibility in behavior that is part of the overall definition of a personality disorder (see discussion of PDNOS in chapter 14). The definition for OBC PD was, therefore, revised in *DSM-IV* to "a preoccupation with orderliness, perfectionism, and mental and interpersonal control, at the expense of flexibility, openness, and efficiency" (APA, 1994, p. 669). These traits provide a broader and clearer description and are closer to the traditional clinical description (Pfohl & Blum, 1991). Emphasizing the impairment to flexibility, openness, and efficiency is also helpful, as the traits of perfectionism, orderliness, and control can be quite adaptive within some contexts.

The *DSM-III-R* criteria for OBC PD consisted of nine items, any five of which were necessary for the diagnosis. Five received only minor (grammatical) changes to wording for *DSM-IV*, two were revised significantly, two were deleted, and one was added. The *DSM-IV* criteria, therefore, consist of eight items (rather than nine), and the threshold was lowered from five to four. All else being equal, this would lower the threshold for the diagnosis (e.g., persons with just four of the nine *DSM-III-R* items would now be given the diagnosis). Consideration was, in fact, given to keeping the threshold at five in order to decrease the prevalence rate, as the *DSM-III-R* criteria had resulted in an increase in diagnosis when compared to *DSM-III* (Blashfield, Blum, & Pfohl, 1992; Morey, 1988b; Pfohl & Blum, 1991). The complete criteria set is presented in Table 10-1.

The major concerns for *DSM-IV* were improving the internal consistency, descriptive validity, and specificity of the criteria set (Pfohl & Blum, 1991). One of the two items that were deleted was indecisiveness, as it obtained the lowest specificity of the OBC PD criteria in the *DSM-IV* MacArthur studies (Phohl & Blum, 1991). Indecisiveness is often seen in dependent, avoidant, paranoid, and passive-aggressive persons. The reasons for this indecisiveness will vary across these personality disorders. One option considered for *DSM-IV* was to revise the item to "making the 'correct' decision often becomes a time-consuming and complicated process that they are loath to entrust to anyone else" (Pfohl & Blum, 1991, p. 374). However, this version would overlap with an existing item (reluctance to delegate tasks, item 6 in *DSM-IV*). It was eventually decided that the poor specificity of indecisiveness may not be correctable.

The second item deleted was "restricted expression of affection" (APA, 1987, p. 356). Difficulty in expressing feelings of warmth and affection is often acknowledged by and troubling to persons with OBC PD, and may represent a major concern or focus of treatment. This item, however, obtained among the lowest specificity rates (Pfohl & Blum, 1991). Restricted expression of affection is very common in schizoid, paranoid, and schizotypal persons. An alternative version considered for *DSM-IV* was a "limited expression of warm emotions" (Task Force, 1991, p. R:14), but this would have increased rather than decreased the overlap and confusion with the schizoid, paranoid, and schizotypal PDs because it replaced the specific reference to feelings of affection with a more general restriction of affectivity. In the interest of furthering the specificity of the clinical diagnosis of OBC PD, the item was deleted.

Table 10-1
DSM-IV Criteria for Obsessive-Compulsive Personality Disorder

A pervasive pattern of preoccupation with orderliness, perfectionism, and mental and interpersonal control, at the expense of flexibility, openness, and efficiency, beginning by early adulthood and present in a variety of contexts, as indicated by four (or more) of the following:

(1) is preoccupied with details, rules, lists, order, organization, or schedules to the extent that the major point of the activity is lost

(2) shows perfectionism that interferes with task completion (e.g., is unable to complete a project because his or her own overly strict standards are not met)

(3) is excessively devoted to work and productivity to the exclusion of leisure activities and friendships (not accounted for by obvious economic necessity)

(4) is overconscientious, scrupulous, and inflexible about matters of morality, ethics, or values (not accounted for by cultural or religious identification)

(5) is unable to discard worn-out or worthless objects even when they have no sentimental value

(6) is reluctant to delegate tasks or to work with others unless they submit to exactly his or her way of doing things

(7) adopts a miserly spending style toward both self and others; money is viewed as something to be hoarded for future catastrophes

(8) shows rigidity and stubbornness

Note. From *Diagnostic and Statistical Manual of Mental Disorders* (4th ed., pp. 672-673), by American Psychiatric Association, 1994, Washington, DC: Author. Copyright 1994 by American Psychiatric Association. Reprinted with permission.

Criterion OBC-1

Is preoccupied with details, rules, lists, order, organization, or schedules to the extent that the major point of the activity is lost.

Revisions and Rationale: This item was essentially unchanged from *DSM-III-R*. It was moved to the top of the list in *DSM-IV* because it was the most diagnostic item in many of the *DSM-IV* MacArthur studies (Pfohl & Blum, 1991). In *DSM-III*, however, it was simply the example provided for the item concerned with perfectionism: "perfectionism that interferes with the ability to grasp 'the big picture,' (e.g., preoccupation with trivial details, rules, order, organization, schedules, and lists)" (APA, 1980, p. 327). It became its own item in *DSM-III-R* because preoccupation with details, rules, order, organization, schedules, and/or lists may, at times, not involve perfectionism, and perfectionism will often involve other acts. An excessive concern with the most minute, trivial details; an insistence on following all rules to the letter; a penchant for indexing, classifying, and compiling lists; a rigid adherence to whatever order has been provided; a tendency to organize and reorganize; and an adherence to a complex, detailed schedule for all of one's every day activities, were all noted in the earliest descriptions of OBC PD (e.g., Abraham, 1921). The purpose of the activity is often lost to the exactitude in managing the process by which the activity is done. Vacations may lose their fun and pleasure, as spontaneous and impulsive decisions that can lead to new, exciting pleasures are squelched for the sake of an adherence to the original plan. Tasks fail to be completed effectively or efficiently as the effort gets distracted, derailed, or otherwise bogged down in bureaucratic details, rules, regulations, or other "points of order."

Rating:

0) Absent
1) Is preoccupied with details, rules, lists, order, organization, or schedules to the extent that the major point of the activity is lost
2) Governs most daily activities (including work and leisure) by specified rules, organizations, schedules, and order

Questions:

a. Do you have a daily schedule? (*If "yes":*) Is it important to stick to it?
b. Do you tend to organize all of your activities? (*If "yes":*) How about when you're on vacation?
c. Do you like to do things impulsively or do you prefer to stick to the plan?
d. Do you ever get stuck or bogged-down on details?
e. How much time do you spend working on your schedules, plans, or lists?

Issues and Problems: This is one of the few OBC PD items that bear an overt resemblance to a symptom of the obsessive-compulsive anxiety disorder. OBC anxiety includes the tendency to engage in repetitive behaviors, such as ordering and checking, according to rules that must be applied rigidly (APA, 1994). Some of the behaviors of a person with OBC PD will resemble closely the acts of a person with OBC anxiety disorder, particularly those that were created by the person for use in daily living (e.g., providing a precise arrangement of the magazines or books in one's office or home, or completing a set order and schedule of ritualistic behaviors before one goes to bed at night). Persons with OBC PD may also become upset or anxious when their rules, order, lists, schedules, or organizations are violated or disrupted. However, their preoccupation tends to be more ego-syntonic than the compulsive rituals of the person with OBC anxiety disorder, which are typically recognized as being excessive and unreasonable. In addition, the person with OBC anxiety disorder often feels driven to perform these acts (usually in response to an obsessive thought), and the acts are done to control or avoid feelings of anxiety (APA, 1994). The ritualistic or rigid behaviors of the person with OBC PD are done because they are the "best," "right," or "correct" way to do things. In addition, anger and annoyance are as (if not more) common in reaction to the bending of the rules than anxiety. An item considered for inclusion in *DSM-IV* was "periods of rigid adherence to authority are punctuated by great irritation or overt anger when authority figures are perceived as 'bending the rules'" (Pfohl & Blum, 1991, p. 374).

An additional issue is distinguishing this item from perfectionism (item OBC-2). As noted above, this item was the example provided in *DSM-III* for perfectionism (APA, 1980). Preoccupation with details will be especially problematic, as an emphasis on detail will often reflect a desire to do every little thing exactly correct. The OBC person will, at times, feel blocked and unable to proceed to the next step until every detail in the first step is completed. A preoccupation with rules, lists, order, organization, and schedules will be less problematic. The OBC person may characterize these obsessions as an effort to do things "right," but they often reflect a rigidity, stubbornness, dogmatism, or control as much as they reflect a perfectionism. The OBC person will often be focused on doing the task "correctly" or "to perfection," but the perfection will often refer to the process or means by which the task is being done (i.e., following all of the rules, order, organization, or schedule), not the outcome of the task. A perfect vacation for the person with OBC PD may be one that was completed exactly on schedule, within budget, and adhering to the original plan; not one that was the most relaxing, pleasant, and fun. When the differentiation between this item and perfectionism is ambiguous (e.g., the person is unable to finish a task because of being bogged down in perfecting every detail), we ask for additional examples, because it is likely that there will be other preoccupations that can qualify for the current item (thus allowing the preoccupation with details to be used for the perfectionism item). Note as well, however, that a rigid adherence to a budget will usually be more appropriately considered as an example of OBC-7 (miserly spending style), discussed below.

Criterion OBC-2

Shows perfectionism that interferes with task completion (e.g., is unable to complete a project because his or her own overly strict standards are not met).

Revisions and Rationale: This item was essentially unchanged from *DSM-III-R*. It was described in *DSM-III* as a "perfectionism that interferes with the ability to grasp 'the big picture'" (APA, 1980, p. 327). The item was changed to an interference with task completion to decrease the subjectivity in judgment regarding what constitutes a successful grasping of the big picture. An interference with task completion also emphasizes a more concrete maladaptivity. Perfectionism is not always maladaptive, and it will contribute to successful, even superior, achievements. However, OBC perfectionism is so excessive that it is debilitating. Persons with OBC PD may have many esteemed accomplishments, but they will just as often be blocked, frozen, or crippled by their perfectionism.

Rating:

0) Absent
1) Shows perfectionism that interferes with task completion (e.g., is unable to complete a project because his or her own overly strict standards are not met)
2) Has been reprimanded or received poor evaluations at work or school due to perfectionism

Questions:

a. Would you say that you're a perfectionist?

b. Do you tend to work and rework projects to get them just right?

c. Did you ever fail to get something done on time because you were trying to get it done just right?

Issues and Problems: A problem that we experience in the assessment of this item is that persons are, at times, unable to assess this trait in themselves. Many people will describe themselves as being perfectionistic, having high or tough standards, or having difficulty completing tasks because they expect or demand so much of themselves. It is particularly important to obtain descriptions of actual examples for this item to determine for oneself whether the person is, indeed, perfectionistic.

Procrastination may qualify for perfectionism when it reflects a reluctance or inability to start a project or task because the person knows how much effort or time it will take to do it right. Passive-aggressive procrastination reflects a hostile resistance, defiance, or opposition to the task. Obsessive-compulsive persons want to do the task, but they just keep putting it off because they know how long and demanding it will be. However, it is important in such cases to determine whether they are the ones that will make the task excessively demanding and effortful.

Examples are relatively easy to find in persons who are within skilled labor, crafts, management, professions, or other jobs that provide a clear opportunity to express perfectionism. The example provided in the *DSM-IV* text is the failure to complete a written report due to many revisions that attempt to achieve perfection (APA, 1994), but many persons are employed within jobs that do not require written reports and many others will be unemployed. However, excessive conscientiousness, in the form of perfectionism, can also be evident within unskilled or everyday tasks (e.g., cleaning, gardening, or maintenance).

Criterion OBC-3

Is excessively devoted to work and productivity to the exclusion of leisure activities and friendships (not accounted for by obvious economic necessity).

Revisions and Rationale: This item was essentially unchanged from *DSM-III-R* (APA, 1987). The only substantial revision from *DSM-III* to *DSM-III-R* was to note that the excessive devotion to work was not due to an obvious economic necessity. Some persons will work through the evenings and weekends, and take no vacations, because of their many debts and/or dependents. The excessive devotion to work of the person with OBC PD is by "choice" or "preference." They live for their career, job, accomplishments, or achievements, sacrificing most other sources of pleasure and gratification, as well as social commitments and responsibilities. The colloquial term for this item is "workaholism." Examples include never taking vacations, bringing work on a vacation in order not to waste time, continually working late into the evening and on weekends, and then bringing the work to bed with them. They may even go to sleep by reviewing the success and failures of that day's efforts and planning the strategy for the next day. They will be acutely aware of deadlines that must be met but will be unaware of the important dates and events in the lives of their family, relatives, or friends (e.g., birthdays, anniversaries, or graduations).

Rating:

0) Absent
1) Is excessively devoted to work and productivity to the exclusion of leisure activities and friendships, not accounted for by obvious economic necessity
2) Loss of relationships due to devotion to work

Questions:

a. How many hours a week do you work?

b. Do you work so hard that you don't have much time for friends or fun? (*If "yes":*) Why?

c. Have friends or family complained that you work too hard?

d. Do you take work with you to bed, on vacations, or just about any place you go?

e. Would you think of yourself as a "workaholic"?

Issues and Problems: A difficulty in the assessment of this item is comparable to one noted for OBC-2. Many persons will consider themselves to be working too hard or to be overworked. Explicit examples are often necessary so that one can assess for oneself whether there is, indeed, an excessive devotion to work. However, what is usually more problematic is that many persons with OBC PD will not describe themselves as being excessively devoted to their work, or they will say that their effort is by necessity rather than by choice or preference. They may describe the many bills, debts, or demands that must be met (excessive work that is secondary to economic necessity does not qualify), and they may complain that their spouse, friends, or relatives do not understand the special demands of their particular career, profession, or job. They may, indeed, have substantial debt and excessive responsibilities, but these are usually also the result of their workaholism (e.g., they rarely decline a request or opportunity for further demands, investments, or tasks).

Complicating the assessment, however, is the fact that it may, at times, involve a degree of value judgment (Wakefield, 1992, 1993). The *DSM-III* wording of this item was rather explicit in this regard, noting that there was an excessive devotion to work to the exclusion of "the value of interpersonal relationships" (APA, 1980, p. 328). Some persons may argue that it is simply a personal value judgment of the extent to which one values work over relationships (Frances, Widiger, & Sabshin, 1991; Spitzer & Williams, 1982). Persons with OBC PD will, at times, say that they are, indeed, devoted to their career or work and have little or no interest in leisure activities or developing a family, but do not feel particularly regretful or impaired. They may enjoy the many hours spent in developing and nurturing their skills, achievements, money, power, or status, and do not perceive this as being excessive, maladaptive, or problematic, particularly when their devotion yields substantial profit, status, power, grants, and other explicit forms of recognition and reward. It is also noted in the *DSM-IV* text discussion of OBC PD that behaviors that are culturally sanctioned should not be included in the consideration of this disorder, noting in particular the emphasis within some cultures on work and productivity (APA, 1994). However, we would also emphasize that consistency with cultural expectations does not necessarily negate or belie the maladaptivity of workaholism (see chapter 14). What is rewarded or valued by the society are not necessarily the optimal or healthiest behavior patterns (Frances et al., 1991). The assessment of this item can then become a difficult clinical judgment of the extent to which the person (and perhaps even the culture) does not (yet) appreciate the maladaptive nature of the lifestyle (i.e., potential costs to relationships or physical health) (Garamoni & Schwartz, 1986; Widiger & Corbitt, in press-b). If the person does have an immediate family or close friends, they will often be helpful in assessing the maladaptivity of the behavior pattern. They may be quite familiar with the personal costs or losses experienced by the person or by themselves.

OBC and schizoid persons may share an absence of close or long lasting personal or sexual relationships, and OBC persons may even appear schizoid in their expression of disinterest and lack of concern for this deficit. However, their apparent disinterest can be readily distinguished from a schizoid indifference. The OBC person will typically attribute the absence of relationships to tough demands and schedules that have not permitted them sufficient opportunity or time. OBC persons will indicate that they do have sexual desires and hope that someday they will find the time for a more stable relationship. They may, in fact, acknowledge periods of time in which they have felt quite alone and worried that someday it may be too late to find somebody.

Narcissistic persons may also evidence an excessive devotion to work and productivity. Their devotion will reflect a drive for status and recognition, rather than just the work itself. Many OBC persons will fail to be particularly narcissistic. They may, in fact, be excessively devoted to a particular activity, hobby, or task that brings no status or recognition. On the other hand, the drive for status and recognition within narcissistic persons will often result in an excessive devotion to work and career (that may represent an important focus of personal and clinical concern). Rather than differentiate between narcissistic and obsessive-compulsive workaholism, it may be best to simply acknowledge when such workaholism is present in both disorders.

Criterion OBC-4

Is overconscientious, scrupulous, and inflexible about matters of morality, ethics, or values (not accounted for by cultural or religious identification).

Revisions and Rationale: This item was essentially unchanged from *DSM-III-R*. It was not included within the *DSM-III* criteria for OBC PD (APA, 1980). However, it was a major aspect of the *DSM-II* criteria, which defined the obsessive-compulsive personality as an "excessive concern with conformity and adherence to standards of conscience" (APA, 1968, p. 43), noting that "individuals in this group may be rigid, over-inhibited, over-conscientious, over-dutiful, and unable to relax easily" (APA, 1968, p. 43). It was also noted within the associated features in *DSM-III* that "individuals with this disorder tend to be excessively conscientious, moralistic, scrupulous, and judgmental of self and others" (APA, 1980, p. 327). This associated feature then became a criterion for diagnosis in *DSM-III-R* (APA, 1987). Persons with OBC PD tend to be rigid, inflexible, and closed-minded with respect to matters of conscience, morality, values, and ethics. They follow ethical or moral standards in the same way they lead their everyday lives: by adhering closely and strictly to a rigid set of explicit rules and regulations (Shapiro, 1965).

Rating:

0) Absent
1) Is overconscientious, scrupulous, and inflexible about matters of morality, ethics, or values, not accounted for by cultural or religious identification
2) Conflicts and disputes with friends, relatives, neighbors, or community have often resulted from this inflexibility

Questions:

a. Do you have a moral code that you tend to live by?

b. How closely do you adhere to such rules of behavior?

c. Are you more devoted than other members of [*insert respective group, affiliation, or community*]?

d. Have you ever gotten into any conflicts or disputes with someone over issues of ethics, values, or morality?

Issues and Problems: An issue in the assessment of this item is the confusion of conscientiousness with closed-mindedness. This item concerns an overconscientiousness with respect to matters of morality, ethics, or values. However, conscientiousness is a general trait of personality that involves the tendency to be dutiful, ordered, deliberate, and disciplined (McCrae & Costa, 1990). Excessive conscientiousness is a major trait of the obsessive-compulsive PD (Widiger & Trull, 1992; Widiger, Trull, Clarkin, Sanderson, & Costa, 1994), as reflected explicitly in the first three items (e.g., preoccupation with organization and schedules, perfectionism, and devotion to work). The management of one's desires and impulses is also major aspect of conscientiousness (Costa, McCrae, & Dye, 1991). However, this item is actually more concerned with closed-minded rigidity than with conscientiousness (i.e., matters of the conscience rather than conscientiousness). For example, an illustration of this item provided in an initial draft of the text to *DSM-IV* was becoming very upset that one forgot to take a dose of medication. We consider this to reflect, instead, OBC-1, or a preoccupation with a schedule (excessive conscientiousness), rather than item OBC-4, an excessive scrupulousness about matters of morality, ethics, or values (closed-mindedness).

It is noted in *DSM-IV* that this item is not accounted for by cultural or religious identification. Some cultural or religious belief systems may appear to be, or may in fact be, rigid and dogmatic with respect to matters of morality, ethics, or values. One should not confuse a belief in or acceptance of such a value system as representing OBC rigidity and dogmatism. Interviewers who disagree with such belief systems may, at times, confuse a conservative value system with being closed-minded. Complicating the assessment, however, is the fact that persons with OBC PD will adhere in a closed-minded and rigid fashion to such religious, moral, or value systems. Membership within such a group does not negate the presence of these personality traits. One approach to this item, comparable to that taken for schizotypal magical thinking, is to assess whether the person is more scrupulous or inflexible than their peers within the particular culture or religion. One should consider whether they have extended the beliefs or practices of this group to a degree that would be considered excessive, and even absurd, to most members of this culture or religion. It is also useful to consider whether the dogmatism and inflexibility have contributed to any stress or strain within relationships (e.g., fights or separations with spouse, relatives, friends, neighbors, colleagues, or the community). Standing up for one's moral values is commendable, but a history of disputes and conflicts with friends, family, relatives, colleagues, and neighbors can suggest a maladaptive inflexibility.

Persons with a paranoid PD will also display a rigid, closed-minded set of values, morals, or ethics. This trait was not included in the *DSM-III-R* (or *DSM-IV*) criteria for paranoid PD, but it was noted in the *DSM-III-R* text that "they tend to be rigid and unwilling to compromise" (APA, 1987, p. 338). In fact, it was even suggested that "because of a tendency of some of them to be moralistic, grandiose, and extrapunitive, people with this [paranoid PD] disorder may be overrepresented among leaders of cults and other fringe groups" (APA, 1987, p. 338) (in *DSM-III*, it was stated that such overrepresentation "seems likely," APA, 1980, p. 308). There are no data to support such a statement, and it is probably quite inaccurate. Nevertheless, it is true that persons with a paranoid PD may be quite rigid, dogmatic, and inflexible with respect to moral, ethical, and other belief systems. One distinction with the obsessive-compulsive PD that may, at times, be useful is that (in our experience) paranoid persons tend to be more judgmental of others than of themselves. Obsessive-compulsive persons are also characteristically quite judgmental and critical of others. However, the judgments of the paranoid person will often reflect a more general antagonistic, cynical, distrustful, and suspicious stance towards others. They are more concerned about the lack of moral strength in others (justifying their lack of trust and respect) than in themselves. Obsessive-compulsive persons, on the other hand, can be somewhat sympathetic with the failings of others, and they are more likely to be as critical or demanding of themselves as they are of others. Thus, paranoid and obsessive-compulsive persons may both adhere rigidly to the same belief system, but this will often reflect the antagonism of the paranoid person and the closed-mindedness of the obsessive-compulsive.

Criterion OBC-5

Is unable to discard worn-out or worthless objects even when they have no sentimental value.

Revisions and Rationale: This item was essentially unchanged from *DSM-III-R*. It was not included within the *DSM-III* criteria for OBC PD, but it was included within the early descriptions of this personality disorder (Abraham, 1921; Freud, 1908; Pfohl & Blum, 1991). This item tends to be among the least sensitive (Pfohl & Blum, 1991). Many persons with OBC PD will not display the tendency to hold onto worthless, worn-out objects. However, the item is very specific to OBC PD. It is rarely seen in the other personality disorders. When it does occur, it can be very diagnostic of the obsessive-compulsive stinginess, rigidity, and parsimony.

Rating:

0) Absent
1) Is unable to discard worn-out or worthless objects even when they have no sentimental value
2) Accumulation of such objects has been a notable strain on relationships

Questions:

a. Do you tend to keep lots of apparently old or unusual things because someday you might want or need them? (*If "yes":*) Is this for sentimental reasons?

b. Do you have difficulty storing all of the things you save?

c. Has anyone ever complained or suggested that you were a "pack rat"?

Issues and Problems: A common difficulty in the assessment of this item is that OBC persons will often fail to characterize the things they hold on to as being worn-out or worthless. The rationale that is commonly provided is that "you never know when you might need it," and, therefore, it could hardly be considered to be worthless (or worn-out). Clothes are not discarded because the fashion may return, one's tastes may change, or, someday, one may lose the necessary weight. Appliances, tools, and other devices are saved because someday one may have the time to repair them. Things that others would discard are saved because someday they may be worth something (e.g., as an artifact of a prior time). Interviews with close friends, spouse, or relatives are often helpful because they may be particularly aware of the trait and the extent to which it has become troublesome and burdensome.

Criterion OBC-6

Is reluctant to delegate tasks or to work with others unless they submit to exactly his or her way of doing things.

Revisions and Rationale: The *DSM-III* version of this item was an "insistence that others submit to his or her way of doing things" (APA, 1980, p. 327). Persons with OBC PD do tend to be controlling (a trait now included within the definition), and it was noted in the text to *DSM-III-R* (and *DSM-III*) that these persons "are always mindful of their relative status in dominance-submission relationships" (APA, 1987, p. 355). "Although they resist the authority of others, they stubbornly and unreasonably insist that people conform to their way of doing things" (APA, 1987, p. 355). The authors of the *DSM-III-R* though were concerned that the *DSM-III* version placed too much emphasis on authoritarianism and domination. Therefore, the item was revised to an "unreasonable insistence that others submit to exactly his or her way of doing things, **or** unreasonable reluctance to allow others to do things because of the conviction that they will not do them correctly" (APA, 1987, p. 356). However, this item has performed poorly (Pfohl & Blum, 1991). The reason for its poor performance is also unclear, given that two options for its attribution are provided (i.e., authoritarian domination and perfectionism). The *DSM-IV* version represents a simplification. Emphasis is given to a stubborn, closed-minded insistence that a task be completed in a particular or exact manner. An example provided in the text to *DSM-IV* is providing excessively detailed instructions that would allow no room for the influence or input of others, and surprise or irritation when useful suggestions are made or each particular instruction is not followed (APA, 1994). Persons with OBC PD will reject offers for help, even when help is needed or desirable, because they find such help to be intrusive and disruptive to their own opinions and plans. They will prefer to do things on their own. When they have to work with others, it will be very difficult for them not to take control.

Rating:

0) Absent
1) Reluctance to delegate tasks or to work with others unless they submit to exactly his or her way of doing things
2) Refusal to delegate tasks or to work with others unless they submit to exactly his or her way of doing things

Questions:

a. Do you often have arguments with people because they disagree with you about how things should be done?
b. Do you ever have trouble delegating responsibility because you're worried that the person won't do it right? (*If "yes"*): Do you then tend to do most things yourself?

Issues and Problems: One difficulty in the assessment of this item is the extent to which the person actually insists or requires that others submit exactly to his or her way of doing things. They are rarely (if ever) this demanding, but their friends and colleagues will often characterize them as being this controlling. The obsessive-compulsive person is often stubborn, picky, petty, or rigid in his or her demands, requirements, or "requests." OBC persons can be very difficult and annoying to work with, but they may not perceive or describe themselves as being excessively demanding or controlling. Note, however, that the item states a reluctance rather than a refusal to delegate responsibility or to work with others. We classify actual refusals at the more severe level of the item.

One approach to the assessment of this item is to ask if others have ever accused the person of being stubborn, picky, petty, or rigid. However, obsessive-compulsive persons may be largely unaware of the extent to which they are perceived this way. Interviews with friends or colleagues are often helpful. One caution is that persons who are currently within an interpersonal dispute will often perceive the other person as the one who has been excessively stubborn and demanding. Confirmation by more than one informant may be necessary.

Passive-aggressive persons will also be very difficult to work with. Resentment of useful suggestions from others and becoming sulky, irritable, and argumentative when asked to do something were two of the *DSM-III-R* diagnostic criteria for the passive-aggressive PD (now provided in the appendix to *DSM-IV*). However, the argumentativeness of passive-aggressive persons will reflect their oppositional antagonism, rather than the need to control or to do things right. Obsessive-compulsive persons can be easy to work with if one is submissive, respectful, and acquiescent. The only thing that might mollify the passive-aggressive person would be to excuse them from the responsibility altogether; this proposal would likely generate only further anger from the obsessive-compulsive person (who would protest the loss of influence, authority, and work).

Criterion OBC-7

Adopts a miserly spending style toward both self and others; money is viewed as something to be hoarded for future catastrophes.

Revisions and Rationale: The *DSM-III-R* version of this item was a "lack of generosity in giving time, money, or gifts when no personal gain is likely to result" (APA, 1987, p. 356). This item obtained among the lowest sensitivity rates (along with OBC-5, inability to discard things) in the *DSM-IV* MacArthur studies (Pfohl & Blum, 1991). The intention of the item was to represent the tendency of the OBC person to be stingy, withholding, and miserly (Widiger et al., 1988). However, the *DSM-III-R* inclusion of a personal gain placed as much emphasis on selfishness, greed, and self-centeredness, which are characteristic of the psychopathic, antisocial, and narcissistic PDs. The *DSM-IV* version refers explicitly to being miserly, and notes that the stinginess applies to oneself as well as to others. Persons with OBC PD will be as reluctant to buy things for themselves as they are for others. They are more miserly than self-centered. They will spend an inordinate amount of time to spend the least amount of money. As noted in the *DSM-IV* text discussion, their standard of living may often suffer because they will hoard for some future unknown or unlikely need (APA, 1994). Spending money on things that would be simply fun, pleasurable, or impulsive would be discouraged, if not abhorred. As noted in OBC-1 (preoccupation with details and organization), they operate within a strict budget and account for every penny.

A difficulty in the assessment of this item for *DSM-III-R* was its substantial social undesirability. Very few persons consider themselves as (or would admit to) lacking generosity with respect to time, money, or gifts just because no personal gain is forthcoming. Few would acknowledge such selfishness (with perhaps the exception of antisocial and narcissistic persons who may lack the empathy to appreciate such blatant selfishness). In addition, even the obsessive-compulsive person will provide some gifts when nothing of equal value will be provided in return. However, the gifts of the obsessive-compulsive person will tend to be more practical than pleasurable (e.g., an appliance for an anniversary). The

DSM-IV revision is helpful in shifting the focus away from a lack of generosity toward others to a more general stinginess.

Rating:

0) Absent
1) Adopts a miserly spending style toward both self and others; money is viewed as something to be hoarded for future catastrophes
2) Has failed to make important and even necessary purchases due to stinginess

Questions:

a. Do you tend to be very frugal, practical, or careful with money?

b. Have you ever been frivolous or impulsive with presents or a major purchase?

c. Have you ever been accused of being stingy or miserly?

Issues and Problems: The shift from selfishness to stinginess does reduce the social undesirability of the item, but it still remains difficult for many obsessive-compulsive persons to acknowledge (or even be aware of) the extent of their stinginess. They will describe themselves as being practical, wise, prudent, frugal, thrifty, or careful, not stingy, penny-pinching, miserly, or tightfisted. However, if one avoids the negative connotations, one can usually obtain forthright descriptions of excessive frugality. Again, interviews with friends and relatives may provide informative examples.

One should also take into consideration cultural variations in spending habits, saving, frugality, and gift-giving. The behavior should be in excess of the frugality normal to the culture in which the person was raised. One indication is the perception of other persons within the same culture that the person is stingy or excessively frugal.

Criterion OBC-8

Shows rigidity and stubbornness.

Revisions and Rationale: This item is a new addition to the OBC PD criteria set. It was obtained from the ICD-10 criteria for the "anankastic" personality disorder (WHO, 1992, p. 206). Freud's (1908) original description of the "anal" character had highlighted the traits of being orderly, parsimonious, and obstinate. Rigidity and stubbornness provide an explicit representation of the trait of obstinacy.

Rating:

0) Absent
1) Shows rigidity and stubbornness
2) Relationships or jobs have been lost due to rigidity and stubborness

Questions:

a. Do you tend to "stick to your guns?"

b. Are you usually reluctant to compromise?

c. Do you like to try new things or new ways of doing things?

Issues and Problems: A difficulty in the assessment of this item is distinguishing it from the prior items. Although obstinacy is not explicitly noted in the description of any of the other items, many of these items do, in fact, involve obstinacy. The authors of the *DSM-III-R* OBC PD criteria set had, in fact, been concerned with the emphasis on obstinacy over orderliness and parsimoniousness in their revision of the *DSM-III* criteria set (Widiger et al., 1988). It is, then, somewhat ironic to add a new item to the *DSM-IV* criteria set to explicitly represent obstinacy. Rigidity and stubbornness are involved in the preoccupation with adherence to a particular rule, order, schedule, or organization (OBC-1), a demand for perfection in everything that one does (OBC-2), an inflexibility with respect to a moral code (OBC-4), a refusal to throw away worthless or worn-out objects (OBC-5), a refusal to delegate or work with others unless the task is done exactly a certain away (OBC-6), and a requirement that a family stay within a miserly, stingy budget (OBC-7). Rigidity or stubbornness is a fairly general trait that can be expressed in a variety of ways. One approach to this item is to assess it after one considers all of the prior items and then include only manifestations of rigidity or stubbornness that were not necessary for the attribution of any of the prior items. If there was a variety of manifestations for a prior item (e.g., clear, nonredundant examples of rigidity and stubbornness with respect to rules, lists, order, organization, and schedules), then it would be appropriate to use one or more of the additional examples for this item. Further examples of rigidity and stubbornness include refusals to consider new activities or interests (i.e., closed-mindedness with respect to aesthetic or leisure activities), inflexibility with respect to politics, or refusal to negotiate or compromise during disputes and disagreements.

11

Paranoid Personality Disorder

Overview: Paranoid (PND) personality disorder has been included in every version of the *DSM*, as far back as the *DSM-I* (APA, 1952). Paranoid PD was defined in *DSM-III-R* as a "pervasive and unwarranted tendency...to interpret the actions of people as deliberately demeaning or threatening" (APA, 1987, p. 339). Paranoid persons will perceive there to be deliberate efforts to demean them, but this perception is not as central or common as perceptions of threat, harm, exploitation, deception, attack, and manipulation (Bernstein, Useda, & Siever, 1993). In addition, passive-aggressive and narcissistic persons will also feel unjustifiably demeaned. They will feel that certain tasks or responsibilities are beneath them or demeaning to their sense of pride. The definition was, therefore, revised in *DSM-IV* to a "distrust and suspiciousness of others such that their motives are interpreted as malevolent" (Bernstein et al., 1993, p. 60) to emphasize that suspiciousness and mistrust of others are the central, defining traits of PND PD. The inclusion of malevolence is also helpful in emphasizing that these persons are not simply apprehensive or wary of others, as in the case of the avoidant, dependent, and schizotypal PDs. They consider other persons to be truly malevolent and, for this reason, not to be trusted.

The *DSM-III-R* criteria for PND PD consisted of seven items. All seven were retained for *DSM-IV* but five received significant revision. Two received just minor revisions in wording. The threshold for diagnosis remains at four of seven. The major concerns for *DSM-IV* were to increase the specificity of the diagnostic criteria, particularly with respect to the PDs that are not within the odd-eccentric cluster, such as the passive-aggressive, borderline, narcissistic, and avoidant (Bernstein et al., 1993).

DSM-IV paranoid PD also contains the expanded exclusion criterion regarding Axis I mental disorders provided for the schizotypal and schizoid PDs, and the qualification that if the criteria were met prior to the onset of schizophrenia, then one should note that the paranoid PD is premorbid. A more detailed discussion of the rationale for this qualification is provided within the chapters on the schizoid and schizotypal PDs. This is likely to be less of an issue for the paranoid PD as there tends to be less comorbidity, co-occurrence, or confusion of paranoid PD with schizophrenia (Bernstein et al., 1993). What will often be problematic in the assessment of each of the *DSM-IV* PND criteria is the extent to which the beliefs and perceptions are delusional. To the extent that a belief is bizarre (i.e., involving situations that clearly cannot occur in real life, or are beyond the realm of accepted reality within that person's culture), one should consider the likelihood of a psychotic diagnosis. Beliefs that one has lost control over one's mind or body (e.g., thought withdrawal or thought insertion) are common examples of bizarre delusions. Delusions, however, need not involve bizarre beliefs, and an Axis I delusional disorder can often be confused with paranoid personality traits. Common nonbizarre delusions are being followed, poisoned, infected, or deceived. Erroneous beliefs are considered to be delusional to the extent that they are held despite clear, contradictory evidence. However, this assessment can be difficult in cases of persons with a paranoid PD. Persons with PND PD will often be quite stubborn, recalcitrant, and firm in their opinions, beliefs, and convictions. This rigidity and recalcitrance may be applied to their suspicions and misperceptions, despite a (privately held) awareness of the illogic and error of the suspicion. It is then important to consider carefully the other indications of a more severe Axis I disorder, such as whether the beliefs are a recent phenomenon (i.e., have not been characteristic of the person since late childhood or adolescence), whether there has been a recent deterioration in functioning, and the presence of a formal thought disorder or hallucinations (see APA, 1994). Table 11-1 presents the complete *DSM-IV* criteria for paranoid personality disorder.

Table 11-1
DSM-IV Criteria for Paranoid Personality Disorder

A. A pervasive distrust and suspiciousness of others such that their motives are interpreted as malevolent, beginning by early adulthood and present in a variety of contexts, as indicated by four (or more) of the following:
   (1) suspects, without sufficient basis, that others are exploiting, harming, or deceiving him or her
   (2) is preoccupied with unjustified doubts about the loyalty or trustworthiness of friends or associates
   (3) is reluctant to confide in others because of unwarranted fear that the information will be used maliciously against him or her
   (4) reads hidden demeaning or threatening meanings into benign remarks or events
   (5) persistently bears grudges, i.e., is unforgiving of insults, injuries, or slights
   (6) perceives attacks on his or her character or reputation that are not apparent to others and is quick to react angrily or to counterattack
   (7) has recurrent suspicions, without justification, regarding fidelity of spouse or sexual partner

B. Does not occur exclusively during the course of schizophrenia, a mood disorder with psychotic features, or another psychotic disorder, and is not due to the direct physiological effects of a general medical condition.

Note: If criteria are met prior to the onset of schizophrenia, add "premorbid," e.g., "Paranoid Personality Disorder (Premorbid)."

Note. From *Diagnostic and Statistical Manual of Mental Disorders* (4th ed., pp. 637-638), by American Psychiatric Association, 1994, Washington, DC: Author. Copyright 1994 by American Psychiatric Association. Reprinted with permission.

Criterion PND-1

Suspects, without sufficient basis, that others are exploiting, harming, or deceiving him or her.

Revisions and Rationale: The *DSM-III-R* version of this item was "expects, without sufficient basis, to be exploited or harmed by others" (APA, 1987, p. 339). This is descriptive of persons with PND PD, but it fails to be sufficiently central or specific to PND PD. Pessimistic persons (e.g., persons with a depressive or self-defeating PD) may expect, without sufficient justification, to be exploited or harmed. Paranoid persons are typically cynical and pessimistic, but pessimism is not central to suspiciousness. "Expects" was, therefore, changed to "suspects" to emphasize the central trait of paranoia (i.e., suspiciousness). "Deceived" was added, along the "harmed," because harm will often imply physical harm, and paranoid persons will suspect conspiracies, deceptions, dishonesty, manipulation, schemes, and trickery more often than actual physical harm.

Unjustifiable suspicion of exploitation or deception is a common trait of the paranoid person. The *DSM-III-R* version of this item obtained among the highest rates of predictive power in the *DSM-IV* MacArthur studies. It was, therefore, maintained at the top of the list for *DSM-IV*.

Rating:

0) Absent
1) Suspects, without sufficient basis, that others are exploiting, harming, or deceiving him or her
2) Preoccupation with these suspicions

Questions:

a. Has anyone (including a company or agency) ever exploited, harmed, or deceived you? (*If "yes":*) Has this happened often?

b. Are you concerned that you might be exploited, harmed, or deceived by somebody?

c. Do you think that most people are basically honest and trustworthy?

Issues and Problems: A difficulty that will, at times, occur in the assessment of this item is verifying whether a suspicion is without sufficient basis. A common approach to this item is to ask if the person feels that anyone has been exploiting or deceiving him or her. However, many people have actually been exploited or deceived, perhaps even a number of times. This is particularly likely to be true for dependent persons, but it may not be an uncommon experience for persons living within dangerous, difficult communities and unstable, hostile relationships.

In addition, many persons with a paranoid PD will not acknowledge their paranoid traits. They will not be aware that they are, in fact, being paranoid. One cannot simply ask them if they tend to be unduly suspicious, distrustful, or paranoid. They suspect that others are, indeed, exploiting or deceiving them; they do not believe that they are being unnecessarily suspicious, accusative, or distrustful. The irrationality of the suspicions may be evident by the unlikelihood of their reality. The beliefs will not be bizarre, but the breadth and extent of the suspicions will appear exaggerated and unrealistic. However, this will, at times, be difficult to judge, and it may require obtaining independent information. Some paranoid persons can be quite convincing and compelling as they spin their tale of conspiracy, which will often have at least a kernel of truth. On the other hand, many paranoid persons will only need a little encouragement to launch into a lengthy diatribe or elaborate exposition, the irrationality of which quickly becomes evident.

Another approach to this item is to ask for opinions regarding the trustworthiness of people in general. Although everyone may have been deceived or exploited at least once, most people believe that people, in general, can be trusted. Paranoid persons, on the other hand, tend to have more general cynical, skeptical attitudes regarding the intentions, trustworthiness, honesty, and integrity of others.

An additional issue is that a valid interview will presume that the paranoid person is being forthright, at least to some extent. However, as noted in PND-3, paranoid persons are typically reluctant to confide in others. It is unusual for them not to be suspicious and wary of a clinical or research interview that is concerned with the assessment of personality traits, particularly one that focuses, in part, on paranoid personality traits. They will be aware that others perceive them as being unduly paranoid, and they will know that it may be best to keep their beliefs to themselves. Reassurance that it is not unusual to have such beliefs, that the results of the interview are, indeed, confidential, and that you are sympathetic to their plight, are often helpful. However, we recall one person whose paranoid traits were clearly documented within the hospital records but who continually and calmly denied any suggestions of suspiciousness during the interview. In fact, he denied the presence of almost anything that might make him "look bad." He described himself, instead, as being quite open, trusting, friendly, and agreeable. We may eventually discuss with such persons inconsistencies and contradictory information that we have obtained elsewhere, but this can, at times, contribute to even more guardedness and withholding. Interviews with colleagues, friends, or relatives are often necessary in such cases, at least to corroborate one's own suspicion that the denials are false. The administration of self-report "validity" scales can also be useful in identifying the occurrence of invalid denial (Widiger & Frances, 1987). We will, at times, discuss with the person their responses to particular items from such validity scales.

Members of minority groups, immigrants, and other persons who are from a different cultural or ethnic group from the interviewer may appear to the interviewer to be unduly suspicious and guarded (Alarcon & Foulks, in press). The interviewer may not appreciate the extent to which experiences of discrimination and exploitation can generate justifiable feelings of suspiciousness and distrust, and the subject may not appreciate the extent to which such suspicions are not justified within some contexts. Confidentiality, which is taken for granted by the interviewer, may not be assumed by the subject, who may be unfamiliar with mental health procedures or may be more generally suspicious of the system. Membership within a minority group does not exclude the presence of paranoid suspiciousness, but it is preferable to assess whether such paranoia is also evident toward other members of the same cultural or ethnic group.

Criterion PND-2

Is preoccupied with unjustified doubts about the loyalty or trustworthiness of friends or associates.

Revisions and Rationale: The *DSM-III-R* version of this item was simply, "questions, without justification, the loyalty or trustworthiness of friends or associates" APA, 1987, p. 339). The *DSM-IV* revision provides a higher threshold for the attribution of this item. At some point, many persons may question the loyalty of their friends (narcissistic persons will often question the loyalty of their subordinates). However, paranoid persons not only question their friends' loyalty but also ruminate excessively about these suspicions. They will have difficulty ignoring, dismissing, or letting go of their suspicions. As noted in the text to *DSM-IV*, they will scrutinize the behavior of their friends and associates, perceiving any deviation, failing, or disappointment as a sign that these persons are abandoning and/or turning against them (APA, 1994). Paranoid persons will often feel that they must rely on themselves, as they are the only person whom they can depend upon and trust.

Rating:

0) Absent
1) Is preoccupied with unjustified doubts about loyalty or trustworthiness of friends or associates
2) Preoccupation with these doubts about friends and associates

Questions:

a. Have your friends or associates been loyal and trustworthy? (*If "no":*) Have you ever discussed with someone, or had to do something about, a disloyal friend?

b. Have your colleagues ever taken your ideas or plans, or revealed your secrets?

Issues and Problems: Many persons may question the loyalty of their friends during times of severe stress, upheaval, and turmoil (which is, itself, not uncommon in persons who are seeking treatment), and such questioning may not be without some validity. One must be careful not to confuse temporary doubts with ongoing personality traits. The *DSM-IV* emphasis on preoccupation is helpful in this regard. It is not enough that a person simply questions the loyalty of others; the person must also be preoccupied with questions of loyalty or trustworthiness. This preoccupation must also have been evident since late childhood or adolescence and prior to any current relationship turmoil.

Note as well that the item concerns doubts about the loyalty of friends or associates, not relatives or sexual partners. A difficulty in the assessment of PND items is that they overlap substantially. This will contribute to excellent internal consistency, but it also contributes to redundant and poorly differentiated assessments. PND-2 is confined to friends and associates because doubts concerning the loyalty or trustworthiness of sexual partner(s) and spouse(s) are covered by PND-7. Doubts about the loyalty or trustworthiness of relatives (other than a spouse) are not covered explicitly by any item. Paranoid suspicions will typically concern friends, associates, and/or sexual partner(s) more than relatives (e.g., siblings, parents, and/or cousins). When preoccupations with unjustified doubts regarding the loyalty or trustworthiness of relatives do occur, we consider whether these suspicions would represent PND-1 (suspicions of exploitation or deception), PND-3 (reluctance to confide), PND-4 (perception of hidden demeaning or threatening meanings), PND-5 (persistently bears grudges), or PND-6 (perceives attacks on his or her character that are not apparent to others).

Criterion PND-3

Is reluctant to confide in others because of unwarranted fear that the information will be used maliciously against him or her.

Revisions and Rationale: The only revision to this item was to insert the word "maliciously" but this does represent an important change. It is not unusual to find patients, prisoners, or research subjects to be reluctant to confide in an interviewer because of an unwarranted fear that something they would reveal might be used against them. They may be reluctant to acknowledge past criminal acts, deviant sexual behavior, or any other humiliating or embarrassing experiences. The withholding of information will often reflect an unwarranted mistrust, but this suspiciousness is below the threshold intended for this item. Paranoid PD suspiciousness includes the belief that the information will be used maliciously (i.e., with evil, cruel, mean, spiteful, or vindictive intent).

This item may, at times, be helpful in distinguishing paranoid persons from schizoid, schizotypal, and avoidant persons. All four of these personality disorders share substantial introversion, but the suspiciousness and mistrust of paranoid persons reflects their antagonism rather than introversion (Widiger, Trull, et al., 1994). Schizoid persons are indifferent toward revealing information, and avoidant persons (yearning for intimacy) may truly enjoy such discussion (although they may feel somewhat insecure and inhibited). Schizotypal persons will be reluctant to confide in others, but this may reflect their more general discomfort and awkwardness with personal intimacy and revelation. Paranoid persons have difficulty becoming close to others because they fear giving away too many secrets, confidences, or anything else that may be used against them. They may be quite willing to obtain personal information from others (unlike the schizotypal person), but they are very reluctant to reciprocate.

Rating:

0) Absent
1) Reluctance to confide in others because of unwarranted fear that the information will be used maliciously against him or her
2) Refusal to confide in others or complete necessary documents due to the above fear

Questions:

a. Is it better not to confide in people?
b. Are you often reluctant to do so? (*If "yes":*) Why?
c. Has anyone ever taken advantage of you by using what you've told them?
d. Have you ever refused to confide in someone or to complete any important documents because of your suspicions?

Issues and Problems: This item will often be evident within the interview itself. Persons with a paranoid PD can be withholding and uncooperative, denying that they have any grudges, suspicions, or preoccupations. However, it is also difficult and risky to infer the presence of paranoid suspiciousness on the basis of excessive denial. It may be correct to infer that a person is being reluctant to confide, but not that this reluctance is due to a paranoid fear that the information will be used against them, let alone used maliciously. The excessive denial may, instead, reflect a borderline, antisocial, or passive-aggressive oppositionalism, or simply fatigue or disinterest. Direct inquiry regarding the reasons for the guardedness is important, but this may also prove to be unsuccessful. Interviews with staff, associates, friends, or relatives may then be useful. Interviews with others who know the person well are also important to confirm one's own impressions. We have, at times, found that interviewers will attribute difficulties during the interview to a trait within the interviewee when, in fact, it reflected difficulties that were confined largely to a particular interview. A reluctance to confide should be evident within relationships outside of the clinical setting (or at least be evident in prior therapeutic relationships).

Interviewers may also experience guardedness and reticence in members of minority, ethnic, immigrant, or religious groups that are different from their own. As we noted in our discussion of the first item, they may not appreciate the confidentiality of the interview, particularly if they are from a cultural perspective that substantially stigmatizes mental disorders or mental illness. Illegal immigrants, or any persons who have good reasons for not being forthright or open, may also appear unduly guarded or secretive. Until one knows the reason for the reticence, one must be careful not to presume that it reflects a paranoid guardedness.

Criterion PND-4

Reads hidden demeaning or threatening meanings into benign remarks or events.

Revisions and Rationale: The only revision to this item was to delete the example of suspecting that a neighbor put out trash early to annoy him or her. It is common for persons with a paranoid PD to develop paranoid suspicions and fantasies concerning their neighbors. However, this particular example was neither prototypic nor even common. It would not apply to persons within apartment buildings who place their trash in bins or receptacles. Nor is putting the trash out early to annoy someone really demeaning or threatening.

The relationship of paranoid persons with their neighbors, however, is often antagonistic, replete with a history of accusations, acrimony, and disputes. The neighbor is someone who is within close, immediate space and who could then potentially observe private and personal activities. Neighbors can intrude upon and violate one's sense of personal space. Thus, it is common for paranoid persons to read hidden demeaning, hostile, or threatening meanings into benign remarks or events involving their neighbors. This may include a paranoid fantasy regarding the morning trash, but it could just as well concern a fleeting remark, an open curtain, a changed lock, a mowed lawn, or a revision to a name on a mailbox.

In addition, this item is not confined to issues with neighbors. Paranoid persons will read demeaning or threatening meanings into remarks or events at work, on the street, at parties, and anywhere else, with anyone else. The paranoid person has the basic assumption that people cannot be trusted, and he or she will often perceive an intent to use, exploit, harm, humiliate, insult, or demean in what was actually a harmless remark or event.

Rating:

0) Absent
1) Reads hidden demeaning or threatening meanings into benign remarks or events
2) Preoccupation with these suspicions

Questions:

a. How do you like your neighbors?

b. Have you been suspicious regarding their motives or intentions?

c. Do your neighbors or people at work ever do subtle things that seem to be intentionally hostile, demeaning, or even threatening to you?

d. Do you know someone else who has continually or often insulted or threatened you in some subtle, underhanded way, or in some way that you just couldn't put your finger on?

Issues and Problems: We begin with inquiries regarding neighbors because the innocent neighbor is a common foil for paranoid fantasies and suspicions. The neighbor is a good source for misinterpretations and exaggerations of harmless incidents or events that have been blown way out of proportion. However, in the assessment of this item, it is important to determine the extent to which any suspicions are justified. A neighbor may not, in fact, be benign, and a deteriorated relationship is often mutually interactive.

In addition, it is also useful to assess whether the trait is evident within other relationships. Examples provided in the *DSM-IV* text discussion concern the suspicion that a store clerk was deliberately attempting to cheat them or that a casual remark from a coworker was an attack on their character (APA, 1994; however, see discussion of these examples below). Paranoid persons will perceive hidden demeaning or threatening meanings in casual, benign remarks they encounter in any everyday setting or situation. Cross-situational assessment is important to ensure that the suspicions are not confined to just one relationship. The paranoia of a person with paranoid PD will, at times, be expressed primarily within one particular relationship, just as dependency or borderline affectivity will often be felt primarily with respect to one significant person. Nevertheless, one should observe at least some degree of paranoia with respect to a variety of persons with whom the individual currently interacts, as well as significant problems with a variety of persons in the past.

An additional issue that is particularly relevant for interviewers who are assessing each item in turn is that persons with a paranoid PD can become increasingly suspicious, wary, and circumspect within the interview. Paranoid persons can become sensitive to the fact that one is asking a series of questions that concern false suspicions, preoccupations, concealments, misinterpretations, grudges, and accusations. It may, in fact, become quite difficult for paranoid persons to remain open, relaxed, comfortable, and forthright under such circumstances. They may feel that they are being misinterpreted, misrepresented, misunderstood, manipulated, and/or interrogated. At times, we have found it helpful to alter temporarily the structure of the interview when this begins to occur. We may make a minor change in the order of the items (e.g., move to a more benign section of the interview), take a break, engage in small talk, or discuss any concerns, reactions, or feelings they might be having. Self-report inventories may also be useful, as some paranoid persons will find it easier to acknowledge their suspicions on a seemingly anonymous (or at least impersonal) questionnaire.

A final note concerns the examples provided in the text to *DSM-IV* (APA, 1994) that were presented above. These examples illustrate the difficulty in differentiating among the paranoid PD items. We would consider the suspicion that a store clerk was deliberately attempting to cheat the person as a representation of PND-1 (suspects that one is being exploited or deceived). A perception that a store clerk was being critical or insulting of the purchase would be a better representation of a hidden demeaning remark. Likewise, the example of interpreting a casual remark from a coworker as an attack on one's character may be better thought of as an example of PND-6 (perceives attacks on one's character or reputation) than as an example of a perceived threat. Differentiation among the items will often be difficult, but to minimize redundancy and maximize comprehensive assessments, it is important to consider carefully which item the behavior best represents.

Criterion PND-5

Persistently bears grudges (i.e., is unforgiving of insults, injuries, or slights).

Revisions and Rationale: We have considered the revision to this item to be only minor, but it could, in fact, represent a significant revision. *DSM-IV* added injuries along with insults and slights. This revision was largely for compatibility with ICD-10 (Bernstein et al., 1993; Task Force, 1991). It is a useful revision because a persistent grudge is as readily maintained in response to an injury as it is to a slight or an insult. The revision is not intended to represent a significant change in meaning or content. It is possible that a person will have exhibited a persistent grudge with respect to an injury but not to a slight or an insult. An injury is more severe than a slight or an insult (e.g., it may involve actual physical harm or loss), and thus, a persistent grudge is perhaps more likely to occur. A common example would be a history of petty, failed, or threatened lawsuits for perceived injuries. However, the item also specifies a plurality of grudges, and it is unlikely that a person will have a history of grudges in response to injuries and not also display persistent grudges in response to perceived insults or slights.

DSM-IV also now specifies that the person *persistently* bears grudges (to be compatible with the ICD-10 wording). However, this revision as well does not really change the item, because the persistence of this behavior pattern has always been assumed. It was presumed in the *DSM-III-R* criterion of bearing a grudge that it was, indeed, persistent. As noted in the *DSM-III-R* text description of this item, "they may bear grudges for a long time, and never forgive slights, insults, or injuries" (APA, 1987, p. 337).

This was a new item to *DSM-III-R* (although the litigious nature of persons with paranoid PD was noted in *DSM-III*; APA, 1980), and it may be the only PND PD item that does not explicitly involve suspiciousness or mistrust. However, the persistence of resentment, anger, bitterness, or any other expression of a persistent grudge will usually reflect an inherent distrust, suspiciousness, and cynicism of others. Any perceived slight, injury, or insult confirms what has always been suspected to be true, that "people cannot be trusted," or that "they have it in for you."

Rating:

0) Absent
1) Persistently bears grudges (i.e., is unforgiving of insults, injuries, or slights)
2) Persistently bears grudges in response to imagined, accidental, or misperceived insults, injuries, or slights

Questions:

a Have you ever felt slighted or insulted by someone?

b. Do insults or slights tend to bother or irritate you for some time?

c. Have you ever sought revenge sometime later for such an injury, insult, or slight?

d. Is there someone you have not forgiven, even to this day?

e. Have you ever threatened to sue somebody?

Issues and Problems: The item does not specify whether the insult, injury, or slight was real or imagined. Either would be sufficient for the item to be considered present. The essence of the item concerns the persistence of a grudge. The paranoid person does not forgive and forget. The insult, slight, or injury could have been real and intentional, as well as accidental, unintended, or even nonexistent. However, we would consider the persistence of a grudge to be more indicative of a paranoid PD to the extent that the slight, insult, or injury did not, in fact, occur, was misinterpreted, or was entirely accidental and unintended.

One will also need to exclude persistent resentment, bitterness, or anger that is quite understandable given the severity of an actual injury, insult, or slight (e.g., sexual or physical abuse, or a severe and intended injury, attack, or insult for which the perpetrator provided no apology, restitution, or remorse). On the other hand, the longstanding feuds of many paranoid persons will often have elements of justification for at least some degree of resentment, anger, or bitterness. The tendency of paranoid persons to search for confirmation of their biases and to perceive malicious injury, slights, and insults where they do not exist, as well as their inability to forgive and forget, will be a significant factor in the perpetuation and escalation of these feuds.

Criterion PND-6

Perceives attacks on his or her character or reputation that are not apparent to others and is quick to react angrily or to counterattack.

Revisions and Rationale: The *DSM-III-R* version of this item was being "easily slighted and quick to react with anger or to counterattack" (APA, 1987, p. 339). This item was found to be the least specific to PND PD in the *DSM-IV* MacArthur studies (Bernstein et al., 1993). Feeling easily slighted and being quick to react angrily or to counterattack is characteristic of persons with a borderline or antisocial PD, and feeling easily slighted is characteristic of the avoidant, narcissistic, and schizotypal PDs (e.g., hypersensitivity). Perceiving an attack on one's character or reputation that is not apparent to others, on the other hand, is more consistent with and specific to the distorting suspiciousness of the paranoid PD.

Rating:

0) Absent
1) Perceives attacks on his or her character or reputation that are not apparent to others and is quick to react angrily or to counterattack
2) Has reacted to such perceptions with an actual or threatened physical counterattack

Questions:

a. Has anyone ever attacked your character, integrity, or reputation?

b. What did you do about it?

c. Has this happened often?

Issues and Problems: This is one of the few complex items in *DSM-IV* with its requirement that two conditions must be met: a misperception of an attack on one's character or reputation and a quick reaction of anger or counterattack. At times, we may observe just the false perception of attacks on one's character (with no reaction of anger or counterattack, let alone a quick reaction), or we may find a history of anger and attacks on others that are not in response to false perceptions of slurs on one's character or reputation. Both aspects of the item must be present to consider the trait to be present. Quick reactions of anger (or counterattack) to actual attacks on one's character (or reputation) would also fail to qualify, even if the response was quite severe and extreme. We also provide a higher rating if the attack/counterattack involves threat of or actual physical harm to the person or property.

It is also important to note that the perceived attacks concern one's character or reputation (e.g., perceived slurs, slander, libel, criticism, questions, or slights with respect to one's fidelity, morality, sexuality, sobriety, spirituality, honesty, trustworthiness, integrity, sanity, or other desirable traits of character or reputation). Persons with a paranoid PD will also be quick to counterattack a perceived exploitation, deception, conspiracy, scheme, disloyalty, or threat, but these are more appropriately considered within PND-1, PND-2, or PND-4. This item will also overlap with PND-5, as a perceived insult or slight may concern an attack on one's character or reputation. We would consider such instances to represent both items if there is both a quick reaction of anger or counterattack (e.g., threats of a lawsuit) and a persistent grudge thereafter (e.g., continuation of suit despite failure to succeed).

Criterion PND-7

Has recurrent suspicions, without justification, regarding fidelity of spouse or sexual partner.

Revisions and Rationale: The revision to this item was comparable to PND-2, wherein questioning was replaced with preoccupation. In this case, unjustified questions were replaced with recurrent (and unjustified) suspicions. The purpose of this revision is to emphasize "the intensity and pervasiveness of the paranoid individual's pathological jealousy with the aim of increasing the item's sensitivity" (Bernstein et al., 1993, p. 60). This item was among the least frequently seen in cases of paranoid PD in the *DSM-IV* MacArthur studies (Bernstein et al., 1993). However, a revision that provides a higher threshold for its attribution may result in the item being assessed even less frequently (rather than more frequently) within persons with a paranoid PD. It has been our experience that the revision is increasing the item's specificity rather than its sensitivity. The original (*DSM-III-R*) version's low sensitivity may have been due to the implicit requirement that there be a history of spouses and/or sexual partners. Persons with a paranoid PD tend to be introverted and are less likely than other persons to have obtained, sustained, and developed a relationship to the point of a marriage, or even a sexual relationship. As noted in the text to *DSM-III-R*, "these people usually avoid intimacy except with those in whom they have absolute trust" (APA, 1987, p. 338). However, when they do become involved in a sexual relationship, they will often be very jealous, controlling, and suspicious. They will search for and perceive signs of infidelity in a failure to answer the phone, smiles at someone else, a decrease or change in sexual interest, late arrivals, or in any other innocent or benign event, incident, or remark.

Rating:

0) Absent
1) Recurrent suspicions, without justification, regarding fidelity of spouse or sexual partner
2) Has left, divorced, or physically attacked partner due to these recurrent suspicions

Questions:

[*About current or past boyfriend/girlfriend:*]

a. Do you think your [*current/past boyfriend/girlfriend/lover/spouse*] has ever had any affairs or been unfaithful to you?

   (*If "yes":*) What makes you think so?

   Why do you think he or she did this?

   What did you do about it?

b. Has a past [*insert partner*] ever complained that you were too jealous?

Issues and Problems: Avoidant and dependent persons will also question the fidelity of a spouse or lover. However, their suspicions will reflect their own insecurity and pessimism rather than doubts regarding the integrity or reliability of their partner. Their suspicions arise from their doubts regarding their own attractiveness, desirability, or ability to hold their partner, and their accusations will have a more pleading, helpless, and pathetic quality than the bitter, derogatory, and hostile quality of the paranoid accusations. In addition, it is clearly necessary to determine whether the suspicion or jealousy was justifiable.

This item specifies that there are recurrent suspicions. However, an entrance into treatment may be at the peak of an explosive, volatile conflict when such accusations and suspicions are rampant. It is important not to misinterpret the intensity of a current episode as suggesting that there has been a chronic history of pathological jealousy. Borderline (and, to a lesser extent, antisocial) persons may also appear quite paranoid in their episodes of rage and anger. Inquiries with respect to the past history may fail to be helpful because it will often be difficult for currently angry, jealous persons to acknowledge a history of false accusations. They may also express the general opinion that "men" or "women" cannot be trusted, or that they are all "pigs" or "sluts." Such derogatory opinions of the opposite (or same) sex and past lovers will not be that unusual in persons who are in the middle of a bitter, volatile divorce or dispute. Interviews with colleagues, associates, or other persons who have known them or their history can be helpful in the assessment of this item.

12

Schizoid Personality Disorder

Overview: The schizoid (SZD) personality disorder was defined in *DSM-III-R* as a "pervasive pattern of indifference to social relationships and a restricted range of emotional experience and expression" (APA, 1987, p. 340). SZD PD is defined in *DSM-IV* as a "pervasive pattern of detachment from social relationships and a restricted range of expression of emotions in interpersonal settings" (APA, 1994, p. 638). Indifference was replaced by detachment for a more overt, behavioral description rather than an inferred trait (Kalus, Bernstein, & Siever, 1993). The second modification was to emphasize the interpersonal context for the disorder.

The initial draft of this disorder for *DSM-III* was given the name of "introverted" (Task Force, 1978, p. K:6) to distinguish it from the prior versions of this disorder. The title of introverted is rather descriptive, as the schizoid PD is almost a pure representation of an extreme version of the personality trait of introversion (Widiger, Trull, et al., 1994). The final decision for *DSM-III* was to retain the name of schizoid for historical continuity. However, the *DSM-III* version of SZD PD was rarely diagnosed (Widiger, 1991; Widiger & Rogers, 1989). It was so infrequently diagnosed that consideration was given to deleting it from *DSM-III-R*. The infrequency of its diagnosis, however, was attributed to the restrictiveness of its diagnostic criteria rather than to an absence of validity or utility to clinical practice. *DSM-III-R* shifted from requiring all four of four criteria to any four of seven criteria (Widiger et al., 1988). As a result, the prevalence of the diagnosis has increased substantially (Blashfield, Blum, & Pfohl, 1992; Morey, 1988b).

The major issues for *DSM-IV* were the differentiation of SZD from the schizotypal and avoidant PDs (Kalus et al., 1993). Four of the seven criteria were revised significantly, two were unchanged from *DSM-III-R*, and one received only minor revision for clarification. The threshold for diagnosis has remained at four of seven.

The most substantial revision may have been to the exclusion criterion. SZD is one of the few PDs with an exclusion criterion. In *DSM-III-R*, it could not be diagnosed if the behaviors occurred exclusively during the course of schizophrenia or a delusional disorder. This was broadened in *DSM-IV* to include a mood disorder with psychotic features, any other psychotic disorder, a pervasive developmental disorder, or a general medical condition (e.g., an apathetic personality change due to a general medical condition; APA, 1994, p. 172) because the flat affect, withdrawal, and emotional detachment of SZD PD is readily confused with these Axis I mental disorders.

It is also indicated in *DSM-IV* that one should note that SZD PD is "premorbid" if the behavior pattern was evident prior to the onset of schizophrenia. Premorbid schizoid traits might have prognostic significance for the course and treatment of the schizophrenia (Siever, 1992) but, more importantly, it might not even be meaningful to suggest that the person had a schizoid personality disorder that was independent of or unrelated to the eventual schizophrenia. Once a person develops schizophrenia, a diagnosis of schizoid PD can become rather pointless. All of the schizoid PD symptoms are readily understood as symptoms of schizophrenia. Negative and residual symptoms of schizophrenia closely resemble schizoid personality traits. Perhaps the only time in which it would be meaningful to diagnose schizoid PD would be when schizoid traits preceded the onset of schizophrenia. However, even in these cases the schizoid traits could represent the prodromal phase of schizophrenia. It would not be difficult to confuse schizoid PD traits with a lengthy and insidious prodromal phase of schizophrenia (resulting in the failure to provide early and aggressive treatment of the schizophrenia). Differentiating schizoid personality traits from a prodromal phase of schizophrenia in someone who is currently within the active (or any) phase of schizophrenia can be exceedingly difficult (e.g., requiring a retrospective assessment of the onset and duration of symptoms of detachment and withdrawal in someone who is currently detached, withdrawn, and perhaps psychotic, and was possibly detached and withdrawn for a substantial but unclear amount of time prior to the active phase). Even if one can document a distinct onset of a rapid progression of withdrawal, detachment, and deterioration (i.e., a clear worsening of the schizoid traits prior to the onset of the active phase) the schizoid traits that preceded this apparent prodromal phase could ultimately be shown to represent a more subtle, subthreshold schizophrenic pathology. Therefore, if one does diagnose SZD PD in someone who is also suffering from schizophrenia, then it should be noted that it is (at best) a premorbid personality disorder. The complete *DSM-IV* criteria set for the diagnosis of SZD PD is presented in Table 12-1.

Table 12-1
DSM-IV Criteria for Schizoid Personality Disorder

A. A pervasive pattern of detachment from social relationships and a restricted range of expression of emotions in interpersonal settings, beginning by early adulthood and present in a variety of contexts, as indicated by four (or more) of the following:
   (1) neither desires nor enjoys close relationships, including being part of a family
   (2) almost always chooses solitary activities
   (3) has little, if any, interest in having sexual experiences with another person
   (4) takes pleasure in few, if any, activities
   (5) lacks close friends or confidants other than first-degree relatives
   (6) appears indifferent to the praise or criticism of others
   (7) shows emotional coldness, detachment, or flattened affectivity

B. Does not occur exclusively during the course of schizophrenia, a mood disorder with psychotic features, another psychotic disorder, or a pervasive developmental disorder, and is not due to the direct physiological effects of a general medical condition.

Note: If criteria are met prior to the onset of schizophrenia, add "premorbid," e.g., "schizoid personality disorder (premorbid)."

Note. From *Diagnostic and Statistical Manual of Mental Disorders* (4th ed., p. 641), by American Psychiatric Association, 1994, Washington, DC: Author. Copyright 1994 by American Psychiatric Association. Reprinted with permission.

Criterion SZD-1

Neither desires nor enjoys close relationships, including being part of a family.

Revisions and Rationale: This item was unchanged from *DSM-III-R*. It was one of two items that obtained both high sensitivity and specificity in the *DSM-IV* MacArthur studies (Kalus et al., 1993) and high prototypicality ratings in surveys of clinicians (Blashfield & Haymaker, 1988; Livesley, Reiffer, Sheldon, & West, 1987) (the other item was, "almost always chooses solitary activities," APA, 1987, p. 340). It was, therefore, placed at the top of the list in *DSM-IV*. Neither desiring nor enjoying close relationships is obviously central to the construct of a schizoid PD. It also provides a major distinction from avoidant PD. Both schizoid and avoidant persons are introverted, withdrawn, and socially isolated, but persons with avoidant PD desire close relationships (APA, 1980) whereas schizoid persons are indifferent to any such opportunities and appear to lack a desire for intimacy or involvement (APA, 1994; Widiger & Frances, 1988).

Rating:

0) Absent
1) Neither desires nor enjoys close relationships, including being part of a family
2) Explicitly indicates no desire for or enjoyment in close relationships

Questions:

a. Have you had a close relationship with someone during your adult life? [*If "yes," assess whether he or she enjoyed this relationship for at least some of the time.*]

b. Do you desire or enjoy having a close friend?

c. Do you often wish that people would just leave you alone?

d. Are you now close to anyone within your family? Would you prefer that your family would just leave you alone? (*If "yes":*) Would you rather not be part of any family?

Issues and Problems: A difficulty that will, at times, arise in the assessment of this item is a misunderstanding of what is meant by "desire" or "enjoy." Many persons who say they neither desire nor enjoy being part of their family are expressing an anger, resentment, or bitterness. It is not unusual to find persons from severely dysfunctional families who express no desire or enjoyment in being close to their relatives. Some persons who have recently experienced a bitter ending to a love relationship, or who have in fact been abused, assaulted, or traumatized within a recent relationship, may also claim to have no desire or interest in becoming closely involved with someone else. We, therefore, ask whether they have had any close relationships with someone during their adult life, and whether they ever enjoyed this relationship. If they have not been in any such relationship, we then ask whether they desire a close friendship, whether they are close to any family member, or whether they would prefer just to be left alone. By a close relationship, we mean a friend, relative, or lover with whom one regularly confides or shares personal concerns, fears, regrets, wishes, interests, and pleasures. We do not include a therapeutic (treatment) relationship (a schizoid person may desire this relationship, but it is a professional relationship for treatment, not a mutual friendship).

Criterion SZD-2

Almost always chooses solitary activities.

Revisions and Rationale: This item was unchanged from *DSM-III-R*. It was one of two items that obtained both high sensitivity and specificity in the *DSM-IV* MacArthur studies (Kalus et al., 1993) and high prototypicality ratings in surveys of clinicians (Blashfield & Haymaker, 1988; Livesley et al., 1987) (the other item was "neither desires nor enjoys close relationships," APA, 1987, p. 340). Schizoid persons will prefer to be by themselves, or will, at least, be indifferent to the presence of others. They will often prefer activities or hobbies that do not involve social interactions or involvements, such as computers, mathematics, or other abstract, mechanical tasks (APA, 1994). They will often go to movies, events, restaurants, or vacations by themselves, expressing little interest in and making no effort to have any company.

Rating:

0) Absent
1) Almost always chooses solitary activities
2) Actively rejects the company of others

Questions:

a. Do you usually do things by yourself?
b. How often do you go to a movie, restaurant, vacation, or some other event by yourself?
c. Do you prefer to do things by yourself?

Issues and Problems: Schizoid persons who are open and aware will acknowledge that they almost always choose solitary activities and prefer to be by themselves. However, we often find that they are not particularly insightful, reflective, or open. And, it is not really the case that they are almost always or even often <u>choosing</u> solitary activities. They may, at times (or often) decline an opportunity to socialize or join others, but most of the time there will be nobody to invite. The isolation of schizoid persons will, at times, feed on itself, to the point that there are very few opportunities. Therefore, in addition to asking what they choose or prefer, we also ask what typically happens. However, the issue of choice or preference is important and necessary to consider. There are many other reasons for being socially isolated that will not involve a matter of choice or preference (e.g., social ostracism).

An additional issue in the assessment of this item is its distinction from the first item, "neither desires nor enjoys close relationships." The distinction is that the current item involves doing things with others, whereas the first item involves getting close to others. Some persons may desire or enjoy intimacy or closeness, but still prefer to be alone.

Criterion SZD-3

Has little, if any, interest in having sexual experiences with another person.

Revisions and Rationale: This item received only minor revisions and was, therefore, essentially unchanged from *DSM-III-R*. *DSM-III-R* used the term "desire" rather than "interest." The revision was made to be compatible with the wording used in the ICD-10 (Kalus et al., 1993; WHO, 1992). This revision is not intended to have any effect upon its assessment. *DSM-IV* also deleted the word "indicates" from "indicates little, if any desire," to emphasize that there is, in fact, little to no interest (not simply an indication of little to no interest). The *DSM-III-R* parenthetical remark that age should be taken into account was deleted because it was considered to be largely obvious, and it appeared to suggest, by omission, that there were no other issues to be taken into account.

Rating:

0) Absent
1) Has little, if any, interest in having sexual experiences with another person
2) No interest in having sexual experiences with another person

Questions:

a. Have you enjoyed the sexual relationships you have had?
b. Some people aren't really interested in getting sexually involved with someone; has this been the case with you?
c. Would it trouble you if you went through your entire life with no sexual relationships?

Issues and Problems: This item is often difficult to assess because it involves personal issues and behavior. Extremely schizoid persons may be quite indifferent to discussing their sex lives (as they are indifferent to almost everything) but many persons, including schizoid persons, will find it difficult, awkward, and/or embarrassing to discuss the extent and quality of their interest in sex. Self-report questionnaires may be helpful in this respect, but it is important to follow up their responses on these questionnaires to clarify whether they, indeed, have little or no interest in having sexual experiences with another person.

It is also important to be sure that the person has understood the intention of the item. We ask if the person is interested in becoming sexually involved "with someone" rather than "with another person" as a literal application of the *DSM-IV* phrasing can imply an interest in having sex with somebody other than a current lover (i.e., "another" person). It is also important not to imply that the interest has to be heterosexual. Interviewers will, at times, ask male subjects about a history of "girlfriends" or female subjects about "boyfriends," not realizing that this reflects a presumption that the person is heterosexual. We recommend keeping the inquiries neutral with respect to sexual orientation in case the person prefers to keep his or her sexual orientation confidential. Finally, it is important to recognize that the item concerns sexual experiences with a person. Extremely schizoid persons may have little interest or pleasure in any sexual activity (consistent with an extreme anhedonia assessed in SZD-4), but this item is confined to an interpersonal context. Some schizoid persons will have an active sex life but it won't involve sex with another person (e.g., they may masturbate frequently), or the relationship may be entirely impersonal (e.g., sexual relationships that are confined to prostitutes with whom there is no sense of intimacy, relatedness, or emotional feeling).

Interest in having sexual experiences only with prostitutes would not technically qualify for this item (because it clearly does involve sex with another person). In such cases, we inquire as to the reason for this specific preference. If the person emphasizes the impersonal nature of the relationship (i.e., no need to talk, no shared feelings, and no possibility of emotional involvement or commitment), then we might consider it to be an example of this item. However, a reliance or emphasis on prostitutes may also occur for other reasons (e.g., an interest in a particular type of sexual activity, denigration of a sexual partner, or insecurity in approaching potential sexual partners).

An additional assessment issue is what is meant by "interest" and/or what is the basis for an apparent disinterest. Persons who are sexually inhibited or repressed, or whose moral values are inconsistent with a very active sex life, may convey little overt or apparent interest in sex. They may have had few (or no) sexual relationships prior to or even during a marriage, and may indicate that they are largely indifferent to any increase in sexual activity. To the extent that the disinterest reflects a moral or value judgment, it should not be included. Anxious or inhibited persons may also deny any interest, but this is often assessed by asking if it would trouble them if they went their entire lives without ever becoming sexually involved with another person. Finally, some persons may be sexually active but indicate little interest in the physical sexual experience. To such persons, interest may imply substantial physical pleasure. They may enjoy the intimacy and closeness but obtain little sexual satisfaction (e.g., persons with an Axis I psychosexual dysfunction). Some schizoid persons may, indeed, have an Axis I psychosexual arousal disorder (APA, 1994), but if a person does enjoy or desire the intimacy and closeness of a sexual relationship, we would not consider this to reflect a schizoid personality trait.

Criterion SZD-4

Takes pleasure in few, if any, activities.

Revisions and Rationale: This item replaces the *DSM-III-R* item of "rarely, if ever, claims or appears to experience strong emotions, such as anger and joy" (APA, 1987, p. 340). This *DSM-III-R* item obtained among the lowest sensitivity and specificity rates (Kalus et al., 1993). A difficulty with the earlier version of this item was its suggestion that schizoid persons rarely become upset, or never become angry, sad, or anxious. The affect of schizoid persons is severely constricted, but this feature was already captured by item SZD-7 (constricted affect). The *DSM-IV* revision emphasizes the trait of anhedonia or a significantly reduced experience of pleasure (Kalus et al., 1993; Siever, 1992). Examples given in the *DSM-IV* text discussion of SZD PD include "a reduced experience of pleasure from sensory, bodily, or interpersonal experiences, such as walking on a beach at sunset or having sex" (APA, 1994, p. 638).

Rating:

0) Absent
1) Takes pleasure in few, if any, activities
2) Takes pleasure in no activities

Questions:

a. What are some of the things that give you pleasure?

b. Do you really enjoy doing [*insert answer to a*]?

c. Do you find that you just don't seem to get much sense of enjoyment out of most everything?

Issues and Problems: This criterion states that the person takes pleasure in few (if any) activities. A person could then (if the item was interpreted literally) obtain intense pleasure in one particular activity but no other activities. However, the intention of the item is not to identify persons who have limited spheres of activity that give them pleasure, but persons who have limited abilities to experience pleasure. We would not consider this item to be present if the person found any activity to be intensely pleasurable. Anhedonia implies an impairment in the ability to experience pleasure in all activities (Chapman & Chapman, 1985, 1987; Chapman, Chapman, & Raulin, 1976; Mishlove & Chapman, 1985). Persons whose pleasures are limited to just one or two activities (e.g., sex or drugs) are more appropriately considered to be "obsessed" or "dependent" upon these activities rather than anhedonic.

The reduced sense of pleasure will usually be evident in all activities of schizoid persons. They may describe themselves as enjoying some activities, but the level of enjoyment is invariably lower than for others who share the same pleasure. For example, they may say that they enjoy reading, walks, or sex, but they would not say (with any substantial enthusiasm) that they "really enjoy," "love," or "have a fantastic time" doing these things. This reduced experience of pleasure is, at times, evident by their indifference as to whether the activity might continue. They might say that they enjoy going to movies or reading, but it wouldn't really matter if they couldn't do the activity for a while, even if it was their major source of pleasure. However, it is important to note that some schizoid persons will use drugs (or sex) to experience a degree of arousal and pleasure that is not normally available to them. They may, then, be very concerned about losing this only source of pleasure. However, one will often be able to determine that the person is relying on an activity to avoid a general sense of anhedonia if there is an indication that they have had substantial difficulties with feelings of boredom, emptiness, or emotional flatness prior to this activity.

In the assessment of this item, it is also important to document that the absence of interest or pleasure in activities has been characteristic throughout the person's adult life. Persons who are depressed, or who have recently experienced a traumatic event, may describe themselves as having little pleasure or interest in most to all activities. Determining that the loss of interest is secondary to a mood disorder will be particularly difficult in cases of chronic dysthymia (see the discussion for the depressive PD). In addition, as noted in the *DSM-IV* text discussion, persons who have moved from rural to metropolitan environments or immigrants from other countries may exhibit an emotional "freezing" that might include the appearance of being cold, indifferent, and socially isolated (APA, 1994).

An additional issue in the assessment of this item is its differentiation from the prior items of neither desires nor enjoys close relationships (SZD-1), almost always chooses solitary activities (SZD-2), and little (if any) interest in having sexual experiences with another person (SZD-3). We will typically give priority to items 1 and 3 when there is difficulty in their differentiation, as they concern a specific form of pleasure or interest (i.e., intimacy and sexual relationships with another person, respectively). In order for the current item to be considered present, there must be an absence of pleasure in other activities that are typically enjoyed by people (e.g., reading, movies, games, sports, or music; Chapman et al., 1976). The differentiation from item SZD-2 (almost always chooses solitary activities) is less problematic, as persons can enjoy intensely the activities they do by themselves.

Criterion SZD-5

Lacks close friends or confidants other than first-degree relatives.

Revisions and Rationale: The *DSM-III* version of this item was "close friendships with no more than one or two persons, including family members" (APA, 1980, p. 311). The item was revised in *DSM-III-R* to "has no close friends or confidants (or only one) other than first-degree relatives" (APA, 1987, p. 340). It was revised for *DSM-IV,* in part, to be congruent with the ICD-10 version (which combines this item with SZD-1, by indicating a "lack of close friends or confiding relationships...and of desire for such relationships;" WHO, 1992, p. 203) (Kalus et al., 1993). However, more importantly, the *DSM-III-R* version was not particularly realistic. The prototypic schizoid person would have virtually no close friends or confidants (including first-degree relatives), but many schizoid persons may have one or two. The 1978 draft version of this criterion was, perhaps, preferable to the final *DSM-III* version, as it required simply "few, if any, close friends" (Task Force, 1978, p. K:8).

The requirement of a virtual absence of close friends or confidants has probably been ignored in many studies. This item obtained the highest sensitivity in the *DSM-IV* MacArthur studies (it was very common in schizoid persons) but among the lowest specificity (it also occurred in many persons who did not have a schizoid PD). This finding of substantial sensitivity but moderate to weak specificity is surprising if SZD-5 is interpreted as meaning virtually no close friends or confidants. However, if the item has, in fact, been interpreted as indicating a severe deficit in the quantity or quality of close relationships, then the findings are not surprising. A person who neither desires nor enjoys close relationships (item SZD-1) will likely have few (if any) close friends or confidants. The item describes the obvious behavioral or interpersonal consequence of lacking the desire. Schizoid persons will be socially isolated loners (APA, 1994). Many other persons may also have few close friends or confidants, but this will be for reasons other than a lack of desire.

Rating:

0) Absent
1) Lacks close friends or confidants other than first-degree relatives
2) No close friends or confidants other than first-degree relatives

Questions:

a. How many close friends (other than relatives) do you have?
b. How often do you invite them over, call them up just to talk, or ask them to go out and do something?
c. Do you confide in them or tell them about any troubles, problems, or fears?
d. Would it be important for you to keep in touch with them if they moved away?

Issues and Problems: As indicated in the discussion of this item for the schizotypal criteria set, a difficulty in its assessment is interpreting what is meant by "lacks" or "close" friends. *DSM-III-R* was quite specific, defining it as none or only one (other than a first-degree relative). However, this specificity was not really helpful. A common difficulty was that schizoid persons will often describe themselves as having more than one close friend or confidant. People will have approached them, and they may have passively acquiesced to invitations. Schizoid persons will interact with others at work, and they may often "confide" in these people (or at least tell them things about themselves). They may then describe these colleagues or acquaintances as close friends. In other words, it is not so much the number of relationships that is important but the superficiality or depth of these relationships. Therefore, we ask how often they invite people to their apartment/house, how often they suggest to someone that they go and do something together, how often they call someone on the phone just to talk, and whether it has been important to them to keep in touch with close friends who have moved away. We find these questions to be useful in assessing the passivity and superficiality of their apparent friendships. As noted in *DSM-III-R*, relationships with relatives (and therapists) would not qualify.

It is noted in the *DSM-IV* text discussion that schizoid persons will have no close friends or confidants other than a spouse or a first-degree relative (APA, 1994). Marriage would be unusual in someone who neither desires nor enjoys a close relationship (including being part of a family), has little (if any) interest in sexual experiences with another person, and lacks close friends or confidants. The presence of a marriage that involves emotional intimacy should question the presence of many of the schizoid PD items. It was noted in the *DSM-III-R* text discussion for SZD PD that "males with this disorder are usually incapable of dating and rarely marry" (APA, 1987, p. 339). It is possible for some schizoid persons to get married out of convenience, passive (or indifferent) acquiescence, and/or simply because it appeared to be the normal thing to do. They may, in fact, confide in this spouse, describe themselves as being close, and perceive the marriage as being satisfying and successful. On the other hand, the marriage is unlikely to be satisfying or successful to the spouse, unless schizoid traits are (for some reason) desirable to this spouse.

Persons with an avoidant PD may also lack close friends or confidants (*DSM-III-R* had included the earlier version of this criterion with the criteria set for the avoidant PD; APA, 1987). However, avoidant persons intensely desire such relationships (in contrast to SZD-1) and may eventually develop a very close relationship upon which they may become quite dependent. The presence of the strong desire and the disappointment in being so alone will readily differentiate avoidant and schizoid persons with respect to this item (Trull, Widiger, & Frances, 1987).

However, as we noted with respect to this item within the schizotypal criteria set, we make no distinction between the schizotypal and schizoid PDs with respect to this item. It is our clinical impression that schizoid persons will have fewer relationships than schizotypal persons, as their anhedonic indifference will be more debilitating toward obtaining and sustaining a relationship than the schizotypal discomfort and anxiety. However, this distinction is more appropriately made with respect to the items that directly concern the desire, manner, or quality of relatedness (e.g., SZD-1 and SZD-6, and SZT-9) rather than the number of relationships. Both schizoid and schizotypal persons will have few to no close friends or confidants.

A final issue in the assessment of this item is the consideration of situational reasons for the absence of close friends or confidants. New arrivals to a country, city, or community may appear and describe themselves as having no close friends or confidants. Differentiation of such cases is readily addressed by the documentation that the isolation has (or has not) been characteristic throughout the person's adult life. What is, at times, more problematic is the isolation experienced by persons as they age and experience the death of close friends and relatives. Some may be resigned to and appear to prefer the solitude. However, it may not be appropriate to consider an adjustment to their aging and isolation as reflecting an actual change in their personality. Also, *DSM-IV* does not actually recognize an adult onset schizoid PD (see chapter 2). All of the PDs must have been evident since late childhood or adolescence. One is free to reject this requirement, but it should be explicitly documented as a deviation from the *DSM-IV* when this is done.

Criterion SZD-6

Appears indifferent to the praise or criticism of others.

Revisions and Rationale: The *DSM-III* version of this item was "indifference to praise or criticism or to the feelings of others" (APA, 1980, p. 311). It was revised in *DSM-III-R* to simply "indifferent to the praise and criticism of others," (APA, 1987, p. 340) to reduce its complexity. This item has been useful in differentiating schizoid PD from avoidant and schizotypal PDs because these latter personality disorders involve considerable social anxiety and hypersensitivity. However, the item consistently obtained the lowest sensitivity rates in the *DSM-IV* MacArthur studies, occurring in at most 34% of the schizoid subjects and within one study in none of the schizoid subjects (Kalus et al., 1993). It is rare to find someone who is truly indifferent. It was, therefore, revised in *DSM-IV* "to include individuals who appear indifferent to praise or criticism, but who do, indeed, have an underlying sensitivity" (Kalus et al., 1993, p. 51). Clinicians have often indicated that once a facade of schizoid indifference is broken, one finds substantial suffering, loneliness, and insecurity (Guntrip, 1968). It is noted in the *DSM-IV* text discussion of schizoid PD that schizoid persons may acknowledge having painful feelings, particularly related to social interactions, when they become (at least temporarily) comfortable within a relationship (APA, 1994).

Rating:

0) Absent
1) Appears indifferent to the praise or criticism of others
2) Appears indifferent, with no apparent underlying sensitivity to praise or criticism

Questions:

a. Have people often hurt your feelings? (*If "no":*) Are your feelings rarely hurt?

b. Are you often self-conscious? (*If "no":*) Are you rarely self-conscious?

c. Are you largely indifferent to what other people think of you?

Issues and Problems: The revision to this item is useful because few schizoid persons are ever entirely or truly indifferent. However, a difficulty in the assessment of this item is the differentiation from avoidant PD. If a schizoid person does not have to be indifferent, and may, in fact, be quite sensitive, there may be little difference between schizoid and avoidant persons in their response to this item. However, to the extent that the person appears overtly self-conscious, timid, or sensitive (i.e., avoidant), he or she would not be given this criterion. Schizoid persons will at least present an appearance of indifference, and will, in fact, be much less sensitive to praise or criticism than even the average (normal) person. They may not be entirely indifferent, and, at times, they will acknowledge having been pleased by some praise or hurt by some criticism, but they will appear to be detached from and indifferent to the praise and criticism (and feelings) of others. Avoidant persons, on the other hand, will be overly sensitive.

Persons who have suffered a recent trauma or stress may also appear temporarily indifferent to the praise or criticism of others. Thus, it is particularly important in the assessment of this item to document that this indifference has been characteristic throughout the adult life. As we noted earlier in the discussion of SZD-4 (takes pleasure in few activities,) persons who have moved from rural to metropolitan environments or immigrants from other countries may exhibit an emotional "freezing" that might include the appearance of being cold, indifferent, and socially isolated (APA, 1994).

Antisocial and narcissistic persons will also be indifferent to the feelings of others, but this typically reflects a lack of empathy or a tough-minded, antagonistic coldness. Narcissistic persons will, in fact, be quite sensitive to praise or criticism (high self-consciousness) at the same time that they are indifferent to the feelings of others (low empathy). Narcissistic persons will, at times, appear indifferent to praise or criticism, but this will usually reflect a disdainful arrogance (i.e., devaluing the worth or significance of the opinions of others) or a facade of self-confidence (i.e., insecure denial). Schizoid persons are not conflicted over how important the opinions of others are (or should be) to their own self-esteem. They are struggling with how little other people actually mean to them; the opinions of others actually mean very little to them.

Criterion SZD-7

Shows emotional coldness, detachment, or flattened affectivity.

Revisions and Rationale: The *DSM-III-R* version of this item was "displays constricted affect, e.g., is aloof, cold, rarely reciprocates gestures or facial expressions, such as smiles or nods" (APA, 1987, p. 340). The purpose of this item was to portray the behavioral presentation of schizoid emotional detachment. Constricted affect, however, does not describe sufficiently the extent of the affective detachment, as persons with obsessive-compulsive PD will also be constricted in their expression of feelings (APA, 1987, 1994). The *DSM-IV* revision was derived largely from the ICD-10 criterion that specified an "emotional coldness, detachment, or flattened affectivity" (WHO, 1992, p. 203). This revision implies a higher threshold for attribution than simply a constricted affect. The *DSM-IV* revision also returns somewhat to the *DSM-III* version, which stated an "emotional coldness and aloofness, and absence of warm, tender feelings for others" (APA, 1980, p. 311).

Rating:

0) Absent
1) Shows emotional coldness, detachment, or flattened affectivity
2) Shows emotional coldness, detachment, <u>and</u> flattened affectivity

Questions:

a. [*If the respondent did not smile (laugh, nod, etc.) much during the interview:*] I noticed that you didn't smile [*laugh, nod, etc.*] much during this interview; is this usually the case?

b. Do you tend to always keep a straight face? Do you rarely express much feeling in the way you look?

c. Have you ever felt warm, tender, or sentimental about someone? Have you ever been in love?

Issues and Problems: A difficulty in the assessment of this item is that it is quite broad. The presence of almost any one of the prior items will often qualify for this item. Neither desiring nor enjoying close relationships (SZD-1), always choosing solitary activities (SZD-2), taking pleasure in no activities (SZD-4), having no close friends or confidants (SZD-5), or being indifferent to praise and criticism (SZD-6), would each imply an emotional coldness and/or detachment. Therefore, we do not consider this item until all of the others have been considered, and we then confine its assessment to material not previously covered. As a result, we tend to give most of the emphasis to the flattened affectivity. To the extent that this occurs, this item becomes simply a more severe variant of the *DSM-III-R* version (i.e., rather than assessing for a constricted affect, one assesses for a flattened affect).

Flat affect can also be difficult to assess (Andreasen, 1979a). Its assessment will usually be based on one's observations of the person (i.e., no change in facial expression, never smiling or nodding, consistently bland, monotone voice, and failure to reciprocate gestures or facial expressions). Our questions, in fact, emphasize observations during the interview.

However, it is important to make additional inquiries regarding the person's usual level of expressivity, because the appearance of flattened affectivity may also reflect a (depressed) mood disorder, pharmacologic treatment, or some other factor (Andreasen, 1979a).

Inquiries regarding whether the person has ever felt warm, tender, or sentimental toward someone, or ever been passionately in love, are also helpful, unless this assessment was included in a previous item (e.g., lacking the desire for a close relationship, or a lack of close friends). Schizoid persons will lack feelings of warmth, tenderness, love, and sentimentality (as indicated in the *DSM-III* version of this item; APA, 1980). It would be unusual for them ever to feel very sad or tearful as they discuss how they lost or missed someone. However, some persons who are not schizoid may deny such feelings because they are inconsistent with their pride in independence or emotional strength (e.g., antisocial, psychopathic, or narcissistic persons). In addition, as we have noted previously, persons who have moved from rural to metropolitan environments or immigrants from other countries may exhibit an emotional "freezing" that might include the appearance of being cold and indifferent (APA, 1994).

Restricted affectivity is also characteristic of persons with schizotypal, paranoid, and, to a lesser extent, obsessive-compulsive PD. Constricted affect is one of the *DSM-IV* criteria for schizotypal PD (APA, 1994). "Restricted ability to express warm and tender emotions" was a *DSM-III* criterion for the obsessive-compulsive PD (APA, 1980, p. 327), "restricted expression of affection" was a *DSM-III-R* criterion for OBC PD (APA, 1987, p. 356), and it is noted in the *DSM-IV* text for OBC PD that the expression of affection is usually highly controlled or stilted and that the person may be very uncomfortable in the presence of others who are being emotionally expressive (APA, 1994). Finally, restricted affectivity, as indicated, for example, by the appearance of being cold and unemotional, and the absence of passive, soft, tender, and sentimental feelings, was included in the *DSM-III* criteria for paranoid PD (APA, 1980) and is noted within the associated features in *DSM-III-R* and *DSM-IV* (APA, 1987, 1994). The deletion of restricted affectivity from the obsessive-compulsive and paranoid PD criteria sets in *DSM-IV* is helpful in reducing artifactual co-occurrence, but persons with obsessive-compulsive, paranoid, and schizotypal PDs will, in fact, display a restricted affectivity. At times, a distinction may be made on the basis of the extent of the affective impairment. Range of affect can be distinguished along four levels: broad (normal), restricted (or constricted), blunted, or flat (APA, 1987, 1994). Normal expression of affect will include variability in facial expression, voice pitch, and gestures. Constricted or restricted affect involves a clear reduction in the expression and intensity of affect, but in flat affect there is essentially no expression (e.g., the voice is a monotone, there is little to no arm or hand movement, and the face is immobile with no change in expression). Only the schizoid PD is characterized by flat affect. In addition, the restriction of affect for the obsessive-compulsive PD is typically associated with excessive intellectualization, particularly in regard to feelings of warmth, affection, and sentimentality. There is often an effort on the part of the obsessive-compulsive person to express feelings, but this is done in a stilted, formal, or awkward manner. Both obsessive-compulsive and paranoid persons may also exhibit substantial anger (APA, 1994). Finally, the presence of both flat and inappropriate affect would be diagnostic of the schizotypal PD rather than the schizoid PD.

13

Schizotypal Personality Disorder

Overview: Schizotypal (SZT) personality disorder was a new addition to *DSM-III* (APA, 1980). The original criteria set was derived from cases of "borderline schizophrenia" diagnosed in the biological relatives of persons with schizophrenia (Siever & Klar, 1986; Spitzer et al., 1979; Stone, 1993). SZT PD was defined in *DSM-III-R* as a pervasive pattern of "deficits in interpersonal relatedness and peculiarities of ideation, appearance, and behavior" (APA, 1987, p. 341). The only revision to this definition for *DSM-IV* was to specify that these social and interpersonal deficits consist of acute discomfort with and reduced capacity for close relationships (APA, 1994).

A proposal considered for *DSM-IV* was to provide a preamble to the SZT criteria stating that "these signs and symptoms should not be limited to discrete periods of mood symptomatology (e.g., depression, anxiety, anger)" (Task Force, 1991, p. R:4). The purpose of this general exclusion criterion was to facilitate the differentiation of SZT PD from the borderline PD, with which there has been substantial co-occurrence and problematic differentiation (Pfohl et al., 1986; Siever, Bernstein, & Silverman, 1991; Siever & Klar, 1986; Spitzer et al., 1979; Widiger et al., 1986). However, a *DSM-IV* MacArthur-funded pilot study of this proposal found that it resulted in little improvement in the differentiation from borderline PD, although it did reduce substantially the number of persons who would receive the diagnosis (e.g., from 43 to 25) (Silverman et al., in press). The PD Work Group and *DSM-IV* Task Force were then concerned that the revision would have a substantial effect on the diagnosis and the construct of a schizotypal PD without actually addressing the problem it was intended to address. There was also a concern that such a general exclusion criterion would not be used reliably. It was applied reliably in the pilot study, but this effort might not generalize to clinical practice or other studies that were not specifically focused on the exclusion criterion or supported by a semistructured interview.

The *DSM-III-R* criteria for SZT PD consisted of nine items, any five of which were necessary for its diagnosis. Only three of these items received significant revision for *DSM-IV*, two remained unchanged, and four received only minor revisions in wording or clarification (the threshold for diagnosis remains at 5 of 9). The major issues for *DSM-IV* were the differentiation from borderline and avoidant PDs and the relationship of SZT PD to schizophrenia (Siever, Bernstein, & Silverman, 1991).

A proposal considered for *DSM-IV* was to move SZT PD from Axis II to the schizophrenia section of Axis I (Siever et al., 1991). SZT PD is considered by most theorists, researchers, and clinicians to represent a characterologic variant of schizophrenic pathology, its historical precedent in *DSM-II* was latent schizophrenia (APA, 1968, p. 34), and ICD-10 includes it among the schizophrenic rather than the personality disorders (i.e., schizotypal disorder; WHO, 1992, pp. 95-96). However, it is likely that some of the other

DSM-IV personality disorders also represent characterologic variants of Axis I disorders (Siever & Davis, 1991; Widiger & Shea, 1991). It would be inconsistent to move just one, and it is not at all clear which others to move nor even, necessarily, where to move them. In addition, even if SZT PD does represent a characterologic of schizophrenia, it is still a disorder of personality (character) and, therefore, belongs with the other personality (character) disorders. A genetic association with schizophrenia provides an explanation for its etiology, and *DSM-IV* is organized with respect to phenomenology rather than etiology.

However, *DSM-IV* does provide an additional exclusion criterion to clarify the diagnosis of SZT in the context of schizophrenia. *DSM-IV* indicates that one should note that SZT PD is "premorbid" if the behavior pattern was evident prior to the onset of schizophrenia. Premorbid schizotypal traits would have prognostic significance for the course and treatment of the schizophrenia, and such traits should then be noted (Siever, 1992). However, it might not even be meaningful to suggest that the person had a schizotypal personality disorder that was independent of or unrelated to the eventual schizophrenia. Once a person develops schizophrenia, a diagnosis of schizotypal PD can become rather pointless. All of the schizotypal PD symptoms are readily understood as symptoms of schizophrenia. The only time it might be meaningful to diagnose schizotypal PD would be when the traits preceded the onset of schizophrenia, but even in these cases, the schizotypal traits could represent the prodromal phase of schizophrenia.

This issue is noted as well in the discussion for the schizoid PD, but it is particularly problematic for SZT PD because the schizotypal criteria set closely resembles the criteria for the prodromal/residual phase of schizophrenia. In fact, a proposal considered for *DSM-III-R* was to make the criteria for SZT PD equivalent to the prodromal/residual phases of schizohrenia (Widiger et al., 1988). If this revision had occurred, then the differentiation of SZT PD from the prodromal phase of schizophrenia would concern simply the time of onset of the symptomatology; if the prodromal symptoms had appeared by late childhood or adolescence, there might not be any meaningful distinction.

The distinctions that do exist between SZT PD and the prodromal phase of schizophrenia can be quite subtle and difficult to assess reliably (e.g., markedly peculiar behavior for the prodromal phase vs. peculiar behavior for SZT, and marked lack of initiative, interests, or energy for the prodomal phase vs. no indication of such decrease for SZT). One can readily confuse schizotypal PD traits with a lengthy and insidious prodromal phase of schizophrenia (resulting in the failure to provide early and aggressive treatment of the schizophrenia). Differentiating schizotypal personality traits from a prodromal phase of schizophrenia in someone who is currently within the active (or any) phase of schizophrenia can be exceedingly difficult (e.g., requiring a retrospective assessment of the onset and duration of symptoms). Even if one can document a distinct onset of a more rapid progression of withdrawal, detachment, and deterioration (i.e., a clear worsening of the schizotypal traits prior to the onset of the active phase) the schizotypal traits that preceded this apparent prodromal phase could ultimately be shown to represent subtle, subthreshold schizophrenic pathology. Therefore, if one does diagnose SZT PD in someone who is also suffering from schizophrenia, it should be noted that it is (at best) a premorbid personality disorder. Table 13-1 presents the *DSM-IV* criteria set for the schizotypal PD diagnosis.

Table 13-1
DSM-IV Criteria for Schizotypal Personality Disorder

A. A pervasive pattern of social and interpersonal deficits marked by acute discomfort with, and reduced capacity for, close relationships as well as by cognitive or perceptual distortions and eccentricities of behavior, beginning by early adulthood, and present in a variety of contexts, as indicated by five (or more) of the following:

(1) ideas of reference (excluding delusions of reference)

(2) odd beliefs or magical thinking that influences behavior and is inconsistent with subcultural norms (e.g., superstitiousness, belief in clairvoyance, telepathy, or "sixth sense"; in children and adolescents, bizarre fantasies or preoccupations)

(3) unusual perceptual experiences, including bodily illusions

(4) odd thinking and speech (e.g., vague, circumstantial, metaphorical, overelaborate, or stereotyped)

(5) suspiciousness or paranoid ideation

(6) inappropriate or constricted affect

(7) behavior or appearance that is odd, eccentric, or peculiar

(8) lack of close friends or confidants other than first-degree relatives

(9) excessive social anxiety that does not diminish with familiarity and tends to be associated with paranoid fears rather than negative judgments about self

B. Does not occur exclusively during the course of schizophrenia, a mood disorder with psychotic features, another psychotic disorder, or a pervasive developmental disorder.

Note: If criteria are met prior to the onset of schizophrenia, add "premorbid," e.g. "schizotypal personality disorder (premorbid)."

Note. From *Diagnostic and Statistical Manual of Mental Disorders* (4th ed., p. 645), by American Psychiatric Association, 1994, Washington, DC: Author. Copyright 1994 by American Psychiatric Association. Reprinted with permission.

Criterion SZT-1

Ideas of reference (excluding delusions of reference).

Revisions and Rationale: This item was unchanged from *DSM-III-R*. The only change from *DSM-III* had been the specification that delusions of reference are excluded. Ideas of reference are beliefs, impressions, or feelings that incidents, events, objects, or other people within the person's immediate environment are expressing a particular and unusual meaning or relevance to oneself (APA, 1987, 1994). These beliefs are not held with a firm conviction that does not yield to further reflection, review, reassurance by others, or other form of reality testing. Otherwise, they would be considered delusions of reference (a delusion is defined as a false personal belief that is firmly sustained in spite of what almost everyone else believes and in spite of what constitutes incontrovertible, obvious proof to the contrary; APA, 1987, 1994). A common example of an idea of reference would be the incorrect sense that persons nearby are taking special notice of oneself in some important, odd, vulgar, meaningful, or significant way (beyond simply a passing comment or reaction). For example, the person might believe that others are talking about his or her sexuality, recent divorce, or ethnicity. A more severe example would be the belief that something in the news, a novel, or song lyrics have some special significance or importance for them. In each case, they would be aware that the belief makes little sense and is, perhaps, unlikely to really be true, but they would either have difficulty shaking the sense that it might be true or repeatedly have such experiences.

The placement of ideas of reference at the top of the list in *DSM-IV* should not be interpreted as indicating that it is the most diagnostic item. It was among the most diagnostic items in the *DSM-IV* MacArthur studies, along with odd beliefs or magical thinking and odd speech. Prior research has also reported excellent findings for the predictive power of unusual perceptual experiences and paranoid, suspicious ideation (Widiger, Frances, & Trull, 1987).

Rating:

0) Absent
1) Ideas of reference (excluding delusions of reference)
2) Preoccupation with ideas of reference

Questions:

a. Have you ever experienced any odd coincidences or occurrences that might have had some special significance for you?
b. Have you ever received any special guidance from some unusual or odd event?
c. Have you often had the idea or sensed that people on a bus or in a restaurant were talking about you?
d. Have you often thought that a comment you overheard was purposely directed at you, or that it referred to you?

Issues and Problems: A difficulty in the assessment of this item is distinguishing it from delusions of reference. Complicating this boundary is the fact that schizotypal persons will, at times, have brief psychotic experiences (Siever, 1992) during which their ideas of reference may become delusions of reference. And, persons who have been delusional in the past may now deny that they held these beliefs with any real confidence or conviction. However, to the extent that there is, in fact, a suggestion that the person may be or has been delusional, attention should then be given to ruling out schizophrenia. If this is done, then emphasis should be given to assessing the chronicity of the ideation. A history of the occurrence of ideas of reference since adolescence would not be negated by occasional, brief episodes of delusional proportions.

The boundary with normal functioning can be equally problematic. Many persons will have had a fleeting sense, for example, that some stranger(s) were talking about them. It is always important to assess how often this has happened and how deviant or aberrant was the experience. Few persons will be able to describe (or remember) repeated experiences, and some examples are more deviant than others (e.g., a fleeting sense that a group of strangers are talking about oneself is less pathological than believing that a grand jury investigation reported on the news may be concerned with oneself). Members of certain religious groups may also believe that "God spoke to them" through coincidences or signs that have a personal significance. Such persons may interpret these incidents as providing a divine guidance to assist them with an important personal decision. In most cases, such beliefs will occur within a shared framework of religious meaning and should not be considered pathological. Pathological elaborations of spiritual ideas of reference will usually seem odd, exaggerated, or misguided to other adherents of the same belief system.

An additional issue is the distinction between an idea of reference and magical thinking. Some ideas of reference are also readily classified as magical thinking (covered in SZT-2) such as the appearance of a magical or spiritual number during a lottery broadcast that is then interpreted as having some special significance for oneself. If the magical thinking involves the belief that the event, incident, or occurrence has some special significance or meaning to oneself (e.g., the number is a sign or in response to something one did) then we would consider this to represent an idea of reference. When the judgment is ambiguous, we favor considering it as an idea of reference because odd beliefs and magical thinking encompass a much wider range of aberrant cognitions.

Criterion SZT-2

Odd beliefs or magical thinking that influences behavior and is inconsistent with subcultural norms (e.g., superstitiousness; belief in clairvoyance, telepathy, or "sixth sense"; in children and adolescents, bizarre fantasies or preoccupations).

Revisions and Rationale: This item was essentially unchanged from *DSM-III-R*. The only revision was a grammatical change in wording and the deletion of the example that "others can feel my feelings" (APA, 1987, p. 342) because it was too aberrant and approached the level of a delusion. The only revision to this item from *DSM-III* to *DSM-III-R* had been the addition of odd beliefs alongside magical thinking. Magical thinking is defined as a belief that thoughts, words, or actions might or will, in some manner, cause or prevent a specific outcome in a way that is contrary to known laws of cause and effect (APA, 1987, 1994). Odd beliefs and magical thinking have long been a part of the description of the schizotypal personality disorder (Meehl, 1964). They are among the more diagnostic symptoms of SZT PD.

Rating:

0) Absent
1) Odd beliefs or magical thinking that influences behaviors and is inconsistent with subcultural norms (e.g., superstitiousness, belief in clairvoyance, telepathy, or sixth sense [*In children and adolescents consider bizarre fantasies or preoccupations.*]
2) Preoccupation with a variety of odd beliefs and magical thinking

Questions:

a. Do you have any unusual superstitions?

b. Do you believe in telepathy? clairvoyance? precognition? a sixth sense? ESP? [*Ask each in turn, not all at once.*] or anything else along these lines? (*If "yes":*) Have these beliefs ever had a significant effect on what you do?

Issues and Problems: The examples provided in *DSM-IV* are helpful, but they also demonstrate the breadth of the item. Included within this item are almost any and all odd beliefs that one might have (e.g., superstitions, clairvoyance, telepathy, sixth sense, reincarnation, astrology, occultism, the supernatural, transcendentalism, exorcism, paranormal events, cabalism, voodoo, satanism, fortune-telling, shamanism, and magical prayer). The range of beliefs could extend from a mild superstition to the boundary of a delusion.

However, normative superstitions and magical behaviors should not be included, even when they influence behavior. Taking a lucky charm to the race track, throwing salt over one's shoulder, or some magical algorithm for selecting a number to play in the lottery are not inconsistent with cultural norms. Many persons will follow superstitions and, on occasion, display magical thinking, but they usually do not take these behaviors too seriously. We do include common superstitions when the person has acted upon many of them, perhaps to the point that everyday behavior is closely and continually guided by such superstition or magical thinking.

A more difficult problem in assessment is the consistency of certain magical beliefs with subcultural norms. Many religious traditions accept apparently superstitious behavior as a means of imploring divine intervention (e.g., lighting candles in a church to secure the intercession of a saint, speaking in tongues, or praying for healing by laying on of hands). Such beliefs will appear aberrant and magical to members of other religious or cultural groups, whose own beliefs may appear magical to still other persons. This will be particularly problematic in the assessment of persons from religious or cultural groups that are a minority or atypical within the society of the interviewer. On the other hand, many of the magical beliefs held by a particular subculture will be adopted by schizotypal persons. And, to the extent that a schizotypal person does take these beliefs seriously and acts on them (i.e., the beliefs influence behavior), the person is likely to be drawn to a subculture that would accept, endorse, or encourage such beliefs. Inconsistency with a subcultural norm to which the person currently belongs could be indicated by (a) adhering to additional aberrant, bizarre beliefs that are beyond or rejected by this particular group, (b) a history of developing but then just as quickly abandoning them, or (c) a history of joining, then leaving, esoteric groups.

However, in the absence of such a history, we may still consider the item to be present when the beliefs are consistent with a subcultural group. The purpose of the exclusion criterion is to avoid labeling all aberrant or deviant beliefs as schizotypal (e.g., Christian Science, astrology, and transcendentalism). Nevertheless, groups which advocate deviant, unusual belief systems will attract schizotypal persons, and it is clinically advisable not to deny this fact or avoid ever making the diagnosis of members of such groups. We may consider the item to be present if the persons joined or entered the group after they had developed the deviant, aberrant belief system. They would, in fact, have an odd belief that has significantly influenced their behavior (e.g., prompted them to change their religious orientation). This has the potential of including persons who are not schizotypal, but they would not receive a diagnosis of SZT PD unless they have four of the remaining eight criteria. However, we do adhere to the subcultural norm exclusion criterion in that we usually exclude persons who were raised within the particular subculture.

A final point is that some persons are reluctant to acknowledge aberrant, peculiar, or superstitious beliefs, particularly those schizotypal persons with suspicious, paranoid ideation (SZT-5). Interviews with staff, relatives, colleagues, or friends can be helpful in the assessment of this item. We have also found self-report inventories to be helpful (Bailey, West, Widiger, & Freiman, 1993; Eckblad & Chapman, 1983). Some persons are more willing to acknowledge these beliefs in response to a questionnaire than during a face-to-face interview, and their responses to the questionnaire can be used in a subsequent interview to initiate more detailed discussion and clarification.

Criterion SZT-3

Unusual perceptual experiences, including bodily illusions.

Revisions and Rationale: This item was essentially unchanged from *DSM-III-R*. The only revision (other than grammatical) was to move the examples from the criteria set to the text and to indicate that the perceptual experiences include bodily or somatosensory illusions. Unusual perceptual experiences have always been part of the description of the schizotypal PD (Meehl, 1964). The experiences fall just short of psychotic hallucinations, in the same manner that the odd beliefs, magical thinking, ideas of reference, and paranoid ideation described in other items fall short of delusions. Examples of this item include sensing the presence of a force or person not actually present; hypnagogic experiences; perceiving that part of one's body has been detached or misshapen (e.g., change in shape of face, or legs seem longer than usual); sensitivity to color, sounds, or light; hearing a voice murmur one's name; noticing sounds on records that were not there before; or feeling detached, unreal, or depersonalized.

Rating:

0) Absent
1) Unusual perceptual experiences, including bodily illusions
2) Preoccupation with unusual perceptual experiences

Questions:

a. Some people have unusual or peculiar experiences. For example, did you ever sense the presence of a dead relative?
b. Did you ever sense the presence of a force or a person that wasn't there?
c. Did you ever feel that things seemed unreal, in only 2 dimensions, or that everything was part of some unreal game?
d. Have you experienced anything else unusual like this?

Issues and Problems: A difficulty in the assessment of this item is distinguishing the experiences from psychotic hallucinations. One of the examples provided in the text to *DSM-IV* is hearing a voice murmur one's name (APA, 1994), which itself appears to be over the boundary of a psychotic hallucination. To the extent that the person is convinced that the experience was real and cannot be shaken from this conviction, it is more likely to represent an hallucination. However, presence versus absence of insight into the reality of the experience is not always decisive. The *DSM-III-R* definition of a psychosis required an incorrect evaluation of the accuracy of the perception (or absence of insight into its pathological nature), but it is now recognized that many persons who are psychotic do acknowledge that they are hallucinating (e.g., a person on LSD who knows it is a drug-induced hallucination or a chronic schizophrenic who knows the vividly heard voice of Jesus is not actually real) (APA, 1994). In addition, many schizotypal persons will believe that their unusual perceptual experiences involve real phenomena (e.g., they may believe that ghosts do exist and that the cold draft they often feel in a corner of a room is, in fact, from a spectre).

The distinction should also consider the more subtle points of the intensity, peculiarity (bizarreness), and vividness of the perceptual experience. Sensing the presence of a dead relative in a bedroom is less pathological than actually hearing the voice through the wall, hearing a vague sound of murmuring is less pathological than hearing a distinct and recognizable voice, and shivering at the sensation that an evil force is present is less pathological than scratching or clawing at the bugs that seem to be crawling under one's skin. Illusions (misperceptions or misinterpretations of a real external stimulus) would be less schizotypal than subthreshold hallucinations (e.g., mistaking the sound of leaves rustling as voices murmuring, as opposed to sensing voices murmuring in a silent room).

As noted above, this issue is comparable to distinguishing ideas of reference (SZT-1) and paranoid ideation (SZT-5) from delusions, and odd thinking (SZT-4) from a formal thought disorder. Complicating this assessment is the fact that schizotypal persons can have fleeting, brief psychotic experiences during which their unusual perceptual experiences become hallucinatory. Also, schizophrenic persons who have had vivid and severe hallucinations in the past may now minimize their description of these experiences, referring to them as unusual perceptual experiences. As indicated above, to the extent that the person may now be or has been hallucinating, attention should be given to ruling out schizophrenia or other psychotic disorders. If this is done, then consideration should be given to assessing the chronicity of the aberrant perceptual experiences. A history of unusual perceptual experiences in someone who does not suffer from schizophrenia would not be negated by occasional, fleeting hallucinatory experiences.

An additional issue is distinguishing schizotypal aberrant perceptual experiences from borderline PD quasipsychotic dissociative experiences. There is little in the content or intensity of the aberrant perceptions that will help in this differentiation (depersonalization and derealization are explicitly cited within this schizotypal item for ICD-10; WHO, 1992). As noted above, a proposal considered for *DSM-IV* was to require that all of the SZT items not be "limited to discrete periods of mood symptomatology (e.g., depression, anxiety, anger)" (Task Force, 1991, p. R:4). This assessment would have been quite similar to that made for a diagnosis of schizoaffective disorder, where it is determined whether schizophrenic-like psychotic symptoms occur only during episodes of a mood disorder (Siever et al., 1991). The proposal was rejected, in part, because there were insufficient data to indicate that this assessment would be made reliably or that schizotypal traits are not closely associated with mood states. The schizoaffective assessment of the association of psychotic symptoms to mood disorders is itself difficult, complex, and controversial (Blacker & Tsuang, 1992; Kendler, 1991) and such an assessment for quasipsychotic symptoms and mood states would likely be even more problematic. Nevertheless, this is the major distinction between this particular SZT item and the borderline criterion of quasipsychotic experiences (BDL-9). To the extent that the aberrant perceptions occur independently of mood or stress, the experience would represent a schizotypal symptom; to the extent that the experience was transient and clearly associated with stress, it would represent a borderline symptom. If the assessment is ambiguous, we consider it to represent a symptom of both disorders. If a distinction must be made in cases that cannot be resolved, we would advise erring in the direction of SZT PD, given that this would be more consistent with the tradition established by *DSM-III* and *DSM-III-R*. The one exception to this rule would concern chronic feelings of depersonalization or derealization (i.e., quasipsychotic extension of feelings of emptiness) that would be considered to represent borderline feelings of emptiness.

We have also found some schizotypal persons to be reluctant to acknowledge their aberrant perceptual experiences, particularly those schizotypal persons with suspicious, paranoid ideation (SZT-5). Interviews with relatives, friends, or colleagues can be helpful, but these individuals will often be unaware or uninformed, and they may base their judgments on questionable speculations concerning things they have seen the person do. As in the case with SZT-2, we have found the use of self-report measures helpful for this item. Some persons are more willing to acknowledge these experiences in response to a questionnaire than during a face-to-face interview. In addition, some inventories, such as the Perceptual Aberrations Scale (Chapman & Chapman, 1987; Chapman, Chapman & Raulin, 1978), present an extensive list of experiences that will help convey the intention of this item and provide a basis for a more detailed inquiry.

As noted in the prior discussion concerning odd beliefs, one must also be careful not to confuse perceptions that are largely normative within particular cultural or religious groups with schizotypal perceptual experiences. Beliefs, perceptions, and practices of groups that are unfamiliar to the interviewer may appear very aberrant (e.g., dissociative experiences or visions of a deceased), particularly if the subject being interviewed is an active member of this spiritual or religious group. One should become familiar with this group's culture and practice before concluding that the person is demonstrating schizotypal perceptions.

A final point is to exclude aberrant perceptual experiences that are secondary to drug usage. Extensive use of hallucinogens, amphetamines, and other substances can result in the appearance of schizotypal symptoms. Aberrant perceptual experiences that occur prior to drug usage or remain long after the acute effects of the drug have ended should be emphasized (a duration considered for *DSM-IV* was 6 months after cessation of drug usage). This assessment, however, will be difficult if the person is reluctant to acknowledge the extent of illicit, illegal drug usage. In addition, some schizotypal persons will be attracted to such substances because they help stimulate psychotic and quasipsychotic experiences.

Criterion SZT-4

Odd thinking and speech (e.g., vague, circumstantial, metaphorical, overelaborate, or stereotyped).

Revisions and Rationale: This item received substantial revision. The *DSM-III-R* version was simply "odd speech" (APA, 1987, p. 342). It was revised to "odd thinking and speech" (APA, 1994, p. 645) to be congruent with the respective criterion from the ICD-10 schizotypal diagnosis (Task Force, 1991; WHO, 1992). *DSM-III-R* was confined to odd speech only because one rarely (if ever) has information regarding the thought process other than through the speech (i.e., one observes or hears speech, not thought). However, the purpose of the item is to assess formal thought process rather than problems with articulation or verbal skills. The revision also allows the clinician or researcher to include reports or observations of odd thinking that are not clearly evident from speech alone. In most cases, however, the assessment of this item will be based on the odd manner of speaking.

More important, perhaps, is the fact that the examples of impoverished, digressive, and inappropriately abstract speech that were included in *DSM-III-R* were deleted, and circumstantial, metaphorical, overelaborate, and stereotyped thinking and speech were added. This revision was, again, for compatibility with ICD-10, but it also represents a return to the list that was provided in *DSM-III* (APA, 1980). Many of the ICD-10 criteria were derived from *DSM-III* (see chapter 3). Thus, it is then somewhat ironic that the effort to obtain international compatibility resulted in a return to *DSM-III*. In any case, these new examples may encourage a higher threshold for the attribution of the item.

Rating:

0) Absent
1) Odd thinking and speech (e.g., vague, circumstantial, metaphorical, overelaborate, or stereotyped)
2) Speech contains a variety of odd metaphors, circumstantial reasoning, and peculiar words, to the point that it becomes difficult at times to understand the meaning or follow the train of thought

Questions:

[*There are no questions for this item. Its assessment is based primarily on the person's speech during the interview. One observes for odd speech, but without loosening of associations or incoherence. Speech is unusually metaphorical, circumstantial, or overelaborate. Speech is not so unusual or distorted that you cannot understand or follow it, but there are often peculiar, idiosyncratic, or confusing words, stereotyped expressions, or odd associations. For example, the person expresses concepts oddly, or uses words in a variety of inappropriate contexts, or abstract concepts are often referred to despite their lack of relevance or applicability. Associations may be meaningful and can be followed, but they result in inappropriately lengthy or detailed responses that are often off the subject.*]

Issues and Problems: The odd thinking of this item should be distinguished from the odd beliefs and magical thinking of SZT-2. SZT-2 refers to the content of thinking (i.e., an odd belief or irrational reasoning), whereas this item refers to the presentation or process of thinking. The distinction is equivalent to that between a delusion and a formal thought disorder. Magical thinking may, at times, suggest odd thinking (or subthreshold formal thought disorder), but magical thinking refers to a particular belief that was, perhaps, derived from irrational presumptions rather than a disturbance in the processing or presentation of thought (e.g., a belief that numbers have magical powers or that a chain of unrelated events has a supernatural connection).

We often find this item to be the most difficult to assess. It is one of the least sensitive items (it is one of the least common to schizotypal persons), but when it is clearly present, it can be very diagnostic. The difficulty is that its assessment relies heavily on one's judgments of what constitutes vague, circumstantial, metaphorical, overelaborate, or stereotyped speech (Andreasen, 1979b). The most obvious, apparent, and clear examples will often cross the boundary into a schizophrenic formal thought disorder. For example, as noted in the *DSM-IV* text discussion (and included within the *DSM-III-R* criterion itself), one must assess whether the speech is loose but not to the point of a loosening of associations.

Echolalia, clanging, and incoherence are indicative of a (schizophrenic) formal thought disorder. However, we do include neologisms in the assessment of this item (in the absence of other indicators of a more psychotic thought disorder).

It is helpful to emphasize that one is assessing for odd, peculiar, strange, eccentric, or weird speech, not simply vague speech. Histrionic persons can be very vague and overelaborate; retarded persons will be concrete (and stereotyped); very intelligent persons may use many metaphors; obsessive-compulsive persons will be circumstantial; and depression, medication, exhaustion, and other factors can result in impoverished speech. Simply being vague, circumstantial, metaphorical, overelaborate, or stereotyped is not sufficient. The speech must convey an impression of being odd, peculiar, or weird.

It is also important to rule out unfamiliarity with the language. A person who is unfamiliar with the language may use certain phrases in an odd and/or repetitive manner. Some persons may also adopt a vernacular that is common to a subculture or ethnic group that can appear stereotyped or odd to someone who is unfamiliar with this style of speech. The mentally retarded and poorly educated may also speak in a manner that appears odd or peculiar to an interviewer.

Criterion SZT-5

Suspiciousness or paranoid ideation.

Revisions and Rationale: This item was unchanged from *DSM-III-R* and *DSM-III*. Suspicious, paranoid ideation is often present in persons with schizotypal PD. Paranoid ideation involves the belief that one is being harassed, persecuted, cheated, or unfairly treated (APA, 1987, 1994). The belief is not held so firmly that it is sustained despite clear evidence to the contrary (i.e., it is not a paranoid delusion). The schizotypal person is often suspicious, distrustful, and wary, but rarely (if ever) delusional.

Rating:

0) Absent
1) Suspiciousness or paranoid ideation
2) Preoccupation with suspicions or paranoid ideation

Questions:

a. Is there anyone you know who was or is treating you unfairly? (*If "yes":*) Is he or she conspiring with others behind your back?

b. Are there people you just can't trust?

c. Do you typically find that you just can't trust people?

Issues and Problems: This item overlaps with the first item, as ideas of reference will often involve paranoid ideation, (e.g., a belief that the persons they see talking in a bar may be planning on mugging them, or that construction in a street is being done purposely to annoy and trouble them). If a belief concerns strangers within their immediate environment, it would usually suggest an idea of reference; beliefs that concern people one knows will typically involve paranoid ideation. Paranoid ideation often involves persons, agencies, institutions, or organizations with whom one has interacted or is familiar. Ideas of reference often involve reactions to an immediate stimulus (event, remark, stranger, or object) within one's immediate environment. However, if a belief is readily considered to represent both items, then preference should be given to ideas of reference because paranoid, suspicious ideation is a broader item that can include many other indicators.

This trait, when present, can often be observed during the interview. For example, the person may ask repeatedly many questions about the reason for the interview, the precautions that have been taken for ensuring confidentiality, and the possible uses to which the results may be put. Schizotypal persons will often become very wary and guarded when the questions are personal.

Persons with a paranoid PD will invariably display suspicious, paranoid ideation. Most of the items for the diagnosis of paranoid PD provide illustrations of paranoid ideation that may be seen in schizotypal persons (e.g., suspects that others are exploiting or deceiving them, preoccupied with doubts about the loyalty or trustworthiness of friends or associates, reads hidden demeaning or threatening meanings into benign remarks or events, fears that information given to others will be used maliciously against them, and recurrent suspicions regarding fidelity of spouse or sexual partner). We consider the presence of any one of these paranoid PD traits to qualify for this schizotypal item. The distinction between these two personality disorders will involve other SZT PD items and the pervasiveness of the paranoid traits (i.e., persons with just SZT PD may meet the criteria for just one or two paranoid PD criteria, but persons with a paranoid PD must have at least four of the paranoid features).

Suspicious, paranoid ideation is also characteristic of the borderline PD (BDL-9). However, in this case, it is transient and confined to periods of severe stress and intense mood states (e.g., anger). If the paranoid ideation occurs only when the person is intensely angry or suffering from severe stress, then we would consider it to reflect borderline PD rather than SZT PD. *DSM-IV* does not require this exclusion criterion, but it is consistent with the borderline PD criterion and was considered for inclusion for *DSM-IV* (Siever et al., 1991). Schizotypal paranoia tends to be more enduring, and it will be evident when the person is calm, dispassionate, or only mildly anxious.

To the extent that the paranoid ideation appears to be delusional (i.e., it is held with a strong conviction and confidence, and it is sustained despite evidence to the contrary), one should then consider whether the more appropriate diagnosis would be schizophrenia (or a delusional or other psychotic disorder), as discussed above. The interviewer should also refer to the discussion of the assessment of suspiciousness and mistrust within members of minority groups in the chapter concerned with the paranoid PD items.

Criterion SZT-6

Inappropriate or constricted affect.

Revisions and Rationale: This item received only a minor revision. The examples provided in *DSM-III-R*, of being silly, aloof, or rarely reciprocating gestures or facial expressions (such as smiles or nods), have been moved from the criteria set to the text. In *DSM-III*, this item was described as "inadequate rapport in face-to-face interactions due to constricted or inappropriate affect" (APA, 1980, p. 313). The revision for *DSM-III-R* was to emphasize the actual phenomenology of the person rather than any difficulties one might have with the person. It is a common experience to have difficulty establishing a sense of rapport with schizotypal persons. One will often have a sense that the interaction was rather odd, strange, or weird. However, difficulties in establishing or sensing rapport can easily depend on one's own personality traits. The assessment of the SZT trait should focus on the characteristics within the subject that contribute to the apparent difficulty in establishing rapport.

Affect is considered inappropriate when it is discordant with what is being said or thought (e.g., laughing when discussing something that is depressing or horrifying). Range of affect can be distinguished along four levels: broad (normal), restricted (or constricted), blunted, or flat (APA, 1987, 1994). Normal expression of affect will include variability in facial expression, voice pitch, and gestures. Flat affect is the most severe, wherein there is virtually no expression (e.g., the voice is a monotone, there is little to no arm or hand movement, and the face is immobile with no change in expression). Constricted affect is less severe, but it is characterized by a clear reduction in the expression and intensity of affect. Blunted affect involves a marked or severe reduction.

Rating:

0) Absent
1) Inappropriate or constricted affect
2) Inappropriate and constricted affect

Questions:

[*There are no questions for this item. Its presence is assessed on the basis of observations of the person. Observe for constricted affect (a clear reduction in the expressive range and intensity of emotion). The person will appear unusually aloof, cold, or unemotional. Tragic or intense experiences are discussed blandly. No humor or emotional spontaneity is expressed. Gestures, such as smiles or nods, are rarely reciprocated. Or, the person displays inappropriate affect (i.e., affect is discordant with the content of the person's speech or thoughts). One example would be a person smiling, giggling, or laughing when discussing something sad or tragic. This does not include mild laughter that expresses an embarrassment or nervousness, unless it is unusually loud or explosive. Giggling or smirking throughout the interview would qualify.*]

Issues and Problems: Either inappropriate or constricted affect are sufficient for this item to be considered present. However, we prefer that both be present, as the presence of just constricted affect is not as compelling or differentiating as the presence of both. Constricted (or restricted) affect is also characteristic of the obsessive-compulsive and paranoid PDs, and flat, blunted affect is characteristic of the schizoid PD, but schizoid, paranoid, and obsessive-compulsive PDs are not characterized by inappropriate affect. The presence of inappropriate affect can then be quite helpful in the differentiation of SZT from these other PDs. Inappropriate affect contributes substantially to the odd, peculiar, and even bizarre presentation (and poor rapport) that often distinguishes the schizotypal from the simply schizoid person. Moreover, one should not often observe markedly inappropriate affect (e.g., raucous, uncontrolled laughter when discussing the death of one's mother).

This would, in fact, suggest a more severe disorder (e.g., schizophrenia). However, one may observe a frozen grin or a repetitive cackling.

Nervous laughter is not uncommon in persons without SZT PD (e.g., brief chuckling when discussing something that is making the person anxious or self-conscious) and should not be confused with inappropriate affect. The "nervous" laughter of schizotypal persons is more sustained and driven. The laughter will appear uncontrollable; if asked to stop, the person will keep having fits of giggling. In any case, observations of nervous or inappropriate laughter should be confirmed by additional observations or reports at other times or in other situations to ensure that it is, in fact, characteristic of the person and not confined to a particularly stressful interview.

The presence of blunted or flat affect should not be considered as ruling out this item, particularly when it occurs in the company of inappropriate affect, but even when it occurs by itself. Schizotypal persons can appear to be very detached, cold, stiff, and aloof to the point that one would characterize their affective expression as blunted or flat, and not simply constricted. The criterion only requires constricted affectivity, but more severely dysfunctional schizotypal persons may display the more severely dysfunctional blunted or flattened affectivity. This is, then, helpful in distinguishing SZT from the obsessive-compulsive PD.

A final issue is that the assessment of this item must rely heavily on one's observations of the person, as noted in the discussion of SZD-7, emotional coldness, detachment, or flattened affectivity (e.g., little to no change in facial expression, rarely smiling or nodding, bland, monotone voice, and/or rarely reciprocating gestures or facial expressions). And, as indicated in the discussion of SZD, it is important to make additional inquiries regarding the person's usual level of expressivity, because the appearance of constricted affectivity may also reflect a (depressed) mood disorder, pharmacologic treatment, or some other factor (Andreasen, 1979a).

Criterion SZT-7

Behavior or appearance that is odd, eccentric, or peculiar.

Revisions and Rationale: The revisions to this item were minor, confined to moving the examples from the criterion to the text and adoption of the wording used in the ICD-10 criteria set (WHO, 1992). This item was not included in the *DSM-III* criteria for SZT PD, which consisted of only eight items (APA, 1980; Spitzer et al., 1979). It was added to the list in *DSM-III-R* to increase the congruency of the SZT PD criteria set with the *DSM-III-R* description of the prodromal/residual phase of schizophrenia that had already included most of the SZT criteria. The only symptoms of the prodromal/residual phase of schizophrenia that were not already included within the SZT criteria set were "markedly peculiar behavior (e.g., collecting garbage, talking to self in public, hoarding food)" (APA, 1987, p. 195) and "marked impairment in personal hygiene and grooming" (APA, 1987, p. 195). The purpose of this item was to represent the same type of odd, peculiar, and eccentric behaviors that are seen in the prodromal/residual phase of schizophrenia (Widiger et al., 1988).

Rating:

0) Absent
1) Behavior or appearance that is odd, eccentric, or peculiar
2) Behavior <u>and</u> appearance is odd, eccentric, or peculiar

Questions:

[*The assessment of this item includes a question, but it may also be based substantially on the observations of the person during the interview. Odd or eccentric behavior or appearance would include, for example, disheveled appearance that is typical of the person and not simply the result of a recent depression, psychosis, or economic impoverishment; unusual mannerisms, facial expressions, or gestures; peculiar rituals during the interview; talking to oneself out loud; never combing hair or combing hair in an odd manner (even for subculture); rarely washing; rarely ironing clothes; or wearing clothes that don't fit or are grossly mismatched (despite being able to afford better). Odd or eccentric behavior reported elsewhere (e.g., hoarding a certain object or product or engaging in a markedly unusual hobby or ritual) would also qualify.*]

a. Do you dress, appear, or do things that others would find peculiar, odd, or weird?

Issues and Problems: This item can be difficult to assess reliably because, like SZT-4 (odd thinking and speech), its assessment relies substantially on one's own judgment of what is odd, eccentric, or peculiar. In the extreme cases, it will be obvious, but often it may not be so apparent or blatant. Appearance, dress, and behavior can also be constrained considerably within an institutional setting. An example given in the text to *DSM-IV* is ink-stained and ill-fitting clothes (APA, 1994), but one will often observe such an appearance in the impoverished, alcoholic, retarded, or homeless. An additional example provided in *DSM-IV* is a manner of dress that doesn't quite fit together (APA, 1994). This is a good description of what one often observes, but it can be difficult to judge reliably. Complicating the assessment is the fact that some schizotypal persons will be homeless and/or economically impoverished. We emphasize a manner of dress that is clearly odd and peculiar, as if the person may have dressed in the dark and selected randomly from a warehouse collection of different fashions, periods, tastes, and even sizes. The point is that the manner of dress is blatantly peculiar and unusual.

One must, of course, consider the possibility that a deviant or aberrant appearance is intentionally odd for aesthetic, fashion, or subcultural expression. Schizotypal persons may, at times, claim that their odd appearance reflects an intentionally unique, cutting-edge, or superior perspective, but further inquiry may demonstrate that the rationale is itself odd, aberrant, and eccentric. They are also unlikely to be able to describe how their dress or appearance is consistent with a particular group or subculture (e.g., they may indicate that it is consistent with a particular group, when they are not, in fact, active, involved, or accepted members of this group). Many schizotypal persons will join fringe and esoteric groups (as discussed under the odd beliefs or magical thinking SZT-2), but their odd appearance may fail to be characteristic of this group (e.g., they may share the esoteric belief system, but the group does not share the schizotypal's odd manner of appearing or behaving).

Interviews with colleagues, friends, or relatives may be particularly helpful to assess the extent to which any peculiarities do reflect cultural, aesthetic, or economic factors. Some schizotypal persons will be unaware of how odd their behaviors or habits may appear to others, or they may be reluctant to acknowledge them. Interviews with colleagues, friends, or relatives will then be helpful because these persons may be quite aware of the schizotypal person's peculiarities.

The presence of unusual mannerisms, unusual hobbies, or eccentric behavior patterns is also included within this item: often talking to oneself, peculiar hand gestures or expressions that are used repeatedly and to excess, odd or eccentric collections, or very unusual rituals that are done in some habitual manner for no apparent reason or for a bizarre reason (i.e., excluding compulsive rituals to control anxiety; APA, 1994). Extremely bizarre behaviors or appearance (e.g., collecting garbage, wearing aluminum foil, and engaging in a loud conversation with oneself in public) are likely to reflect a psychotic deterioration (i.e., delusional or hallucinatory experiences) and/or schizophrenic symptomatology.

Criterion SZT-8

Lack of close friends or confidants other than first-degree relatives.

Revisions and Rationale: The *DSM-III-R* version of this item was "no close friends or confidants (or only one) other than first-degree relatives" (APA, 1987, p. 342). In *DSM-III*, it was even stated that social contacts were limited to everyday tasks (APA, 1980; Spitzer et al., 1979). The *DSM-IV* revision allows the presence of a close friend or confidant. The *DSM-IV* revision was made primarily for compatibility with ICD-10 (Task Force, 1991; WHO, 1992) but also in recognition that it is rare for persons, even schizotypal persons, to have virtually no close friends or confidants. The prototypic schizotypal person may have no close friends, but most schizotypal persons will have others who could qualify as a close friend or confidant. The friendship, however, is typically limited, awkward, and stiff, lacking any real intimacy or depth. "Lack of close friends" means that there is a significant deficit in the quantity and quality of friendships. As noted in the text discussion of this item in *DSM-IV*, schizotypal persons (unlike schizoid persons) will "express unhappiness about their lack of relationships" (APA, 1994, p. 642). They are very uncomfortable within, and will therefore avoid, any personal relationship, but they may in fact have a "few close friends or confidants other than a first-degree relative" (APA, 1994, p. 642).

Rating:

0) Absent
1) Lack of close friends or confidants other than first-degree relatives
2) No close friends or confidants other than first-degree relatives

Questions:

a. How many close friends (other than relatives) do you have?
b. How often do you invite them over, call them up just to talk, or ask them to go out and do something?
c. Do you confide in them or tell them about any troubles, problems, or fears?
d. Would it be important for you to keep in touch with them if they moved away?

Issues and Problems: As indicated in the discussion of this item under the schizoid PD criteria set (SZD-5), a difficulty in its assessment is interpreting what is meant by "lacks" and "close" friends. The *DSM-III-R* pseudospecificity of none or only one close friend or confidant is not particularly helpful because what is most important and problematic to assess is the quality or depth of the relationship(s). Schizotypal persons may have friends (or acquaintances) that they describe as being good, close friends but these friendships will typically be awkward, difficult, stiff, and even peculiar. These relationships are unlikely to have much playfulness or pleasure, and they will lack real intimacy and depth. Schizotypal persons rarely (if ever) overcome the anxiety and discomfort they feel when they interact with and relate to others (as indicated in SZT-9). Their closest friends may be comparably odd and peculiar, with the bond based on the sharing of esoteric, peculiar interests or beliefs. Similar to the approach taken for the schizoid item, we ask how often they invite people to their apartment/house, how often they suggest to someone that they go out and do something together, how often they call someone on the phone just to talk, and whether it has been important to them to keep in touch with close friends who have moved away. We find these questions useful in assessing the passivity and superficiality of their apparent friendships. As was the case for *DSM-III-R*, relationships with relatives (or therapists) would not qualify.

A lack of close friends or confidants will also be characteristic of other PDs. Avoidant persons may have few close friends because they are shy, inhibited, and insecure; borderline persons because they have alienated people with their hostility, intensity, and manipulation; narcissistic persons because the friends could not tolerate their self-centered arrogance; and antisocial persons because they have exploited those around them. Homeless persons, immigrants, and those new to a community may lack close friends for at least a period of time. A proposal considered for *DSM-IV* was to add the clause that schizotypal persons lack friendships "due primarily to lack of desire, pervasive discomfort with others, or eccentricities" (Siever et al., 1991, p. 190). This proposal was rejected because of its complexity. However, we do find it useful to attempt to rule out instances in which the lack of close friends is clearly not due to lack of desire, pervasive discomfort, or eccentricities (e.g., due to having exploited or abused past friends). On the other hand, we make no distinction between the schizotypal and schizoid PDs with respect to this item. It is our clinical experience that schizoid persons have fewer relationships than schizotypal persons, and their relationships tend to have even less depth and intimacy. The schizoid anhedonic indifference towards others is more debilitating toward obtaining and sustaining a relationship than the schizotypal discomfort and anxiety. However, this distinction is more appropriately made with respect to items that explicitly concern the desire, manner, and/or quality of relatedness (e.g., SZT-1 and SZT-6, and SZT-9) than the number of relationships. Both schizotypal and schizoid persons will have few to no close friends or confidants.

Criterion SZT-9

Excessive social anxiety that does not diminish with familiarity and tends to be associated with paranoid fears rather than negative judgments about self.

Revisions and Rationale: This item was revised significantly for *DSM-IV*. The *DSM-III-R* version was "excessive social anxiety, e.g., extreme discomfort in social situations involving unfamiliar people" (APA, 1987, p. 341). However, this description was not actually specific to the schizotypal PD. Social anxiety, including extreme discomfort in social situations involving unfamiliar people, is also seen in persons with avoidant and paranoid PDs. The *DSM-IV* criteria set for avoidant PD includes being inhibited in new interpersonal situations (APA, 1994) and the *DSM-III* criteria for paranoid PD included an "inability to relax" within the broader criterion of hypersensitivity (APA, 1980, p. 309). The *DSM-III* version of this schizotypal item was even less specific, requiring only "undue social anxiety or hypersensitivity to real or imagined criticism" (APA, 1980, p. 313) that would be seen in persons with narcissistic and dependent persons, as well as in avoidant and paranoid persons. The *DSM-IV* version establishes a higher threshold by emphasizing that the anxiety does not diminish with familiarity and tends to be associated with paranoid fears rather than with feeling incompetent, unappealing, or inferior (Siever et al., 1991). The social anxiety of avoidant persons does tend to diminish with familiarity, as they gradually feel accepted and liked. The schizotypal person would continue to feel uncomfortable, finding the growing intimacy to be more disconcerting, threatening, and/or undesirable than the superficiality and distance that were present at the beginning of the relationship. This discomfort may also be experienced through feelings of suspiciousness, distrust, and paranoid ideation, which is not characteristic of the avoidant PD.

Rating:

0) Absent
1) Excessive social anxiety that does not diminish with familiarity and tends to be associated with paranoid fears rather than negative judgments about oneself
2) Social anxiety has been so excessive that the person is unable to sustain employment

Questions:

a. Do you tend to feel more comfortable or relaxed as people get to know you, or do you, instead, continue to feel anxious or uncomfortable?

b. Do you find it uncomfortable when you visit a close relative?

c. Does personal or intimate talk make you extremely uncomfortable or nervous?

Issues and Problems: The *DSM-IV* revision was helpful in distinguishing the social anxiety of SZT PD from the social anxiety of the avoidant, dependent, and narcissistic PDs, but it may not be helpful in distinguishing SZT PD from paranoid PD. Social anxiety is not included within the *DSM-IV* diagnostic criteria for paranoid PD but, as noted above, it was included within the *DSM-III* criteria (APA, 1980). Paranoid persons will also be tense and will have difficulty relaxing around others. However, it is also important to note that the reference to paranoid fears in this schizotypal item is primarily to help distinguish schizotypal PD from avoidant PD. The item indicates that the anxiety tends to be (not must be) associated with paranoid fears. The social anxiety of a person with paranoid PD is invariably and solely due to feelings of distrust and suspiciousness. Schizotypal persons may feel simply (but very) uncomfortable and nervous, and they may not be able to articulate any reason or rationale for this discomfort (e.g., "any talk about feelings [love, children, personal things] makes me uncomfortable").

Most importantly, schizotypal social anxiety tends to be pervasive and enduring. Social anxiety has not been included within the *DSM-III-R* or *DSM-IV* criteria for paranoid PD because paranoid persons will often be cold, unemotional, objective, detached, serious, and dispassionate. Many times they will not appear or feel particularly anxious, even with strangers. They may still be suspicious, guarded, and wary, but they will feel cold, detached, and calculating (e.g., analogous to a soldier, detective, or spy who is in danger and must keep a "cool head").

14

Personality Disorder Not Otherwise Specified

Every class of disorders included in *DSM-IV* (e.g., mood, anxiety, and personality disorders) provides a diagnosis of not otherwise specified (NOS). The presence of this diagnosis is a recognition that the nomenclature is not sufficient or comprehensive in its coverage of the respective domain (Frances & Widiger, 1986). There are disorders of personality that are not covered by the 10 officially recognized PDs, and these can be given the diagnosis of personality disorder, not otherwise specified (PDNOS).

There are two recommended usages of PDNOS (APA, 1994). The first is when a person does not meet the *DSM-IV* criteria for any one of the 10 officially recognized PDs but does have features from more than one of them, and, together, these features result in a clinically significant distress or impairment in important areas of functioning. The presence of features from more than one PD is necessary, because if the symptoms were confined to just one PD, that person would (according to *DSM-IV*) be below the threshold for that respective PD diagnosis. For example, a person with three borderline traits (and no features from any other PD) does not have enough borderline traits to be diagnosed with borderline PD. One would, instead, provide the code for the absence of a PD (V71.09, indicating no diagnosis on Axis II) and, at best, note only the presence of borderline traits. One can note the presence of these maladaptive personality traits by simply listing them on Axis II alongside the code for no PD, but one is not, then, diagnosing the presence of a personality disorder.

However, the presence of additional PD traits from other PDs could put the person over the threshold of a clinically significant dysfunction. For example, a person with three borderline traits, two antisocial traits, and three paranoid traits would presumably have more personality dysfunction than the person with just three borderline traits and, perhaps, enough to put him or her over the threshold for a diagnosis (this person could even have more impairment than someone who had five borderline features, enough to meet the *DSM-IV* criteria for a borderline PD diagnosis). One would diagnose this person with PDNOS, mixed, with borderline, antisocial, and paranoid features.

The second recommended usage of PDNOS is when the person has a specific PD that is not officially recognized within *DSM-IV* (APA, 1994). The two examples noted in *DSM-IV* are the passive-aggressive (PAG) and the depressive DPS (discussed in chapters 15 and 16) that appear in the *DSM-IV* appendix for criteria sets provided for further study. However, the clinician and researcher are free to include any other unofficial PD they consider to be present, such as authoritarian, Type A (Garamoni & Schwartz, 1986; Siegman & Dembroski, 1989), self-defeating (Cooper, 1993), sadistic (Gay, in press), delusional-dominating (Pantony & Caplan, 1991), pleonexic or machiavellian (Nikelly, 1992), racist

(Hamlin, 1990), or anything else. The examples provided in *DSM-III* were masochistic, impulsive, and immature (APA, 1980; at this time, PDNOS was labeled "atypical, mixed, or other personality disorder," APA, 1980, p. 329). These were diagnoses considered for official recognition in *DSM-III* but not given final approval (Frances, 1980). The examples provided in *DSM-III-R* were impulsive and immature (continued from *DSM-III*), and the self-defeating and sadistic PDs that were included in the appendix to *DSM-III-R* for proposed diagnostic categories needing further study (APA, 1987) (see chapter 3).

In one respect, PDNOS should be used sparingly because, as noted in the introduction to the PD section of *DSM-IV*, PDNOS is a residual diagnosis that is unlikely to be used reliably. The only reliable application may be with respect to the PAG and DPS diagnoses, whose criteria sets are provided in the appendix. Mixed PD and diagnoses without uniform criteria sets (e.g., authoritarian) are unlikely to be diagnosed reliably. In addition, any PDNOS diagnosis will lack a formal recognition. PAG and DPS are not officially recognized. They do not have their own code numbers. They share the code number of PDNOS (301.90; APA, 1994) with mixed PD or with any other idiosyncratic PD diagnosis (including even phlegmatic from the nomenclature of Hippocrates; Frances & Widiger, 1986).

However, it could also be said that PAG and DPS do have some formal recognition, given the presence of their criteria sets within *DSM-IV* and their being cited within the *DSM-IV* text discussion of PDNOS. They do have more recognition than the phlegmatic, self-defeating, sadistic, pleonexic, or authoritarian PDs. One might consider PAG and DPS (and mixed PD) to have a partial or quasi-official recognition, which is, in part, why the self-defeating and sadistic PDs were removed entirely from the manual in *DSM-IV* (Widiger, in press).

It is also difficult to suggest that PDNOS be used only sparingly. When PDNOS has been included within empirical studies, it has typically been the most prevalent PD diagnosis, being diagnosed more often than even the borderline in the studies by Fabrega, Ulrich, Pilkonis, and Mezzich (1991), Kass, Skodol, Charles, Spitzer, and Williams (1985), Koenigsberg, Kaplan, Gilmore, and Cooper (1985), Loranger (1990), Morey (1988b), and Zimmerman and Coryell (1989). These studies include surveys of clinicians (e.g., Morey, 1988b), clinician ratings (e.g., Kass et al., 1985), chart review (Loranger, 1990), and semi-structured interview assessments (e.g., Zimmerman & Coryell, 1989). PDNOS is clearly an important, or at least often-used, diagnosis.

It is emphasized in *DSM-IV*, however, that when using PDNOS, one should ensure that the behavior pattern meets the overall criteria for a personality disorder (APA, 1994). These criteria have not been emphasized in our discussion of the officially recognized PDs because their individual diagnostic criteria were developed to meet the general definition. Our discussion of the problems and issues in the assessment of individual PD criteria has often concerned aspects of the general criteria for a PD (e.g., presence since adolescence, distinction from an Axis I disorder, or deviation from a cultural expectation). However, in the absence of a specific criteria set for a particular PD, one should ensure that the overall criteria for a PD have been met.

DSM-IV Criteria for a Personality Disorder

DSM-III-R provided only a narrative definition of a personality disorder:

> Personality traits are enduring patterns of perceiving, relating to, and thinking about the environment and oneself, and are exhibited in a wide range of important social and personal contexts. It is only when personality traits are inflexible and maladaptive and cause either significant functional impairment or subjective distress that they constitute Personality Disorders. The manifestations of Personality Disorders are often recognizable by adolescence or earlier and continue throughout most of adult life, though they often become less obvious in middle or old age. (APA, 1987, p. 335)

The impetus for the inclusion of more specific, explicit criteria for the general construct of a personality disorder was provided by the presence within ICD-10 of such a criteria set (WHO, 1992, p. 202). However, significant revisions were made to each of the criteria provided in the ICD-10. Table 14-1 presents the *DSM-IV* criteria. Each of these criteria will be discussed in turn.

Table 14-1
DSM-IV Criteria for a Personality Disorder

A. An enduring pattern of inner experience and behavior that deviates markedly from the expectations of the individual's culture. This pattern is manifested in at least two (or more) of the following areas: (1) cognition (i.e., ways of perceiving and interpreting self, other people, and events), (2) affectivity (i.e., the range, intensity, lability, and appropriateness of emotional response), (3) interpersonal functioning, (4) impulse control.

B. The enduring pattern is inflexible and pervasive across a broad range of personal and social situations.

C. The enduring pattern leads to clinically significant distress or impairment in social, occupational, or other important areas of functioning.

D. The pattern is stable and of long duration and its onset can be traced back at least to adolescence or early adulthood.

E. The enduring pattern is not better accounted for as a manifestation or consequence of another mental disorder.

F. The enduring pattern is not due to the direct physiological effects of a substance (e.g., a drug of abuse, a medication) or a general medical condition (e.g., head trauma).

Note. From *Diagnostic and Statistical Manual of Mental Disorders* (4th ed., p. 633), by American Psychiatric Association, 1994, Washington, DC: Author. Copyright 1994 by American Psychiatric Association. Reprinted with permission.

Criterion A. The requirement of a deviation from cultural expectations is useful in emphasizing that some behavior patterns that appear to be abnormal from one cultural perspective may be normative from another cultural perspective. However, requiring that the behavior pattern represent a deviation from a cultural expectation is likely to be controversial. The issue of maladaptation and cultural norms is difficult and complex (Alarcon & Foulks, in press; Frances et al., 1991; Kirmayer, 1994; Landrine, 1992; Rogler, 1993; Strack & Lorr, in press; Wakefield, 1992, 1993, 1994) and unlikely to be addressed adequately by such a simple requirement. We will illustrate this complexity by offering a series of questions and hypothetical examples.

One would not want to diagnose immigrants to a new culture with a mental disorder simply because they brought with them behavior patterns from their prior culture that are considered to be deviant or aberrant within the new culture. What is considered to be excessively inhibited in one culture may be courteously dignified within another. However, to the extent that such behavior patterns are, indeed, maladaptive within the new culture, they could be said to represent significant impairments in social (and perhaps occupational) functioning. Their development within the prior culture might be said to be comparable to the development of a behavior pattern within one's family of origin that becomes maladaptive when the person leaves home for the broader society. The behavior pattern (e.g., submission, aggression, hostility, or low self-esteem) was adaptive (or normative) within the family of origin but not within the wider society in which the person must now function.

However, one would not want to presume that a person must adapt to the culture or society in order to be considered free of a personality disorder. There is nothing absolute or special about one's own culture, or the culture in which the person is now trying to adapt, that mandates that either should be the final judge. Perhaps it is the new culture or society that should be more flexible or tolerant with respect to its new or deviant members than the members themselves. Perhaps the society should adapt to diversity among individuals rather than require individuals to adapt to the norms of a particular society.

On the other hand, to the extent that the culture in which the person must now function is, in fact, irrelevant, then there is perhaps no point (and it may even be inconsistent) to require the presence of a social deviance to consider a behavior pattern to be disordered. If adaptation to the current culture is not necessary to consider a PD to be present, then neither, perhaps, should a deviance from any cultural expectations be necessary.

A requirement that the behavior pattern represent a deviation from a cultural expectation should not be interpreted to mean that what is valued or encouraged by a culture cannot be maladaptive. It is certainly possible for a cultural expectation to impart clinically significant maladaptive behavior patterns, such as excessive submissiveness (Brown, 1986; Kaplan, 1983) and excessive achievement striving (Garamoni & Schwartz, 1986). Optimal functioning does not necessarily involve adaptation to cultural expectations, and adaptation to cultural expectations does not necessarily ensure the absence of maladaptive personality traits. Many maladaptive behavior patterns will represent excessive or exaggerated expressions of traits that the culture values or encourages. It is within cultural expectations to be conscientious, responsible, diligent, and dedicated to one's work or career, but not to the point that one sacrifices one's physical health, friendships, or family. It is within cultural expectations to be agreeable but not to be docile, meek, and submissive. It is within cultural expectations to be assertive, but not to be domineering, or to be confident but not to be conceited and arrogant. In sum, we would not interpret this criterion to mean that anything encouraged or valued by the culture to a moderate degree cannot be considered to be maladaptive when it is expressed to a more severe degree.

Our discussion of this issue is not meant to provide a final conclusion. On the contrary, rather than to suggest a simple solution, we believe it is best for the clinician and researcher to appreciate the complex and controversial nature of the issue and its assessment. Deviance from cultural expectations is a valid but very fallible indicator of a personality disorder (Frances, Widiger, & Sabshin, 1991; Rogler, 1993; Wakefield, 1992, 1993). It is a useful indicator, but it is not sufficient nor even necessary. Social, occupational, and/or physical impairment or distress are likely to be more valid indicators of a personality disorder (APA, 1987; Widiger & Corbitt, in press-b).

The ICD-10 version of this criterion is, to some extent, preferable to the *DSM-IV*. The ICD-10 states that "for different cultures it may be necessary to develop specific sets of criteria with regard to social norms, rules, and obligations" (WHO, 1992, p. 202), with the decision, then, made on a case-by-case basis. Each case should be informed by an understanding of the issues with respect to that particular culture. To facilitate this effort, we have discussed throughout the PDI-IV the question of cultural expectations as it becomes relevant to individual PD symptoms.

The first criterion specified in Table 1 also indicates that a PD must be manifested in at least two of the following areas: (a) cognition, (b) affect, (c) interpersonal relationships, or (d) impulse control. This is, again, more restrictive than the respective ICD-10 criterion, which indicates only that a PD "usually" involves several areas of functioning (WHO, 1992, p. 202), including affectivity, arousal, impulse control, ways of perceiving and thinking, or style of relating to others. The purpose of this criterion is to ensure that the PD is, indeed, pervasive in its effects. The requirement is useful in differentiating a personality disorder from chronic Axis I disorders that are confined to an impairment in mood, cognition, or impulse control. To the extent that a behavior pattern is confined largely to an impairment within one particular domain of functioning, the more appropriate diagnosis is likely to be an Axis I disorder (Millon, 1986). However, it should also be recognized that many personality traits are confined largely to a particular domain of functioning (e.g., McCrae & Costa, 1989). For example, some personality disorders may be confined largely to disorders of interpersonal relatedness (Benjamin, 1993; Kiesler, 1991).

Criterion B. The second criterion for a PD is that the behavior pattern must be inflexible and pervasive across a broad range of personal and social situations. Maladaptive behavior patterns that are confined to only one area of a person's life are unlikely to be due to a personality disorder. Personality disorders involve the characteristic manner in which the person behaves each day and across most situations (Millon, 1981; Widiger & Frances, 1985, 1988). Some maladaptive behavior patterns may not be evident at all times or in all situations (see chapter 2), and some may even be advantageous within some situations (Widiger & Corbitt, in press-b). However, a disorder of personality should be evident across a range of situations. Documenting the existence of this cross-situational presentation is important as it is not unusual to neglect situational factors in the context of an immediate, florid behavior problem or conflict (Mischel, 1984). As we noted in chapter 2, passive-aggressive PD has probably been overdiagnosed within military, prison, or inpatient settings, and concerns were raised that *DSM-III-R* self-defeating PD would be overdiagnosed in adult victims of abuse (Widiger & Frances, 1989a; Widiger et al., 1989).

Criterion C. The third criterion is that a PD must result in clinically significant distress or impairment. Note that it can be either distress or impairment. Some maladaptive personality traits will involve only minimal impairment but will be of substantial distress to the person, whereas others may be of little concern to the person but result in substantial impairment. The *DSM-IV* criterion also specifies that the impairment is in social, occupational, or other important areas of functioning. The maladaptive nature of a personality trait will typically be evident in both social and occupational functioning, but there are other domains of functioning that may also be affected. For example, some personality traits (e.g., the hostility and time urgency of Type A traits, low conscientiousness) may contribute to an eventual physiological dysfunction (Siegman & Dembroski, 1989).

A difficulty in the assessment of this criterion, however, is the threshold for a "clinically significant" impairment. As noted in the introduction to *DSM-IV*, the purpose of this criterion is to establish the threshold when the symptomatic presentation is not clearly pathological (APA, 1994). The impairment should be neither inconsequential nor minor. However, nowhere in *DSM-IV* is it stated what is meant by a clinically significant impairment or distress. Spitzer and Williams (1982) defined clinically significant as that point at which the attention of a clinician was warranted (whether or not the person was currently the object of this attention). A level of impairment that does not warrant the attention of a clinician is, perhaps, too low to warrant a clinical diagnosis of a mental disorder. However, there are a variety of possible interpretations for the warranting of clinical attention, such as impairments for which treatment by a clinician would be beneficial, impairments for which treatment by a clinician would be necessary, impairments for which treatment is necessary, or impairments for which treatment is desirable (Widiger & Corbitt, in press-b). Each is a viable threshold for a diagnosis of a mental (including personality) disorder. We will emphasize here impairments for which treatment by a clinician would be beneficial and impairments for which treatment would be desirable.

If treatment by a clinician would help to ameliorate an impairment that is secondary to a maladaptive personality trait, then treatment would certainly be warranted. If the level of impairment warrants the attention of a clinician, it is justifiable to conclude that the impairment is clinically significant. However, a difficulty with this threshold is that it could apply to just about any maladaptive personality trait. Most persons can (and perhaps should) be more flexible (e.g., less submissive, more assertive, less dependent, or less aloof), and many (if not most) would benefit from an increased flexibility with respect to these traits. The thresholds for the diagnosis of the 10 officially recognized PDs is substantially higher than this threshold of impairment.

The threshold of impairment that is, perhaps, used by most persons who seek treatment is whether they desire to overcome whatever pathology is causing their distress or impairment. People will seek professional intervention at the point at which they (or others) are sufficiently distressed with their condition in life that they desire a change, and they feel unable to effect this change on their own. However, the degree of impairment that is sufficiently distressful or intolerable to potentiate a desire for treatment will vary substantially across persons.

Distress over the limitations or impairments of one's personality will also fail to be an infallible indicator for the presence of a disorder (Frances et al., 1991). For example, consider a woman who seeks professional assistance because her assertiveness results in vicious anger and abuse from her husband (Walker, 1984). She may already be excessively submissive and deferential, and yet wants the clinician to help her become an even more tolerant and forgiving spouse. Likewise, an absence of distress does not necessarily suggest the absence of a clinically significant impairment. Some persons may be significantly impaired by their personality traits (e.g., suspiciousness, antagonism, anhedonia, or low empathy) but do not find them distressing. They may notice only the few advantages that are derived from these traits (e.g., freedom from guilt and concern for others) rather than the disadvantages (e.g., failure to sustain lasting relationships). These persons may be (appropriately and, at times, inappropriately) referred for treatment by someone else (e.g., by a spouse, employer, or the judicial system).

Because of the fallibility of distress and subjective desire, some have interpreted clinically significant impairment to mean that degree of impairment that a clinician believes should be of concern to the person. Clinicians will often have more experience and knowledge regarding what is optimal, desirable, or adequate functioning. However, it is also the case that a clinician can be very mistaken in such a judgment.

Criterion D. The fourth criterion is that the behavior pattern must be stable, of long duration, and have an onset that can be traced at least to adolescence or early adulthood. In other words, the *DSM-IV* criteria for a PD do not recognize adult-onset PDs (see chapter 2). The onset must be apparent at least by adolescence or early adulthood. The ICD-10 version of this criterion is, in this case, even more stringent, indicating that they "always appear during childhood or adolescence" (WHO, 1992, p. 202), although the ICD-10 does also recognize maladaptive personality change within adulthood (see chapter 2).

The behavior pattern must also be present or stable thereafter, rather than episodic in its appearance. As we discussed in chapter two, one should be very cautious, and perhaps reluctant, to provide a PD diagnosis in a young adult (e.g., age 20) whose maladaptive behavior pattern has been evident only since adolescence (e.g., age 18). Maladaptive behaviors during this brief period of time could reflect situational or developmental reactions that will soon dissipate.

Criterion E. The fifth criterion is that the behavior pattern must not be better accounted for by another mental disorder, including the officially recognized PDs. It is preferable to use an officially recognized PD diagnosis when it is as effective or descriptive in accounting for the behavior pattern (e.g., obsessive-compulsive PD in favor of Type A).

The more common application of this criterion will concern Axis I mental disorders. As discussed in chapter two, it is not difficult to confuse an Axis I mental disorder (e.g., impulse dyscontrol, anxiety, or mood disorder) with a personality disorder. When using a PD diagnosis that is not officially recognized, it is particularly important to first rule out the presence of an Axis I mental disorder that may adequately account for the behavior pattern.

Criterion F. The sixth and final criterion is that the behavior pattern is not due to the direct physiological effects of a substance or a general medical (physical) condition. Note, however, that it is not the purpose of this criterion to suggest that PDs are confined to disorders with a nonphysical, psychosocial etiology. This has been a common misconception (Gunderson & Pollack, 1985; Widiger & Shea, 1991). Biogenetic factors are quite important in most (if not all) of the PDs (Cloninger, 1987; Siever & Davis, 1991). The purpose of this criterion is merely to refer the person to the disorders of personality diagnosed on Axis I (i.e., labile, disinhibited, aggressive, apathetic, and paranoid) (APA, 1994, p. 171). Disorders of personality that are due to a specific and known medical condition are currently classified on Axis I, in part because their age of onset may occur at any point in time.

15

Depressive Personality Disorder

The depressive (DPS) PD is defined in *DSM-IV* as a pervasive pattern of depressive cognitions and behaviors (APA, 1994). These are persons who characteristically display a gloominess, cheerlessness, pessimism, brooding, rumination, and dejection. The original version of the definition for this proposed diagnosis was "excessive negative, pessimistic beliefs about oneself and other people" (Phillips, Hirschfeld, Shea, & Gunderson, 1993, p. 39). It was revised to "simply depressive cognitions and behaviors" (APA, 1994, p. 732) to avoid an explicit overlap with the passive-aggressive PD, which also includes pessimism and whose proposed revision was initially given the label of negativistic PD (Millon, 1993; Task Force, 1991).

A depressive/masochistic PD was considered for inclusion in *DSM-III* but rejected, in part, because of the overlap with the Axis I mood disorder of dysthymia (Widiger & Frances, 1989a). Many criticisms of this decision, however, subsequently appeared (e.g, Frances & Cooper, 1981; Gunderson, 1983; Kernberg, 1984b). Frances (1980) noted, for example, how there was a characterologic variant of schizophrenia in *DSM-III* (schizotypal PD) and a characterologic variant of depression in ICD-9 (affective PD, depressive type), but no characterologic variant of depression in *DSM-III*. Frances suggested that the diagnosis of Axis I dysthymia should be confined to vegetative symptoms. "Nonvegetative chronic depression should have appeared separately under one or another title (I would have preferred depressive or masochistic personality) in the personality disorders section" (Frances, 1980, p. 1052).

The proposal to include a masochistic PD in *DSM-III-R* was an effort to resolve this dispute (Widiger et al., 1988). The proposal to emphasize masochism was helpful in differentiating the PD diagnosis from dysthymia, but the construct of masochism had its own opposition and controversy (e.g., Caplan, 1991; Walker, 1987) and was eventually abandoned by the *DSM-IV* PD Work Group (see chapter 3 and Widiger, in press). However, the proposal for a depressive PD was pursued again with *DSM-IV* (Phillips et al., 1993), given the support within the clinical, empirical, and theoretical literature (Akiskal, 1989; Akiskal & Akiskal, 1992; Klein, 1990; Klein & Miller, 1993; Phillips, Gunderson, Hirshfeld, & Smith, 1990).

The major issues for *DSM-IV* were its overlap with Axis I dysthymia, overlap with existing PD diagnoses (e.g., passive-aggressive, dependent, obsessive-compulsive, and self-defeating), and absence of empirical support for a particular criteria set (Phillips et al., 1993). The overlap with dysthymia was further complicated by the expansion of the dysthymic criteria set in *DSM-III-R* to include an early-onset subtype that subsumed explicitly what had been traditionally diagnosed as a characterologic depression (Keller, 1989). In addition, ICD-10 abandoned the diagnosis of a depressive PD, also subsuming it within the mood disorder of dysthymia (WHO, 1992).

The *DSM-IV* PD Work Group developed an initial draft of a criteria set (Task Force, 1991), based, in large part, on Akiskal's (1983, 1989) research criteria for a dysthymic temperament that was, in turn, derived largely from Schneider's (1959) description of the "depressive psychopath" (psychopath was a general term used at that time to refer to a personality disorder). The *DSM-IV* proposal for DPS PD placed particular emphasis on cognitive traits to facilitate its distinction from the mood disorder of dysthymia. *DSM-III-R* dysthymia, in contrast, includes such vegetative symptoms as sleep and appetite changes. The proposed criteria set was included in the *DSM-IV* mood disorders field trial and was fairly successful in identifying persons who failed to meet the *DSM-III-R* criteria for dysthymia (Hirschfeld, Shea, Holzer, & Scott, 1992). However, the Mood Disorders Work Group was also impressed with the conceptual relationship of the DPS items to the construct of dysthymia and, therefore, deleted many of the vegetative symptoms of dysthymia and incorporated some of the DPS items into the *DSM-IV* criteria for dysthymia (Task Force, 1993).

However, the final decision of the *DSM-IV* Task Force was to retain most of the original criteria for dysthymia, to include the proposed criteria for dysthymia in the appendix to *DSM-IV* for proposed criteria sets (diagnoses) needing further study, to also include within this appendix the proposed criteria for depressive PD, and to note the controversy regarding the differentiation of DPS PD from early onset dysthymia in the text discussion. For example, it is indicated that "it remains controversial whether the distinction between depressive personality disorder and dysthymic disorder is useful" (APA, 1994, p. 732). DPS may represent an "early-onset, persistent, trait-like variant of the depressive disorders" (APA, 1994, p. 732). Some may prefer to continue to use the diagnosis of early-onset dysthymia, but the PD Work Group felt that a dysregulation in mood does not adequately explain why some persons are characterized by chronic attitudes of pessimism, negativism, hopelessness, and dejection.

The DPS criteria set consists of seven items, any five of which are necessary for the diagnosis. The rank order of the criteria was based, for the most part, on clinical theory and prior literature (Phillips et al., 1993). The threshold for diagnosis was derived, in part, from data provided by the mood disorders field trial. Table 15-1 presents the *DSM-IV* criteria for the proposed depressive PD diagnosis.

Criterion DPS–1

Usual mood is dominated by dejection, gloominess, cheerlessness, joylessness, unhappiness.

Revisions and Rationale: This criterion is clearly central to the construct of a depressive PD. The characteristic mood of the depressive person is gloomy, unhappy, glum, sullen, oppressed, joyless, and morose.

Rating:

0) Absent
1) Usual mood is dominated by cheerlessness, joylessness, sullenness, and seriousness
2) Usual mood is dominated by dejection, gloominess, and unhappiness, as well as cheerlessness, joylessness, sullenness, and seriousness

Table 15-1
DSM-IV Criteria for Depressive Personality Disorder

A. A pervasive pattern of depressive cognitions and behaviors beginning by early adulthood and present in a variety of contexts, as indicated by five (or more) of the following:
   (1) usual mood is dominated by dejection, gloominess, cheerlessness, joylessness, unhappiness
   (2) self-concept centers around beliefs of inadequacy, worthlessness, and low self-esteem
   (3) is critical, blaming, and derogatory toward self
   (4) is brooding and given to worry
   (5) is negativistic, critical, and judgmental toward others
   (6) is pessimistic
   (7) is prone to feeling guilty or remorseful

B. Does not occur exclusively during major depressive episodes and is not better accounted for by dysthymic disorder.

Note. From *Diagnostic and Statistical Manual of Mental Disorders* (4th ed., p. 733), by American Psychiatric Association, 1994, Washington, DC: Author. Copyright 1994 by American Psychiatric Association. Reprinted with permission.

Questions:

a. What is your typical mood?
b. Are you usually very serious or sullen?
c. Do you usually feel gloomy, dejected, or unhappy? (*If "yes":*) How long have you felt that way?
d. Have you ever felt really happy, cheerful, humorous, or playful?

Issues and Problems: The major issue in the assessment of this criterion is its distinction from the depressed mood of someone with major depression or dysthymia. Note, however, that the mood of the person with a depressive PD is typically sullen, somber, gloomy, or cheerless, rather than tearful, suicidal, hopeless, or agitated. Persons with a depressive PD are usually described (by themselves and others) as being overly serious, dull, joyless, or humorless, rather than depressed. The mood of the person with depressive PD will also fail to exhibit the fluctuating or episodic course of a mood disorder. Persons with a depressive PD will not experience their mood as a disorder that has come upon them or developed in reaction to a particular event or stress. Their gloominess will be ego-syntonic. They will state that this is how they have always felt and they can hardly imagine feeling any different. They may realize that others are more cheerful, playful, humorous, or pleasant, but they will not necessarily consider this an admirable or desirable feature. Such joyfulness and cheerfulness may even seem foreign or unusual to them, as they lack a history of experiencing such gaiety or joy.

It may not be possible to distinguish the mood of depressive PD from the ongoing mood of someone with dysthymia, particularly those with the early-onset subtype. Dysthymia can become a fairly chronic disorder that the person eventually accepts and experiences as the natural, everyday manner of functioning. However, to the extent that the mood has represented the characteristic manner of functioning almost everyday throughout the adult life and for as long as the person can remember, then it likely represents a trait of the personality (Akiskal, 1989; Widiger, 1989). To the extent that a distinct onset later in life can be identified (i.e., a change occurred in the characteristic mood), then it would reflect a dysthymic mood disorder. Interviews with others who have known the person in childhood and adolescence may be useful in this respect, as persons who have been dysthymic for long periods of time may no longer have an accurate memory for the mood that preceded the onset of their dysthymia.

Note as well that this is one case when our 0-1-2 rating does not correspond precisely to the *DSM-IV* criterion. A rating of 1 is not synonymous with the presence of the *DSM-IV* criterion. We have made this one exception because the criterion includes a variety of moods that vary in the extent of their DPS severity, and we have difficulty defining a more severe variant of the item that would not be readily confused with a mood disorder. The presence of a rating of 1 would indicate the presence of the *DSM-IV* criterion (i.e., cheerless and joylessness), but the presence of the *DSM-IV* criterion may, at times, be more severe than a rating of 1 (i.e., due to the presence, perhaps, of chronic dejection, gloom, and unhappiness).

Criterion DPS–2

Self-concept centers around beliefs of inadequacy, worthlessness, and low self-esteem.

Revisions and Rationale: Consistent with the gloomy, glum, and dejected mood will be a negative self-image. Persons with a depressive PD have a very low opinion of themselves. They will feel inadequate, incompetent, unattractive, undesirable, and unworthy. This low self-esteem will often be a major focus of treatment (although the depressed mood and pessimism may also represent a central focus, particularly for pharmacologic and cognitive approaches, respectively). Depressive persons may be very conscientious, dutiful, and disciplined (Akiskal, 1989), but they may not consider themselves to be particularly competent, dutiful, or conscientious. They would be much more productive, effective, and successful if their confidence and esteem were higher.

Rating:

0) Absent
1) Self-concept centers around beliefs of inadequacy, worthlessness, and low self-esteem
2) Significant social or occupational decisions have been made as a result of a the feeling of inadequacy or worthlessness (e.g., failure to pursue job or career, or acceptance of exploitation, abuse, or victimization)

Questions:

a. How do you feel about yourself?

b. Do you generally feel positive or negative about yourself?

c. How would you describe your abilities, competency, or attractiveness?

d. Have you ever felt really good about yourself?

Issues and Problems: This can be a relatively straightforward item to assess in that one will rarely need to infer its presence or provide indirect inquiry because it is the person's subjective opinion that is of interest. Also, persons with a depressive PD will typically be quite open and forthright in their self-description. They will rarely deny or withhold their low self-esteem.

However, an issue that will often arise in the assessment of this item (and every other DPS item) is whether the low self-esteem reflects a characteristic level of esteem or a currently depressed mood. As noted in Table 1, an exclusion criterion for depressive PD is that the features have not occurred exclusively during the course of a major depressive episode nor dysthymia. Persons who are suffering from a major depression or a dysthymia will also display a very low self-esteem, and they may not be able to provide an accurate description of their level of self-esteem prior to the onset of their mood disorder. The low self-esteem of a person with depressive PD is virtually indistinguishable from the low self-esteem of a person with a depressive mood disorder. The distinction will require an assessment of the duration, stability, and chronicity of the low self-esteem. This will be particularly problematic for persons suffering from a double depression (i.e., the development of major depression during a long episode of dysthymia; Hirschfeld & Goodwin, 1988). One should be very cautious and even reluctant to assess this item, or any other depressive PD item, in someone who is currently suffering or recovering from a severe depressive mood disorder (Hirschfeld et al., 1989). Interviews with someone who has known the person since childhood, however, may be particularly helpful.

An additional issue in the assessment of this item is the differentiation of a situational reaction from the trait disposition. Persons who have recently experienced (or are currently experiencing) a severe loss, failure, injury, victimization, or other trauma, may feel inadequate or worthless (Belle, 1990; Koss, 1990; Walker, 1984, 1987). Thus, it is particularly important in the assessment of this criterion to document that it has been present throughout the person's adult life and prior to the occurrence of any adult trauma.

Criterion DPS-3

Is critical, blaming, and derogatory toward self.

Revisions and Rationale: Consistent with their low self-esteem, persons with depressive PD tend to be self-critical and self-blaming. The depressive and passive-aggressive PDs share a number of traits (e.g., pessimism and critical of others), but the self-criticism and self-blame of the depressive person is helpful in distinguishing these two PDs. Whereas passive-aggressive persons tend to blame others, depressive persons will also blame themselves. They will accept, and even claim, fault and responsibility. They may also passively, and perhaps even actively, suffer the consequences for whatever conflicts or problems have arisen at work, with friends, or at home. They rarely defend themselves and are, therefore, prone to be exploited.

Rating:

0) Absent
1) Is critical, blaming, and derogatory toward self
2) Has been exploited, abused, or in some way taken advantage of as a result of the self-blame, self-criticism, and/or self-derogation

Questions:

a. What have been some of your recent problems or conflicts with persons close to you? [*followed by:*] What has been the reason or source for these troubles? [*followed by:*] Who has been the most to blame?

b. Have you had any major troubles at work or with money? (*If "yes":*) What has been the cause of these problems?

c. Do you tend to blame yourself unfairly for things? Has anyone ever said that you do this?

Issues and Problems: A difficulty in assessing this item is distinguishing it from DPS-2 (low self-esteem) and DPS-7 (feelings of guilt). The depressive PD items obtain substantial internal consistency (i.e., high intercorrelation), but this may, at times, be due to their failure to involve different traits or even different facets of the same trait. Item ratings may not necessarily involve independent assessments. Describing oneself as a failure or as inadequate is being self-critical and derogatory toward oneself, and being derogatory toward oneself (e.g., "I deserve no better") is expressing feelings of worthlessness and low self-esteem. To emphasize the distinction between self-criticism, self-blame and low self-esteem, we ask the person to describe recent and past interpersonal conflicts and to then provide their understanding of the blame or responsibility for the problem. Or, we ask them to describe financial, occupational, or other other problems, and then assess whether they are overly critical, derogatory, or blaming of themselves. The distinction from DPS-7 is discussed below.

Again, it is important in the assessment of this DPS item not to confuse a situational reaction to a stressor, trauma, loss, or failure with a more chronic, long-lasting characteristic of the person (see chapter 2). For example, victims of abuse may be prone to blame themselves for their victimization (Browne, 1993; Strube, 1988; Walker, 1984, 1987). One should be especially careful in the assessment of this item to document that the self-blame and self-criticism have been present throughout adult life and prior to any adult trauma (Widiger & Frances, 1989b). This may, at times, be difficult, as some persons who have been abused or exploited will be reluctant to openly acknowledge or discuss these experiences, particularly with members of the opposite sex or with persons who fail to convey sufficient empathy (Jacobson & Richardson, 1987).

Criterion DPS-4

Is brooding and given to worry.

Revisions and Rationale: Depressive persons tend to brood, mope, sulk, and worry. They dwell on the negative. It is difficult to get them to acknowledge that things have gone or might go well. Their thoughts continually revert to the negative. They will cast a dark cloud over any joyous event, and will ruminate excessively about how things will eventually go wrong. When things do go wrong, they passively accept it as an affirmation of their continued sense of foreboding. When things go well, they will worry about how things will eventually go bad.

Rating:

0) Absent
1) Is brooding and given to worry
2) Preoccupation with failures, losses, and worries

Questions:

a. What are some of your hopes and aspirations regarding [*treatment, career, relationship, health, or finances*]?
b. Do you expect things to turn out well, or do you worry a lot about [*the topic selected*]?
c. Do you tend to brood about what has happened in the past?
d. Is it hard for you to forget about past losses or failures and just move on with your life?

Issues and Problems: This item can be relatively straightforward to assess, as the brooding rumination is usually quite evident during the interview. However, to facilitate the distinction between this item and DPS-6 (pessimism), it is important to document that there is, indeed, a ruminative brooding, not just a pessimistic outlook. We ask persons to describe their hopes and expectations regarding significant aspects of their life (e.g., treatment, career, relationships, health, or finances). Negativistic expectations represent the pessimism of DPS-6. The current item is indicated by excessive or incessant brooding or worrying over the expected failure or loss.

Persons can also brood and worry without being pessimistic, but this will occur more often within the obsessive-compulsive PD than within the depressive PD. The perfectionism of obsessive-compulsive PD will also result in excessive rumination and worrying. Obsessive-compulsive persons will worry excessively over how things may go wrong or how they might fail. However, when asked for their expectations regarding the likely outcome, obsessive-compulsive persons tend to provide a more realistic and accurate portrayal. They may fear the worst rather than expect the worst, displaying an excessive perfectionism rather than negativism.

Depressive persons also tend to dwell on the negative experiences of the past. They will brood incessantly over how things went wrong, in addition to how things will likely go wrong. Brooding over past failures or losses is much more characteristic of the depressive than the obsessive-compulsive person.

It is again important to note the importance of distinguishing between a current state of depressed mood and the personality trait of brooding. Persons who are currently experiencing or suffering from a major depression will also brood and worry, and this may continue for some time after the remission of the more florid symptoms of depression (Widiger, 1993b). Brooding about the past is one of the research criteria for dysthymia obtained, in part, from the *DSM-IV* depressive PD proposal (Phillips et al., 1993). The only distinction here would be whether a clear onset for the brooding can be identified or whether it has been a trait of the person since childhood and adolescence.

Persons who are currently under severe stress or who have experienced a severe disruption to their lives may also worry excessively. However, it would not be characteristic of the average person to also brood about past losses and failures. Nevertheless, it is again important in the assessment of this DPS item to document that the tendency to brood and worry has been characteristic throughout adulthood.

Criterion DPS-5

Is negativistic, critical, and judgmental toward others.

Revisions and Rationale: As indicated by Phillips et al. (1993), "individuals with [depressive PD] tend to judge others as harshly as they judge themselves" (p. 40). They are as likely to rain on the parades of others as on their own. Their descriptions of others tend to focus on negative qualities and features rather than positive. They are sensitive to the foibles, flaws, and failures in others as well as in themselves. They will expect these traits to be or to become predominant and significant in their relationships, and they may often remind others of such traits.

Rating:

0) Absent
1) Is negativistic, critical, and judgmental toward others
2) Friendships or other significant sources of support have been lost as a result of the tendency to be excessively negativistic, critical, and judgmental of others

Questions:

a. Have your friends been supportive or helpful during your times of trouble?
b. Have you usually found friends or colleagues to be disappointing in one way or another?
c. Do you tend to notice the good or the bad in others?

Issues and Problems: The major issue in the assessment of this item is that negativistic criticism of others is also a central trait of the passive-aggressive PD. There may, at times, be no clear distinction between the expression of this trait across these two PDs. A distinction that can be helpful is the fact that depressive persons tend to be less hostile in their criticism. The criticisms of the depressive person reflect their general pessimistic, negative outlook on life (on themselves and on others), rather than an antagonistic attitude towards others. They will be as, if not more, harsh on themselves. They are as likely to blame themselves as to blame others, whereas passive-aggressive persons are much more likely to blame others than themselves. The criticisms of others displayed by the passive-aggressive person will include an impatient annoyance and irritation, whereas such criticism by the depressive person will be more despondent and resigned. Passive-aggressive persons may also be especially (but not exclusively) critical of persons or institutions of authority (see PAG-4).

It is important in the assessment of this item not to confuse a conflict or difficulty with a particular person (e.g., spouse) or set of persons (e.g., therapists or authority figures) with the more general DPS trait. For example, a person may be (excessively or justifiably) judgmental and negative toward his or her spouse, but to be considered as a trait of the depressive PD, the trait should be evident within most current and prior relationships.

Members of minority groups or other victims of discrimination or exploitation may be justifiably judgmental and critical of the group (or person) who has exploited or victimized them. To be considered as a trait of DPS PD, the attitudes should not be confined to any particular group. Similarly, persons with a borderline or a narcissistic PD may be very critical and judgmental regarding a particular person, but a depressive trait will be much more pervasive and less discriminating.

Criterion DPS-6

Is pessimistic.

Revisions and Rationale: Pessimism is perhaps a central, defining feature of the depressive PD. Pessimism was, in fact, included within the definition of the original depressive PD proposal provided to the PD Work Group (Phillips et al., 1993). Persons with a depressive PD expect the worst, and their incessant pessimism can be a major source or reason for their failure to make realistic, optimal, or adaptive life decisions. They may feel that it is pointless and futile to try to improve themselves, their relationships, or any other significant aspect of their lives. This defeatism will often be a principal reason that positive change has not occurred. However, the depressive person would interpret this eventual failure only as an affirmation for his or her defeatism.

Rating:

0) Absent
1) Is pessimistic
2) Pessimism has been major source or reason for failure to make realistic or adaptive life decisions

Questions:

a. [*From criterion DPS-4*] What are your hopes and aspirations?
b. Do you expect things to turn out well or poorly?
c. Would you describe yourself as an optimist or a defeatist?
d. Do you often give up because you know that things won't get any better anyway?

Issues and Problems: The pessimism of persons with depressive PD is usually quite evident and readily assessed by asking them for their expectations of the future. However, in so doing, it is important to inquire with respect to a variety of areas. Pessimism confined to just one area may, in fact, represent a largely accurate or realistic expectation, or at least reflect issues that are confined to this area (e.g., pessimism regarding a marital relationship or employment). On the other hand, the pessimism of the person with depressive PD may, for a period of time, be focused primarily on one area of life.

Another issue in the assessment of this item is its distinction from DPS-4, brooding and given to worry. Persons who brood and worry about the future are typically expressing a pessimism. As we noted in our discussion of DPS-4 though, depressive persons will also brood about the past. In addition, DPS-4 involves not only pessimism regarding the future but also incessant brooding and worrying about this future. However, because of the overlap in these items, we begin the assessment of the current item with a consideration of the response to the questions from DPS-4 (which would not have to be repeated).

Criterion DPS–7

Is prone to feeling guilty or remorseful.

Revisions and Rationale: This is one depressive PD item that was not included among Akiskal's (1989) criteria for his construct of a characterologic depression (or depressive temperament). However, it has been included within other descriptions of characterologic depression (Kernberg, 1984b; Schneider, 1959). Feelings of guilt are also consistent with the tendency to be self-blaming and self-critical. Persons with a depressive PD tend to be excessively apologetic, remorseful, and guilt-ridden. Their sense of guilt will contribute to a willingness and, at times, even a desire to accept punishment, abuse, or exploitation that they do not, in fact, deserve. This does not represent an unconscious enjoyment of such punishment, but rather a belief that such punishment is warranted and may be the only way they can relieve their feelings of guilt. As noted in the text discussion, "they may feel that they do not deserve to have fun or to be happy" (APA, 1994, p. 732).

Rating:

0) Absent
1) Is prone to feeling guilty or remorseful
2) Preoccupation with feelings of guilt and remorse

Questions:

a. With respect to some of the problems we have talked about before [*see criterion DPS-3*] have you felt bad about your responsibility?

b. Do you often feel guilty?

c. Is it difficult for you to get over feelings of guilt, even about little things?

Issues and Problems: The major issue in assessing this item is its distinction from DPS-3 (self-blame, self-criticism). Self-blame and self-criticism will often represent or express underlying feelings of guilt. DPS-3, however, is a somewhat broader trait. Self-blame will usually be associated with feelings of guilt, but self-criticism and self-derogation may concern attributes, mannerisms, acts, or decisions for which feelings of guilt will not arise (e.g., self-criticism regarding one's physical attributes or abilities). However, such attributions might then, in turn, be more appropriately considered to reflect DPS-2 (low self-esteem). In other words, as one differentiates DPS-3 from DPS-7, DPS-3 may then lose some of its distinction from DPS-2.

To facilitate a distinction among the items, we consider self-blame for failures, losses, or problems to represent DPS-3, but the excessive guilt, apology, or remorse that may be associated with this attribution of responsibility to represent the current item. We consider, in particular, the tendency to feel guilty for days, weeks, months, or even years after the event occurred. Persons with a depressive PD will continuously and daily express feelings of guilt for largely trivial, inconsequential errors or accidents.

16

Passive–Aggressive Personality Disorder

The passive-aggressive (PAG) PD was an officially recognized PD in all prior versions of the *DSM*, from *DSM-I* (APA, 1952) to *DSM-III-R* (APA, 1987). However, there has been considerable skepticism regarding the diagnosis in the last two editions of the *DSM*. An exclusion criterion was provided in *DSM-III* such that a person could not be given the diagnosis if he or she met the criteria for any one of the other PDs (APA, 1980, p. 329). Given the prevalence and co-occurrence rate for these other PDs (Widiger & Rogers, 1989), this was a very severe exclusion criterion. It would have had the effect of rarely (if ever) providing the PAG diagnosis. The provision of this exclusion criterion reflected the ambivalence and disagreement among the *DSM-III* PD Advisory Committee members concerning whether the diagnosis should have even been included (Frances, 1980; Gunderson, 1983). As stated in the 1978 draft of *DSM-III*:

> This is a controversial diagnostic category whose ultimate fate will be determined after clinical experience with its use in the *DSM-III* Field Trials. Central issues in the controversy are the extent to which (a) the features of this disorder are in fact maneuvers used by individuals in certain isolated situations rather than pervasive personality traits, and (b) how frequently there is a need for this category. (Task Force, 1978, pp. K:27-28)

Some argued that the passive-aggressive behavior that resulted in a PAG PD diagnosis was either a reaction to being within situations in which more overt assertiveness, objection, and opposition were discouraged or even punished (e.g., the military, prisons, and inpatient hospital settings) or simply a passing stage of normal development (e.g., adolescent rebellion to parental authority) (see chapter 2). It was, therefore, decided that the diagnosis could be given in *DSM-III* only if no other PD diagnosis might apply, thereby discouraging its usage in favor of any other PD, each of which presumably had more validity, or at least credibility.

The *DSM-III* exclusion criterion, however, was usually ignored in both research and clinical practice. The *DSM-III-R* PD Advisory Committee, therefore, decided to delete the exclusion criterion and allow research and clinical experience to decide the ultimate fate of the diagnosis (Widiger et al., 1988). Rather than prevent its usage by fiat, it was preferable to determine whether the diagnosis was used and provided useful information.

Opposition to the diagnosis, however, continued (e.g., Blashfield, Sprock, & Fuller, 1990). One criticism was that the criteria set continued to be too narrowly defined around the single behavior pattern of passive resistance to authority (McCann, 1988). The *DSM-III-R* criteria had been broadened somewhat, including the tendency to be sulky, irritable, resentful, and scornful. However, the definition remained confined to a "passive resistance to demands for adequate social and occupational performance" (APA, 1987, p. 357) which only further complicated the effort to distinguish between a situational passive-resistance and a more pervasive personality style (Millon, 1981, 1993). In addition, PAG PD has only been recognized within the ICD-9 and ICD-10 nomenclatures as one of the residual PD diagnoses (along with the eccentric, immature, narcissistic, psychoneurotic, and haltlose PDs; WHO, 1992, p. 207). The diagnosis was also rarely researched, but this criticism would also apply to many of the other individual PDs (Blashfield, 1993).

A substantial revision to the criteria set and definition was proposed for *DSM-IV*, with a new label, negativistic PD, derived from Millon's formulation of the active-ambivalent personality syndrome (Millon, 1969, 1981). The proposed definition was a pervasive pattern of "argumentativeness, oppositional behavior, and negative and defeatist attitudes" (Millon, 1993, p. 81), and the criteria set provided a further expansion beyond simply resistance to passive-authority, including irritability, negativism, pessimism, complaining, discontent, envy, disgruntlement, and moodiness. All of the *DSM-III-R* criteria received at least a significant revision in this proposal; none remained unchanged. This revision was so substantial, and the validity of the original version was so questionable, that the *DSM-IV* PD Work Group decided to include the diagnosis in the *DSM-IV* appendix for criteria sets provided for further study. The final definition represented a compromise between the *DSM-III-R* and proposed revision, defining PAG PD as a pervasive pattern of negativistic attitudes and passive-resistance to demands for adequate performance.

Seven criteria are provided (see Table 16-1), any four of which are necessary for its diagnosis. The rank order of the criteria could not be based on the *DSM-IV* MacArthur studies due to the extent of the revisions. Studies that had used the *DSM-III-R* criteria had only questionable relevance to the performance of the *DSM-IV* criteria, and no data on the new criteria set were available to the Work Group. The rank order was, therefore, based on the extent to which the criteria were derived from or resembled a *DSM-III-R* criterion (i.e., those with the most historical continuity were given a higher ranking).

Table 16-1
DSM-IV Criteria for Passive-Aggressive PD

A pervasive pattern of negativistic attitudes and passive resistance to demands for adequate performance, beginning by early adulthood and present in a variety of contexts, as indicated by four (or more) of the following:

(1) passively resists fulfilling routine social and occupational tasks
(2) complains of being misunderstood and unappreciated by others
(3) is sullen and argumentative
(4) unreasonably criticizes and scorns authority
(5) expresses envy and resentment toward those apparently more fortunate
(6) voices exaggerated and persistent complaints of personal misfortune
(7) alternates between hostile defiance and contrition

Note. From *Diagnostic and Statistical Manual of Mental Disorders* (4th ed., pp. 734-735), by American Psychiatric Association, 1994, Washington, DC: Author. Copyright 1994 by American Psychiatric Association. Reprinted with permission.

Criterion PAG-1

Passively resists fulfilling routine social and occupational tasks.

Revisions and Rationale: This criterion provides the defining trait of the *DSM-III* and *DSM-III-R* definitions for the PAG PD: the tendency to passively resist fulfilling routine social and occupational demands, obligations, and responsibilities. It represents four of the criteria that were included in *DSM-III-R*: (a) "procrastinates, i.e., puts off things that need to be done so that deadlines are not met" (APA, 1987, p. 357), (b) "seems to work deliberately slowly or to do a bad job on tasks that he or she really does not want to do" (p. 357), (c) "avoids obligations by claiming to have 'forgotten'" (p. 357), and (d) "obstructs the efforts of others by failing to do his or her share of the work" (p. 358). In *DSM-IV*, this passive resistance to the fulfillment of obligations and responsibilities is represented by a single trait rather than a list of the variety of ways in which passive resistance is often expressed. The criterion is placed at the top of the list because it represents four of the nine *DSM-III-R* PAG PD criteria. This single *DSM-IV* criterion, in fact, represents all of the substantive criteria included in *DSM-III*. The *DSM-III* criteria for PAG PD consisted of "resistance to demands for adequate performance in both occupational and social functioning [that is] expressed indirectly through at least two of the following: (1) procrastination, (2) dawdling, (3) stubbornness, (4) intentional inefficiency, [or] (5) 'forgetfulness'" (APA, 1980, p. 329). In other words, the first of the seven *DSM-IV* criteria contains the entire *DSM-III* criteria and almost half of the *DSM-III-R* criteria.

Rating:

0) Absent
1) Passively resists fulfilling routine social and occupational tasks
2) Fails to fulfill many important social and occupational obligations or responsibilities as a result of this passive resistance

Questions:

a. It is sometimes difficult, if not impossible, to tell your boss or some other authority how you really feel about a job or task that was given to you. Do you ever do things to show your resistance or opposition in some indirect way?

b. Do you sometimes just forget you were asked, procrastinate or dawdle, work slowly, work ineffectively or inefficiently, or even get in the way of others' work, to express your objection?

c. Do you ever do these things with your friends or family when they make unreasonable demands or annoy you?

d. Has anyone ever accused you of being passive-aggressive?

Issues and Problems: We assess this item by considering each of the specific ways of passively resisting demands or obligations included in the *DSM-III* and *DSM-III-R* specified above (e.g., procrastination, dawdling, or intentional inefficiency). These earlier criteria do provide valid representations of this trait. Considering them explicitly is also helpful in providing historical continuity.

However, one can and should consider additional ways of passively resisting the fulfillment of routine tasks. It is important to ensure that one has documented the presence of the resistance in both social (e.g., home or leisure) and occupational (e.g., job) activities. This requirement to consider both social and occupational activities was included within the *DSM-III-R* definition for the PAG PD, but not within any of the specific *DSM-III-R* PAG PD criteria. PAG PD has often been diagnosed on the basis of the passive-aggressive behavior observed within an institutional setting in which the person is currently functioning (e.g., hospital or prison) or within the clinical/research interview itself. Passive-aggressive persons will reveal their tendencies through passive resistance to the demands, rules, or responsibilities expected of inpatients or inmates, but the assessment of this item should not be confined to the institutional behavior. This would perpetuate the common error in the overdiagnosis of this PD. In *DSM-IV*, it is required that the passive resistance be present in both social and occupational activities, necessitating a consideration of tasks outside of the institutional setting.

On the other hand, it is often quite difficult to assess these behaviors through direct inquiry. It has been our experience that persons who characteristically procrastinate, work deliberately slowly, claim to have forgotten their obligations, obstruct the efforts of others, dawdle, and are otherwise intentionally inefficient, will usually deny the presence of these traits. Most persons are quite aware of how annoying, irritating, and troublesome such behaviors are to others, and acknowledging the presence of this trait can bring considerable criticism, scorn, and condemnation from others. Such an acknowledgment will also undermine the presumed credibility of the scorn, criticism, and complaints that the passive-aggressive person has of others (e.g., items 2, 4, and 6). It is difficult to complain of being misunderstood and unappreciated while at the same time acknowledging that one does, in fact, characteristically resist responsibilities and obligations through passive-aggressive behavior.

It is for this reason that we use somewhat indirect questions that attempt to provide a degree of approval or support for the passive-aggressive behaviors. One might also consider asking whether others have accused them of being passive-aggressive, and then inquiring as to the respective passive-aggressive behaviors that might be present. In any case, the observation of the behavior within an institutional setting will often be helpful in at least alerting the diagnostician to the potential presence of this disorder, as it will be very difficult for the passive-aggressive person to resist displaying the behaviors within such a setting. Interviews with family, friends, colleagues, or associates, however, will often be more helpful. These persons will be quite aware of these traits and will be particularly helpful in documenting their chronicity and pervasiveness.

Criterion PAG-2

Complains of being misunderstood and unappreciated by others.

Revisions and Rationale: Passive-aggressive persons will typically fail to appreciate the extent to which they are passive-aggressive. Their behavior will generate considerable criticism, annoyance, complaint, frustration, and/or reprimanding from others, but they will be either unaware of or deny their own responsibility for this rebuke. They will, instead, complain of being misunderstood and unappreciated.

This criterion includes two of the *DSM-III-R* PAG PD criteria: (a) "protests, without justification, that others make unreasonable demands" (APA, 1987, p. 357), and (b) "believes that he or she is doing a much better job than others think he or she is doing" (p. 358). Neither of these *DSM-III-R* criteria had been included in *DSM-III*. They were included in *DSM-III-R* to broaden the criteria beyond simply a passive resistance to authority (Widiger et al., 1988). In *DSM-IV,* they have been subsumed within the more general trait of complaining about being misunderstood or unappreciated. This item is listed as the second criterion because it represents two of the remaining five *DSM-III-R* criteria.

Rating:

0) Absent
1) Complains of being misunderstood and unappreciated by others
2) Complains of being misunderstood by friends, relatives, <u>and</u> persons at work

Questions:

a. Do others tend to make unreasonable demands on your time or effort?

b. Do they fail to appreciate your effort, or recognize how good of a job you do?

c. Are your objections or protests regarding your efforts often misunderstood?

d. Do you resent it when people keep telling you how to do things?

e. Do people fail to appreciate or misunderstand you in other ways as well?

Issues and Problems: This is one of the PAG PD items that might be readily assessed within the interview itself, as it usually takes little to stimulate complaints regarding others. Passive-aggressive persons will have many antagonistic relationships, the responsibility for which they typically place on the shoulders of others. Their tendency to externalize blame is one of their more problematic traits, and it will often appear spontaneously during the the interview.

We approach the assessment of this item by first assessing the two *DSM-III-R* criteria that were subsumed by this item (i.e., "protests, without justification, that others make unreasonable demands," and "believes that he or she is doing a much better job than others think," APA, 1987, pp. 357-358). These *DSM-III-R* criteria can provide a good assessment of the tendency to complain of being misunderstood and unappreciated, and their assessment will also facilitate historical continuity. However, complaints of being misunderstood or unappreciated can be expressed in many other ways, and these should be considered as well. For example, the one *DSM-III-R* PAG PD criterion that was deleted, "resents useful suggestions from others concerning how he or she could be more productive," APA, 1987, p. 358) will, at times, represent an expression of this trait. However, a difficulty that can arise with more broadly defined items is their differentiation from other items. Any single statement by a passive-aggressive person can, at times, represent a complaint of being misunderstood (PAG-2), being argumentative (PAG-3), or being critical and scornful (PAG-4). The assessment of the current item should be confined to complaints that their passive-aggressive behavior is being misunderstood and that their efforts to fulfill tasks (responsibilities or obligations) are being unappreciated.

Expressions of this or similar traits will also be evident in persons with other PDs. For example, paranoid persons will complain of being misunderstood and dependent persons will complain of being unappreciated (the latter instances will often be justified). However, it is much less common for paranoid persons to complain of being unappreciated and for dependent persons to complain of being misunderstood. Both complaints are necessary for this item to be considered present for the passive-aggressive PD.

A more problematic differentiation will involve the borderline PD. Persons with borderline PD will often complain of being misunderstood and/or unappreciated by others. We attempt to differentiate between these two PDs by determining whether it is the passive-aggressive behavior assessed in the first item that is being misunderstood and that it is the person's efforts to fulfill responsibilities, obligations, or demands that are not being adequately appreciated. The complaints of persons with borderline PD, on the other hand, will often concern the fights they have had with lovers, spouses, or relatives. They will feel that the value of their relationship, love, or involvement is not being appreciated or that their difficulties in trying to maintain, develop, or resolve the bond are being misunderstood or unappreciated.

Criterion PAG-3

Is sullen and argumentative.

Revisions and Rationale: The *DSM-III-R* version of this item was "becomes sulky, irritable, or argumentative when asked to do something he or she doesn't want to do" (APA, 1987, p. 357). This is a common behavior of persons with PAG PD (Millon, 1981), but it was revised to being more generally sullen and argumentative in order to broaden the trait beyond a resistance to demands for the performance of social or occupational tasks (Millon, 1993). As we noted above, the major concern with this diagnosis has been the confusion of situational resistance with a more general negativism. Passive-aggressive persons will be sullen and argumentative at almost any time and within most situations. They tend to be "sullen malcontents and perennial complainers" (Millon, 1993, p. 83). They can get into an argument over almost any issue, no matter how trivial or inconsequential.

Rating:

0) Absent
1) Is sullen and argumentative
2) Has lost employment or friends due to being argumentative (and sullen)

Questions:

a. We are often asked to do things that are quite unreasonable and perhaps even ridiculous. Do you tend to become rather sullen or argumentative when this happens, or do you just accept it without any expression of annoyance or protest?

b. Do you generally feel discontented or sullen?

c. Do you find that you're getting into arguments almost every day?

d. Have people ever accused you of being excessively sullen or argumentative?

Issues and Problems: We begin the assessment of this item with the *DSM-III-R* version for the sake of historical interest and continuity. However, it is important to emphasize that the *DSM-IV* version is much broader. Even if the person is argumentative and sullen when asked to do something he or she doesn't want to do, one will still need to assess whether the more general and pervasive sullenness and argumentativeness is present. One may observe this trait during a clinical or research interview (e.g., complaints regarding the length, place, or content of the interview) although many passive-aggressive persons will be able to convey a spirit of compliance, cooperation, and agreeableness during the brief period of time required for an interview. One may, at times, solicit the trait by engaging the person in discussions of general issues or events within the news or the local setting. The passive-aggressive person will typically be disagreeable and argumentative, noting the flaws or fallacies of whatever the interviewer might offer. However, to be considered as a manifestation of this PAG trait, there must be a sullen (pessimistic, critical, disdainful, or disparaging) tone. Note, however, that disagreements that involve the criticism of authority (including institutional rules or policies) should be considered for the subsequent item (PAG-4, unreasonably criticizes and scorns authority).

Borderline, histrionic, paranoid, antisocial, and narcissistic persons can also be argumentative. Irritability is a criterion for the diagnosis of antisocial PD, but it is coupled with aggressiveness, as evidenced by physical fights (ATS-2). Passive-aggressive persons are unlikely to become overtly (actively) aggressive, hence the name "passive" aggressive. "Irrational, angry outbursts or tantrums" was a *DSM-III* criterion for the histrionic PD (APA, 1980, p. 315), along with an "overreaction to minor events" (p. 315). However, histrionic persons do not tend to be consistently sullen and argumentative throughout the day, and their arguments tend to be more explosive and volatile. Passive-aggressive persons, on the other hand, tend to be chronically argumentative. They will also convey a negative, hostile tone without necessarily ever appearing really angry. Borderline persons may display a constant anger and argumentativeness, but, in this case, it is usually coupled with temper tantrums and even fights (see BDL-8).

Paranoid persons will be consistently sullen and even argumentative, but their concerns are focused primarily on their suspicions. The passive-aggressive person is more generally and pervasively sullen and discontented. Finally, narcissistic persons will often be argumentative and disdainful, but they can also be quite optimistic and pleasant rather than sullen. Like the passive-aggressive person, narcissistic persons will argue for the sake of arguments, but their arguments will usually reflect their disdain (devaluation) of the opinions of others and their desire to indicate how much brighter and more knowledgeable they are, rather than continually exuding discontent, malcontent, and disagreement.

Criterion PAG-4

Unreasonably criticizes and scorns authority.

Revisions and Rationale: This item received the least revision of the *DSM-III-R* PAG PD criteria. The *DSM-III-R* version was "unreasonably criticizes or scorns people in positions of authority" (APA, 1987, p. 358) (this item was not included among the *DSM-III* criteria set). However, the revision does provide a substantive change in the content or meaning of the item. Passive-aggressive persons are not only critical and scornful of persons in positions of authority, but of authority itself. They will criticize and scorn not only the unit chief of a hospital but also the hospital and its policies and rules. They will not only be excessively and repetitively scornful of their bosses, but also of CEOs, lawyers, doctors, politicians, big business, and other institutions and professions that may have some influence or control. As noted in the discussion of PAG-3, passive-aggressive persons tend to be sullen malcontents and perennial complainers (Millon, 1993). This item concerns their expression of scorn, disdain, derision, and discontent with respect to authority.

One minor note is that the *DSM-IV* version involves criticism and scorn whereas the *DSM-III-R* version involved criticism or scorn. This revision could, at times, have an effect on the attribution of the item's presence, but we have rarely found this to be an issue. All of the *DSM-IV* PAG items, in fact, involve the conjunction "and" rather than the disjunction "or." This preference reflects an interest in making the criteria set more restrictive (i.e., both traits are required rather than either one). However, this will not usually affect whether a person would be assessed with the item. Persons who are scornful are almost invariably critical. Persons who are critical are not necessarily scornful, but we have found that persons who are consistently critical of a variety of persons in positions of authority are almost invariably scornful of this authority as well.

Rating:

0) Absent
1) Unreasonably criticizes and scorns authority
2) Has been formally reprimanded for unnecessary, excessive, or hostile criticism and scorn of authority

Questions:

a. People often seem to be promoted to their level of incompetence. Have you found this to be the case in your experience?

b. Do you think people in authority tend to exploit or abuse their power?

c. What do you think of [*lawyers, doctors, landlords, politicians, psychiatrists, psychologists, professors, administrators; ask about one or more in turn*]? Are these people generally overpaid, pampered, or exploitive?

Issues and Problems: We again begin the assessment of this item with the *DSM-III-R* version. In this case, it is not only of historical interest but also because the *DSM-III-R* version will often provide a sufficient assessment of its presence. Criticism and scorn of persons in positions of authority does qualify as criticism and scorn of authority. It is only when there is no apparent criticism or scorn of any particular individuals that there is a need to consider authority itself (or representative symbols of authority). However, when presented with criticisms of a particular person in a position of authority, it is important to assess whether there is, indeed, scorn for such persons (or authority) in general. Disdain, hostility, or scorn for one particular employer or for one particular therapist, chief nurse, or unit chief would not be sufficient to consider this item to be present. It may, instead, indicate a problem or issue within this particular relationship (or situation). To be considered as a manifestation of a passive-aggressive personality trait, the criticism and scorn must be evident towards people in positions of authority, not just a particular person (note, again, that both criticism and scorn must also be present).

A common problem in the assessment of this item is that PAG persons will, at times, be reluctant to reveal their scorn to a person perceived to be in a position of authority, which may include the clinical or research interviewer. As noted above, they are often aware that they are perceived as complainers, whiners, and malcontents, and they may deny the presence of these attitudes in an interview whose purpose is to document its presence. We, therefore, provide suggestions that such scorn or derision is understandable or realistic to facilitate a willingness to express it. However, it is common for an indication of this scorn to surface spontaneously at some point during the interview.

Borderline and narcissistic persons will also be critical and scornful of persons within positions of authority. For persons with borderline PD, it will often reflect their tendency to devalue at one time (or one person) and to idealize at another time (or another person). If the criticism and scorn is coupled with idealization of other persons in authority (e.g., derision of the father and idealization of the mother, or derision of one therapist and idealization of another), then it is more likely to reflect a borderline than a passive-aggressive trait. In addition, the scorn and derision towards an authority figure will usually involve someone with whom the borderline person has, in fact, had an intense or significant relationship, or at least someone who represents a particular relationship issue. Thus, persons with borderline PD may devalue therapists, but not the psychiatric profession, or if they devalue the psychiatric profession, they may not devalue other professions (or they may idealize the profession at another point in time). The passive-aggressive person's scorn and devaluation of persons in authority tends to be more pervasive and uniform.

Narcissistic persons will also be unreasonably critical and scornful of authority or of persons in positions of authority. However, this will typically reflect their envy and resentment of persons or institutions that are being provided with a recognition or status that the narcissistic person covets (however, see PAG-5). Narcissistic scorn of authority will contain more devaluation than derision, as their concern is to undermine the status and recognition rather than to defy and oppose it. On the other hand, one may, at times, find it difficult (and pointless) to differentiate narcissistic or borderline scorn of authority from PAG scorn, as some narcissistic and borderline persons will, indeed, be scornful and critical of authority.

One additional note concerns the point that the criticism and scorn must be unreasonable. This is particularly important when it concerns individual persons. Many persons, including passive-aggressive persons, will be in relationships in which a superior or boss warrants substantial criticism and scorn. This problem can often be addressed by assessing whether there has been criticism for similar persons in the past or within other situations. However, even criticism or scorn of a series of persons or a profession in general may reflect a not uncommon perspective. It is not unusual, whether or not it is justified, for persons who are not passive-aggressive to be scornful or resentful of a particular profession (e.g., politicians, lawyers, landlords, or doctors). Members of a minority or oppressed group may also be understandably scornful of the group or culture that wields the predominant power within the society or has a history of being discriminatory and abusive.

Criterion PAG-5

Expresses envy and resentment toward those apparently more fortunate.

Revisions and Rationale: This is one of the three new items (which is why it is placed toward the end of the list) obtained from the proposal for a negativistic PD (Task Force, 1991). The item was derived from a review of the literature on the more general construct of a negativistic PD (Millon, 1981, 1993). Passive-aggressive persons will not only be scornful of persons within positions of authority but also resentful of persons who are more fortunate than they are (e.g., people who have an easier job, receive higher pay, or are more healthy). They have difficulty sharing the joy or pleasure of another person's good fortune. Rather than expressing any pleasure, compliment, or delight in another person's success, they will belittle the success, complain that they are never so lucky, suggest that the person is undeserving, or do whatever they can to rain on that person's parade.

Rating:

0) Absent
1) Expresses envy and resentment toward those apparently more fortunate
2) Loss of friendships due to feelings of envy and resentment

Questions:

a. Have any of your friends or colleagues been successful or fortunate in some way? (*If "yes":*) Did they deserve their good fortune?
b. Do you resent their good luck?
c. Do you feel at all envious about their success?

Issues and Problems: One issue in the assessment of this item is its differentiation from the prior item (PAG-4). Persons who are scornful and critical of authority are often resentful and envious (and vice versa), and persons within positions of authority are often more fortunate (and vice versa). The differentiation can often be made with respect to the target of the attitude (persons of good fortune vs. persons of authority) rather than the attitude itself (resentment vs. scorn). In addition, whenever there is envy, resentment, scorn, and criticism toward persons who are in positions of authority, we will consider it to reflect PAG-4 rather than the current item, even if these persons are also perceived as being more fortunate. The negativistic attitudes toward the good fortune of others will often be expressed toward peers and subordinates rather than toward persons in authority (e.g., friends, coworkers, colleagues, or anyone within the general public who experiences good fortune). One exception we make is when the resentment, scorn, criticism, and envy are clearly focused upon and confined to the good fortune of the person(s) in authority (e.g., born to an upper class family) and do not involve the ability, competence, or abuse in the exercise of that authority.

An additional assessment problem is that passive-aggressive persons may willingly reveal their resentment but not their envy. The envy may be expressed more subtly, if at all. It may, in fact, be vehemently denied. The resentment, bitterness, and belittlement of their friends' good fortune can mask their intense feelings of envy. Also, any acknowledgment of envy will undermine their effort to belittle, devalue, or deprecate the other's good fortune. At times, the envy must be inferred.

Narcissistic persons will also express envy and resentment toward those who are apparently more fortunate. One of the criteria for the NAR PD is being envious of others (NAR-8). However, narcissistic envy tends to be more overt and is often directed at others' abilities, successes, and accomplishments rather than simply their good fortune. They may deprecate or belittle the accomplishments and successes of others as being simply a matter of good fortune (luck, connections, or inheritance), but the resentment actually concerns others' accomplishments rather than their good fortune. If a success was clearly and explicitly due to luck, the narcissistic person might feel little need to devalue or diminish that success. In addition, narcissistic persons will express the belief that others are envious of them (see NAR-8). Passive-aggressive persons are more generally pessimistic, disgruntled, and discontented and will not consider others to be envious of them. They are just as likely to rain on their own parade as on the parade of others. An item considered for inclusion within the PAG criteria set was "communicates a pervasive mix of angry and pessimistic attitudes toward numerous and diverse events (e.g., cynically notes the potentially troublesome aspects of situations that are going well)" (Task Force, 1991, p. R:17). Passive-aggressive persons are just as likely to belittle and deprecate their own success and good fortune as that of others, rather than expressing a narcissistic conceit, pride, or satisfaction.

An additional issue in the assessment of this item is a consideration of attitudes and envy that are understandable within particular social groups or cultures. Persons who are a minority within the society may express an envy and resentment towards those in power and control, particularly when this power and control have been used to maintain the good fortune of those in power and to deny comparable success to the minority group. This envy and resentment will, at times, be expressed inappropriately or excessively, and could, indeed, represent an outlet for the expression of a passive-aggressive personality disorder. However, in this case, it would be preferable not to consider the envy and resentment to reflect PAG traits unless they are also directed toward members of the same social, cultural, or ethnic group who have shared that group's discrimination and misfortune.

A final issue in assessment is the fact that tolerance or allowance of the expression of envy or resentment can vary substantially across cultures and societies. In such cases, the diagnosis of PAG PD will need to emphasize other traits of the disorder. For example, we would not encourage lowering the threshold for the attribution of this item to correct for a cultural variation in its expression. We would, instead, consider the cultural variations to reflect an effective inhibition or control of the trait.

Criterion PAG-6

Voices exaggerated and persistent complaints of personal misfortune.

Revisions and Rationale: This item is the second of the three new items. Passive-aggressive persons tend to be characteristically "pessimistic, disgruntled, and disillusioned with life" (Millon, 1993, p. 83). They feel that they are doomed to failure because of their poor luck, misfortune, and mistreatment. An earlier version of this item provided a more vivid description of this characteristic attitude: "claims to be luckless, ill-starred, and jinxed in life; personal discontent is more a matter of whining and grumbling than of feeling forlorn or despairing" (Millon, 1993, p. 84). Passive-aggressive persons externalize blame for their failures, either on others (e.g., PAG-2 or PAG-4) or simply on bad luck and misfortune. The final version of this item was preferred, however, because it would be simpler and easier to use.

Rating:

0) Absent
1) Voices exaggerated and persistent complaints of personal misfortune
2) Complains, grumbles, and whines about (exaggerated) personal misfortunes throughout the interview

Questions:

a. Have you gotten a raw deal in life?

b. Do you generally feel luckless or jinxed?

c. Do things always seem to go wrong for you? (*If "yes":*) Whose fault is it for all of this trouble?

Issues and Problems: An issue in the assessment of this item is its overlap with and differentiation from prior items. As passive-aggressive persons express their resentment of the good fortunes of others (PAG-5), they may also express exaggerated complaints of their own personal misfortune. For example, as they complain of being unappreciated by their employer, they may also complain of their poor luck and misfortune in having such a lousy employer. We consider whining, grumbling, and complaining about misfortune to reflect the current item even if one also infers a resentment toward the good fortune of others. Priority should be given to the more explicit (rather than inferred) representation of the trait. We also consider complaints regarding their perceived mistreatment by others to reflect the current item if the intention or purpose of the complaint is to excuse their own failures or losses. If the purpose of the complaints is to cite or list the faults of their employer (or others), then we would consider it to reflect either PAG-2 (being misunderstood or unappreciated) or PAG-4 (criticism and scorn of authority). However, in many cases, the person will present a series of complaints regarding a person, each of which may follow or relate to the other complaints, but each of which also provides distinct examples of these different items.

Persons with a depressive PD will also express exaggerated and persistent complaints of personal misfortune. This pessimism is so central to the depressive PD that we may not discern any meaningful or useful distinction between the depressive and PAG expressions of this trait. Both depressive and PAG persons will feel luckless, ill-starred, and jinxed in life. However, as noted in the original version of this item presented above (Millon, 1993), the PAG discontent may be expressed more by whining and grumbling than by feeling forlorn or despairing. The PAG person will tend to whine, grumble, and complain, rather than feel lost in a depressive despair. It is more important to passive-aggressive persons for others to continually and repeatedly hear of their misfortune and bad luck. Passive-aggressive complaining is often for the purpose of making excuses for losses and failures, whereas the depressive person is being simply descriptive. The complaints of the depressive person can be equally exaggerated, but not for the purpose of making excuses. The depressive person is more likely to be silently resigned to a perceived (and perhaps actual) misfortune.

A final issue in the assessment of this item is the consideration of the extent to which the complaints are justified. Those within minority, abused, or mistreated groups may present many complaints of misfortune and mistreatment, and an interviewer who is not from the same (socioeconomic, cultural, or ethnic) group may not appreciate the validity of these complaints. This is not to say that PAG PD traits may not be expressed by a minority group member through complaints about the majority group. The minority group status is a useful outlet for the expression of passive-aggressive excuses and complaints. However, in such cases, it will be important to document that the complaints are, indeed, exaggerated and persistent despite evidence to the contrary. The expression of these traits outside of the context of the minority group status is particularly helpful and informative.

A final note concerning this item is the fact that the tendency to complain about personal misfortunes may vary substantially across cultures. Some groups may encourage and foster greater abilities to accept misfortune and maintain a stoic resilience. We would not lower the threshold for the attribution of this item to correct for cultural variation. We would consider these differences to reflect variation in the social-cultural etiology of the trait.

Criterion PAG-7

Alternates between hostile defiance and contrition.

Revisions and Rationale: This is the third of the three new PAG items. An earlier version was "alternates between hostile assertions of personal autonomy and independence, and acting contrite and dependent" (Millon, 1993, p. 84). The presence of both a hostile independence and a submissive dependence has been emphasized within the interpersonal descriptions of this disorder (Benjamin, 1993; Kiesler, 1991). Millon (1993) has noted, as well, an "interpersonal ambivalence, as seen in a struggle between acting dependently acquiescent and being assertively independent" (p. 83). This was a defining trait of Millon's original formulation for the negativistic personality as an active-ambivalent syndrome (Millon, 1969, 1981). However, in the final version of this item, the reference to independence and dependence was deleted for simplification as well as to avoid a confusion with the dependent PD.

Rating:

0) Absent
1) Alternates between hostile defiance and contrition
2) Alternates between hostile assertions of personal autonomy and independence, and acting contrite and dependent

Questions:

a. Have you ever felt guilty about some of your complaints, criticisms, or defiance [*or insert behaviors identified in criteria PAG-1, PAG-3, or PAG-4*]?

b. Have you ever apologized to these people?

c. Do you think that some or much of this behavior represents a difficulty within your own personality?

Issues and Problems: One difficulty in the assessment of this item is documenting that there is, indeed, an alternation. We consider the item to be present only if there is a history of both hostile defiance and contrition toward the same person. This fluctuation must also have been evident in a variety of relationships.

More problematic, however, is the assessment of contrition. Contrition is much less evident than hostile defiance. It tends to be fleeting, if evident at all. We consider hostile defiance to be indicated by the presence of PAG-1, PAG-3, or PAG-4. Each of these can be considered to represent a display of hostile defiance (i.e., passively resists the fulfillment of responsibilities or obligations, is argumentative or sullen towards others, and is critical or scornful of authority). The presence of contrition for this hostile defiance is often an expression of insight into the presence of passive-aggressive traits. However, as noted earlier, acknowledgment of this insight would undermine the presumed credibility of the hostile defiance. The presence of contrition will, then, vary substantially across persons with a passive-aggressive PD and may be more evident as the person grows older or responds to treatment. It has been our experience that this is the least sensitive and most unreliable of the PAG items.

17
Administration and Scoring of the PDI-IV

The preceding chapters presented a substantial amount of instructions, suggestions, and guidelines. The purpose of this brief chapter is to describe the use of the PDI-IV materials and to highlight key points for administering and scoring the PDI-IV. The interview assessment of a personality disorder is often difficult and complex. It does not simply involve the administration of a series of questions and the recording of affirmative or negative responses. The interviewer must also consider a variety of issues, including the establishment and maintenance of rapport; the nosological confusion and overlap among various mental disorders; the effects of situations upon behavior; cultural and gender biases; and distortions in self-description due to the presence of a personality, mood, or other disorder. These issues are discussed in general in chapters 2 and 14 and are discussed in great detail for each individual criterion in chapters 4 through 13, 15, and 16. While the purpose of this chapter is to describe the use of the PDI-IV materials and to highlight key points with regard to the administration and scoring, it is not meant to replace the information contained in the rest of this book. Proper training in administration and scoring of the PDI-IV necessarily involves knowledge of the material presented throughout this book.

APPROPRIATE POPULATIONS

All but the antisocial personality disorder diagnosis can be provided to persons younger than age 18 (APA, 1994). However, as discussed in chapter 2, it is preferable to confine the administration of the PDI-IV to persons above the age of 18. Personality disorder diagnoses can be provided at any age beyond 18 to persons who have had evident symptoms since the age of 18 (i.e., not evident simply during the past 5 years).

The administration of these semistructured interviews presumes the ability of the respondent to understand and respond meaningfully to verbal questions regarding current and past behavior, feelings, relationships, and attitudes. Respondents whose cognitive abilities or motivation are significantly impaired by psychosis, drug intoxication or withdrawal, neurological disorder, or comparable condition are unlikely to provide a valid interview.

Respondents who are significantly depressed, anxious, or angry may have difficulty providing valid responses to PDI-IV questions. However, comparable distortions can also occur as a result of a personality disorder. As indicated throughout the preceding chapters, respondents' answers to PDI-IV questions are not presumed to always be forthright or accurate. Many of the PDI-IV questions are indirect or are phrased in a manner to maximize rapport or to minimize defensive reactions. A general discussion of how to address inaccurate responses that may result from various mental disorders was presented in chapter 2, and specific suggestions for addressing inaccurate responses to individual PD criteria are presented in chapters 4 through 13, 15, and 16.

PROFESSIONAL QUALIFICATIONS

Administration, scoring of respondents' answers, and interpretation of PDI-IV results are solely the province of qualified professionals. Administration, scoring, and interpretation of the PDI-IV requires an understanding not only of the information contained in this manual, but also of the *DSM-IV*, the diagnosis and assessment of mental disorders and psychopathology, and knowledge of the appropriate uses and limitations of semistructured interviews. Clearly, the utility, reliability, and validity of the PDI-IV as a semistructured interview measure of *DSM-IV* personality disorders are directly related to the knowledge and experience of the qualified professional who administers, scores, and interprets the PDI-IV. As discussed in chapter 1, graduate students in clinical or counseling psychology, psychiatric residents, and other professionals are considered qualified users of the PDI-IV, provided they obtain sufficient training in administering and scoring the PDI-IV and continual supervision by an experienced clinician. In addition, a valid administration of the PDI-IV does depend, in part, on the conscientiousness and skills of the interviewer. The PDI-IV will facilitate the obtainment of a valid diagnosis, but it does not guarantee that a valid diagnosis has been obtained.

While the administration of PDI-IV interviews is relatively straightforward, interviewers are encouraged to thoroughly familiarize themselves with the layout of the interviews and the phrasing of the PDI-IV questions. Interviewers should pay particular attention to administrative instructions and prompts that appear in italics in the interview booklets. Interviewers should complete two practice administrations to ensure that they can administer the interviews in a relaxed and fluent manner.

INTERVIEW MATERIALS

Two different interview booklets are provided. The PDI-IV Personality Disorders Interview Booklet presents the diagnostic criteria and corresponding questions according to individual personality disorders. The PDI-IV Thematic Content Areas Interview Booklet presents the diagnostic criteria and corresponding questions according to thematic content areas. The questions for each diagnostic criterion are the same in each interview form. One minor exception is question c of schizoid criterion SZD-7, which asks if the respondent ever felt warm, tender, or sentimental toward someone. This question was deleted in the Thematic Content Areas Interview Booklet because of redundancy with earlier questions in other content areas and inconsistency with other questions in the Appearance and Perception section. Otherwise, the booklets differ only in the order that diagnostic criteria are presented.[1]

The general format for the interview booklets is as follows. Each personality disorder or thematic content area begins at the top of a page and is printed in bold against a shaded background. Labels for the diagnostic criteria are bold (i.e., **ATS-A1**). Diagnostic criteria appear at the right of the criteria labels, framed by horizontal lines. PDI-IV ratings are immediately below the respective diagnostic criteria. Questions labeled with lower case letters (e.g., "a.," "b.") appear below the ratings. Space is provided under each question to record the respondent's answers. *Direct instructions* to interviewers are in italics, enclosed in brackets (e.g., [*Ask about any DUIs*] and [*Ask about any tickets*] for criterion ATS-A5). In contrast, *prompts* to examiners and *suggestions for follow-up questions* are enclosed in parentheses and are typeset in italics [e.g., (*If "yes":*)].

PDI-IV Personality Disorders Interview Booklet

The PDI-IV Personality Disorders Interview Booklet contains 94 semistructured interview items printed in burgundy ink on white paper. It provides spaces for capturing basic demographic information (e.g., name, sex, marital status) about the respondent. Space is also provided on the front page to record the respondent's answer to the general, open-ended question that begins the interview. Diagnostic criteria are presented according to each individual personality disorder, arranged alphabetically, beginning with antisocial personality disorder. Criterion labels reference the order of the *DSM-IV* diagnostic criteria. For example, the avoidant personality disorder criterion that reads "Is unwilling to get involved with people unless certain of being liked" is labeled AVD-2 because it is the second criterion listed by *DSM-IV* for this personality disorder.

PDI-IV Thematic Content Areas Interview Booklet

The PDI-IV Thematic Content Areas Interview Booklet contains 93 semistructured interview items printed in dark gray ink on white paper. It provides spaces for capturing basic demographic information (e.g., name, sex, marital status) about the respondent. Space is also provided on the front page to record the respondent's answer to the general, open-ended question that begins the interview. Diagnostic criteria are presented according to each thematic content area (i.e., attitudes toward self, attitudes toward others, security or comfort with others, friendships and relationships, conflicts and disagreements, work and

[1]Note that schizoid criterion SZD-5 and schizotypal criterion SZT-8 are equivalent in content but differ slightly in phrasing. Criterion SZD-5 reads "*Lacks close friends* or confidants other than first-degree relatives," while criterion SZT-8 reads "*Lack of close friends* or confidants other than first-degree relatives." This wording difference is reflected in the Personality Disorder Interview Booklet. However, these two criteria are assessed simultaneously with the same set of questions in the Thematic Content Areas Interview Booklet, which presents the criterion "*Lacks close friends* or confidants other than first-degree relatives" for both SZD-5 and SZT-8. This wording difference is considered trivial and should not affect ratings assigned to respondents' answers.

leisure, social norms, mood, and appearance and perception). Criteria are numbered sequentially throughout the booklet, with criterion labels that reference how they are ordered in *DSM-IV* included in parentheses to facilitate cross-referencing. For example, the first criterion in the Attitudes Toward Self section of the Thematic Content Areas Interview Booklet is numbered "1 (BDL-3)." The number "1" refers to the sequential order in the Thematic Content Areas Interview Booklet, and "BDL-3" refers to the fact that this is the third diagnostic criterion of the borderline personality disorder.

PDI-IV Score Summary and Profile Booklet

The Score Summary and Profile Booklet facilitates summarizing the responses to individual PDI-IV criteria and plotting the overall dimensional profile. It also provides spaces for capturing basic demographic information about the respondent. The Score Summary for Personality Disorders (page 2 of the Score Summary and Profile Booklet) contains 12 areas that correspond to each of the *DSM-IV* personality disorders. Each area provides spaces to record the PDI-IV criterion scores. The Score Summary for Thematic Content Areas (page 3 of the Score Summary and Profile Booklet) contains nine areas that correspond to each of the thematic content areas assessed by the PDI-IV, with spaces provided to record the PDI-IV criterion scores.

The Dimensional Profile provides a grid for indicating the extent to which each personality disorder exists on a scale of absent, traits, subthreshold, threshold (i.e., presence of the disorder), moderate, and extreme. This coding scheme was proposed for *DSM-IV* to provide uniform criteria and terminology for clinical and research use. The profile was included in the PDI-IV so that it will be available to clinicians and researchers who might find it useful. Chapter 2 provides an extended discussion of potential clinical and research uses of the profile. The purpose of the profile is to encourage clinicians to consider the *extent to which each maladaptive personality syndrome is present* rather than to simply categorize a personality disorder as present or absent, as well as to facilitate the acknowledgement and communication of more complex personality profiles. Specific ways that the profile may be used include assisting the professional to determine the ranking of multiple diagnoses in their order of importance (e.g., relevance or need for treatment, severity of impairment, or predominance of symptoms) and to identify characteristics of the respondent that, while not the focus of treatment, are nevertheless important and relevant to the understanding of the respondent's psychopathology and treatment.

ADMINISTRATION AND SCORING OF RESPONSES

Test Environment

The PDI-IV interviews should be administered individually, face-to-face, and in a private setting. The ability of the respondent to be forthright and open will be compromised in situations in which the responses can be heard by others not involved in the interview. Telephone interviews are unlikely to be as thorough or private as face-to-face interviews.

Selection and Use of Interviews

The Thematic Content Areas Interview Booklet *should be used only when the interviewer wishes to assess all of the personality disorders.* When all criteria will be assessed, the Thematic Content Interview Booklet is preferred over the Personality Disorder Interview Booklet because it minimizes diagnostic halo effects and the unnecessary repetition of questions. Conversely, the Personality Disorders Interview Booklet is most useful when the assessment is confined to only a subset of the 12 personality disorders. However, the Personality Disorder Interview Booklet may be used when the interviewer wishes to assess all of the personality disorders. As was discussed previously in chapter 2, it is recommended that the decision to administer only a portion of the PDI-IV should be guided, in part, by the results of a self-report personality inventory.

All of the questions provided for each criterion should be administered routinely, as well as any additional questions or inquiries that are necessary to render a confident assessment of the criterion. *It is also frequently useful and often necessary to ask for examples and illustrations when a respondent indicates the presence of a symptom.* All of the questions do not need to be administered if the interviewer is confident that they are unnecessary. Deviations from the questions may, at times, be necessary to provide an optimal assessment or to maintain rapport. However, as discussed in chapter 1, any significant deviations in administration should be documented. Interviewers may alter the phrasing of questions to be more consistent with their usual manner of speech. Alterations, however, should not change the meaning or understanding of the questions. *Follow-up questions should be asked whenever they are deemed necessary.* The length of an interview may vary from 1 to 3 hours, with the majority of the interviews requiring approximately 2 hours. As one becomes more experienced with the interviews, one will become more fluent with the questions and more comfortable with skipping questions and/or scoring criteria on the basis of responses to prior questions. Scores may be summarized and profiled in approximately 15 minutes.

General Instructions

Prior to beginning the interview, record the respondent's demographic information in the spaces provided. Begin each interview with the following general question that is printed on the first page of each interview booklet:

> I would like to begin this interview with having you tell me the major events, issues, or incidents that you have experienced since late childhood or adolescence. I realize that this is a very open-ended question, but I want to know what you believe are the major events or episodes of your life. I want to be aware of them as I ask you more specific questions about your personality.

Record the respondent's answer to this question in the space provided. Proceed to the first personality disorder or thematic content area that will be assessed. If the entire personality disorders interview will be administered, the first personality disorder to assess is antisocial personality disorder. If the entire thematic content interview will be administered, the first content area to assess is Attitudes Toward Self.

Each interview proceeds in the following manner. Administer the questions that are listed under each criterion. Record the respondent's answers. Based upon the respondent's answers to the questions, record the score for the criterion in the box printed next to the criterion. If the criterion is absent, assign a score of 0; if it is present, assign a score of 1; if it is present to a severe degree, assign a score of 2. An extended discussion of the scoring of each criterion is provided in the chapter that concerns the respective personality disorder for that criterion. However, several points warrant emphasis. The respondent may provide answers that contradict answers to previous questions. When that happens, return to the earlier question to obtain clarification. It is very important to assign the score to the criterion immediately after the questions have been asked. This allows the interviewer to ask follow-up questions to clarify the criterion rating if necessary.

Several criteria require a slight modification to the general format. The antisocial personality disorder criterion ATS-C assesses the presence of 15 characteristic behaviors that are associated with conduct disorder and the score is assigned on the basis of the number of these 15 behaviors that are present. The 15 behaviors are categorized according to seven questions that are used to elicit the pertinent information. After recording the respondent's answers to questions a through g, place a check mark in the circles next to the behaviors to indicate the presence of that behavior. The score for criterion ATS-C can then be quickly determined by summing the number of circles that are checked.

The assessment of the schizotypal personality disorder criteria that deal with odd thinking and speech (criterion SZT-4) and inappropriate and constricted affect (criterion SZT-6) are based primarily upon behavioral observations of the respondent during the interview. No questions are provided for these two criteria. The schizotypal personality disorder criterion that deals with odd, eccentric, or peculiar behavior or appearance (criterion SZT-7) is also based primarily upon behavioral observations, although one question is provided to facilitate the assessment of this criterion. Finally, it should be noted that the schizotypal personality disorder criterion SZD-5 is identical in content to the schizoid personality disorder criterion SZT-8. This duplication mirrors the symptom overlap of these two *DSM-IV* personality disorders.

SUMMARIZING AND PROFILING OF SCORES

Transfer the respondent's demographic information from the interview booklet to the front page of the PDI-IV Score Summary and Profile Booklet. Next, open the booklet to reveal the Score Summary for Personality Disorders, which is printed on page 2 of the booklet, and the Score Summary for Thematic Content Areas, which is printed on page 3 of the booklet.

When the Thematic Content Areas Interview Booklet is used, scores may be summarized in the following manner. As a first step, transcribe the criterion scores (i.e., 0, 1, or 2) from the interview booklet to the corresponding spaces on the Score Summary for Thematic Content Areas. Next, transfer the scores from the Score Summary for Thematic Content Areas to the corresponding spaces on the Score Summary for Personality Disorders. On the Score Summary for Personality Disorders, the number of criteria necessary to diagnose each *DSM-IV* personality disorder is presented in the space directly above the criterion scores. Criteria with scores of 1 or 2 are considered to be "present" for the purpose of assigning a personality disorder diagnosis. For each personality disorder, mark an "X" in the small box next to the name of the disorder if the diagnostic threshold for that personality disorder was met or surpassed (i.e., if the respondent manifests a sufficient number of diagnostic criteria to warrant assignment of that personality disorder diagnosis). It is recognized that not all professionals will wish to summarize scores using the Score Summary for Thematic Content Areas. Therefore, the professional may wish to transcribe the criterion scores from the Thematic Content Areas Interview Booklet directly to the Score Summary for Personality Disorders (page 2 of the Score Summary and Profile Booklet).

Note that the Antisocial personality disorder departs slightly from this format. In order to meet the *DSM-IV* diagnostic criteria for antisocial personality disorder, the respondent must have a history of conduct disorder spanning a 12-month period, beginning prior to age 15 (i.e., must obtain a score of 1 or 2 on Criterion ATS-C) *and* must obtain a score of 1 or 2 on at least three of Criteria ATS-A1 through ATS-A7.

When the Personality Disorder Interview Booklet is used to administer the PDI-IV, regardless of whether the entire interview or only a subset of the interview was administered, transfer the criterion scores (i.e., 0, 1, or 2) from the interview booklet to the corresponding spaces on the Score Summary for Personality Disorders (page 2 of the Score Summary and Profile Booklet). If the entire personality disorders interview is administered, the professional may elect to also summarize scores according to thematic content areas. To do this, transfer the scores from the Score Summary for Personality Disorders to the corresponding spaces on the Score Summary for Thematic Content Areas. It is recognized that not all professionals will want to take this extra step and summarize scores in this manner. In order to facilitate the process of transferring scores from the Score Summary for Personality Disorders to the Score Summary for Thematic Content Areas, Table 17-1 presents the PDI-IV criteria and the corresponding numbers within the Thematic Content Areas Interview Booklet. If only a subset of the personality disorders interview is administered (e.g., only the Cluster A personality disorders), then the Score Summary for Thematic Content Areas will not be meaningful and should not be used. That is, all diagnostic criteria must be administered in order to make meaningful comparisons of responses among different thematic content areas.

On the Dimensional Profile that is printed on the front page of the Score Summary and Profile Booklet, circle the appropriate number to indicate the number of diagnostic criteria for each personality disorder that were scored 1 or 2. Although the Dimensional Profile may be useful when only a subset of the personality disorders interview is administered (e.g., only the Cluster A personality disorders), the Dimensional Profile should not be used in conjunction with the Thematic Content Areas Interview Booklet unless the *entire* thematic content interview was administered. That is, comparisons of dimensional aspects of personality disorders can only be accomplished when all of the criteria for each of the personality disorders under consideration are administered.

Table 17-1
PDI-IV Criteria and Thematic Content Areas Interview Booklet Numbers

PDI-IV criteria	Thematic Content Areas Interview Booklet number	PDI-IV criteria	Thematic Content Areas Interview Booklet number	PDI-IV criteria	Thematic Content Areas Interview Booklet number	PDI-IV criteria	Thematic Content Areas Interview Booklet number
ATS-C	74	DEP-1	20	OBC-1	62	SZT-1	87
ATS-A1	75	DEP-2	22	OBC-2	63	SZT-2	88
ATS-A2	76	DEP-3	57	OBC-3	61	SZT-3	90
ATS-A3	69	DEP-4	5	OBC-4	73	SZT-4	92
ATS-A4	54	DEP-5	49	OBC-5	89	SZT-5	42
ATS-A5	65	DEP-6	44	OBC-6	19	SZT-6	93
ATS-A6	60	DEP-7	52	OBC-7	67	SZT-7	85
ATS-A7	78	DEP-8	51	OBC-8	58	SZT-8	46
						SZT-9	36
AVD-1	64	HST-1	33	PND-1	40	DPS-1	79
AVD-2	31	HST-2	72	PND-2	29	DPS-2	2
AVD-3	34	HST-3	82	PND-3	30	DPS-3	14
AVD-4	37	HST-4	35	PND-4	41	DPS-4	7
AVD-5	32	HST-5	24	PND-5	43	DPS-5	27
AVD-6	4	HST-6	81	PND-6	39	DPS-6	6
AVD-7	66	HST-7	21	PND-7	56	DPS-7	15
		HST-8	48				
BDL-1	50	NAR-1	3	SZD-1	47	PAG-1	25
BDL-2	53	NAR-2	8	SZD-2	45	PAG-2	12
BDL-3	1	NAR-3	9	SZD-3	71	PAG-3	26
BDL-4	70	NAR-4	10	SZD-4	68	PAG-4	23
BDL-5	84	NAR-5	11	SZD-5	46	PAG-5	16
BDL-6	83	NAR-6	77	SZD-6	38	PAG-6	13
BDL-7	80	NAR-7	59	SZD-7	86	PAG-7	28
BDL-8	55	NAR-8	17				
BDL-9	91	NAR-9	18				

References

Abraham, K. (1921). *On character and libido development.* New York: Basic.

Akiskal, H. S. (1983). Dysthymic disorder: Psychopathology of proposed chronic depressive subtypes. *American Journal of Psychiatry, 140,* 11-20.

Akiskal, H. S. (1989). Validating affective personality types. In L. Robins & J. Barrett (Eds.), *The validity of psychiatric diagnosis* (pp. 217-227). New York: Raven.

Akiskal, H. S., & Akiskal, K. (1992). Cyclothymic, hyperthymic, and depressive temperaments as subaffective variants of mood disorders. In A. Tasman & M. B. Riba (Eds.), *Review of Psychiatry* (Vol. 11, 43-62). Washington, DC: American Psychiatric Press.

Alarcon, R. D., & Foulks, E. F. (in press). Cultural factors and personality disorders: A review of the literature. In T. A. Widiger, A. J. Frances, H. A. Pincus, M. B. First, R. Ross, & W. W. Davis, (Eds.). *DSM-IV sourcebook* (Vol. 3). Washington, DC: American Psychiatric Press.

Alterman, A. I., & Cacciola, J. S. (1991). The antisocial personality disorder diagnosis in substance abusers: Problems and issues. *Journal of Nervous and Mental Disease, 179,* 401-409.

American Psychiatric Association. (1952). *Diagnostic and statistical manual of mental disorders.* Washington, DC: Author.

American Psychiatric Association. (1968). *Diagnostic and statistical manual of mental disorders* (2nd ed.). Washington, DC: Author.

American Psychiatric Association. (1980). *Diagnostic and statistical manual of mental disorders* (3rd ed.). Washington, DC: Author.

American Psychiatric Association. (1987). *Diagnostic and statistical manual of mental disorders* (3rd ed., rev.). Washington, DC: Author.

American Psychiatric Association. (1994). *Diagnostic and statistical manual of mental disorders* (4th ed.). Washington, DC: Author.

American Psychological Association. (1993). Guidelines for providers of psychological services to ethnic, linguistic, and culturally diverse populations. *American Psychologist, 48,* 45-48.

Ames-Frankel, J., Devlin, M. J., Walsh, B. T., Strasser, T. J., Sadick, C., Oldham, J. M., & Roose, S. P. (1992). Personality disorder diagnoses in patients with bulimia nervosa: Clinical correlates and changes with treatment. *Journal of Clinical Psychiatry, 53,* 90-96.

Andreasen, N. C. (1979a). Affective flattening and the criteria for schizophrenia. *American Journal of Psychiatry, 136,* 944-947.

Andreasen, N. C. (1979b). The clinical assessment of thought, language, and communication disorders: I. The definition of terms and their reliability. *Archives of General Psychiatry, 36,* 1315-1321.

Bailey, B., West, K. Y., Widiger, T. A., & Freiman, K. (1993). The convergent and discriminant validity of the Chapman scales. *Journal of Personality Assessment, 61,* 121-135.

Barnett, P., & Gotlib, I. (1988). Psychosocial functioning and depression: Distinguishing antecedents, concomitants, and consequences. *Psychological Bulletin, 104,* 97-126.

Belle, D. (1990). Poverty and women's mental health. *American Psychologist, 45,* 385-389.

Benjamin, L. S. (1993). *Interpersonal diagnosis and treatment of personality disorders.* New York: Guilford.

Ben-Porath, Y. (1994, April). *Assessment of personality disorders with the MMPI-2.* Paper presented at the 2nd Annual Kentucky Conference on Advanced Studies in Psychopathology, Lexington, KY.

Bernstein, D. P., Useda, D., & Siever, L. J. (1993). Paranoid personality disorder: Review of the literature and recommendations for *DSM-IV. Journal of Personality Disorders, 7,* 53-62.

Berry, D. T. R., Wetter, M. W., & Baer, R. A. (in press). Detecting malingering in clinical personality testing. In J. N. Butcher (Ed.), *Foundations of clinical personality assessment.* New York: Oxford University Press.

Blackburn, R. (1988). On moral judgments and personality disorders: The myth of psychopathic personality revisited. *British Journal of Psychiatry, 153,* 505-512.

Blacker, D., & Tsuang, M. (1992). Contested boundaries of bipolar disorder and the limits of categorical diagnoses in psychiatry. *American Journal of Psychiatry, 149,* 1473-1483.

Blashfield, R. K. (1984). *The classification of psychopathology. Neo-Kraepelinian and quantitative approaches.* New York: Plenum.

Blashfield, R. K. (1988). [Similarity matrix for personality disorders]. Unpublished raw data.

Blashfield, R. K. (1993, September). *Growth of the personality disorder literature from 1975 to 1991.* Poster presented at the 3rd International Congress on the Disorders of Personality, Cambridge, MA.

Blashfield, R. K., Blum, N., & Pfohl, B. (1992). The effects of changing Axis II diagnostic criteria. *Comprehensive Psychiatry, 33,* 245-252.

Blashfield, R. K., & Breen, M. (1989). Face validity of the *DSM-III-R* personality disorders. *American Journal of Psychiatry, 146,* 1575-1579.

Blashfield, R. K., & Haymaker, D. (1988). A prototype analysis of the diagnostic criteria for *DSM-III-R* personality disorders. *Journal of Personality Disorders, 2,* 272-280.

Blashfield, R. K., & McElroy, R. (1987). The 1985 journal literature on the personality disorders. *Comprehensive Psychiatry, 28,* 536-546.

Blashfield, R. K., Sprock, J., & Fuller, A. (1990). Suggested guidelines for including/excluding categories in the *DSM-IV. Comprehensive Psychiatry, 31,* 15-19.

Briere, J., & Conte, J. (1993). Self-reported amnesia for abuse in adults molested as children. *Journal of Traumatic Stress, 6,* 21-31.

Brown, L. (1986). Gender-role analysis: A neglected component of psychological assessment. *Psychotherapy, 23,* 243-248.

Browne, A. (1993). Violence against women by male partners. *American Psychologist, 48,* 1077-1087.

Caplan, P. J. (1991). How do they decide who is normal? The bizarre, but true, tale of the *DSM* process. *Canadian Psychology, 32,* 162-170.

Chapman, L. J., & Chapman, J. P. (1985). Psychosis proneness. In M. Alpert (Ed.), *Controversies in schizophrenia* (pp. 157-174). New York: Guilford.

Chapman, L. J., & Chapman, J. P. (1987). The search for symptoms predictive of schizophrenia. *Schizophrenia Bulletin, 13,* 497-503.

Chapman, L. J., Chapman, J. P., & Raulin, M. L. (1976). Scales for physical and social anhedonia. *Journal of Abnormal Psychology, 85,* 374-407.

Chapman, L. J., Chapman, J. P., & Raulin, M. L. (1978). Body image aberration in schizophrenia. *Journal of Abnormal Psychology, 87*, 399-407.

Clark, L. A. (1992). Resolving taxonomic issues in personality disorders. *Journal of Personality Disorders, 6*, 360-378.

Clark, L. A. (in press). *Manual for the Schedule for Normal and Abnormal Personality (SNAP).* Minneapolis: University of Minnesota Press.

Clark, L. A., & Livesley, W. J. (1994). Two approaches to identifying the dimensions of personality disorder: Convergence on the five-factor model. In P. T. Costa & T. A. Widiger (Eds.), *Personality disorders and the five-factor model of personality.* Washington, DC: American Psychological Association.

Clark, L. A., Watson, D., & Mineka, S. (1994). Temperament, personality, and the mood and anxiety disorders. *Journal of Abnormal Psychology, 103*, 103-116.

Clark, L. A., Watson, D., & Reynolds, S. (in press). Diagnosis and classification of psychopathology: Challenges to the current system and future directions. *Annual Review of Psychology.*

Clarkin, J. F., Hull, J. W., Cantor, J., & Sanderson, C. (1993). Borderline personality disorder and personality traits: A comparison of SCID-II BPD and NEO-PI. *Psychological Assessment, 5*, 472-476.

Clarkin, J. F., Hull, J. W., & Hurt, S. W. (1993). Factor structure of borderline personality disorder criteria. *Journal of Personality Disorders, 7*, 137-143.

Cleckley, H. (1941). *The mask of sanity.* St. Louis, MO: Mosby.

Cloninger, C. R. (1987). A systematic method for clinical description and classification of personality variants. *Archives of General Psychiatry, 44*, 573-588.

Cooper, A. M. (1987). Histrionic, narcissistic, and compulsive personality disorders. In G. Tischler (Ed.), *Diagnosis and classification in psychiatry* (pp. 290-299). New York: Cambridge University Press.

Cooper, A. M. (1993). Psychotherapeutic approaches to masochism. *Journal of Psychotherapy Practice and Research, 2*, 1-13.

Cooper, A. M., & Ronningstam, E. (1992). Narcissistic personality disorder. In A. Tasman & M. B. Riba (Eds.), *Review of psychiatry* (Vol. 11, pp. 80-97). Washington, DC: American Psychiatric Press.

Corbitt, E. M. (1994). *Sex bias and the personality disorders: a reinterpretation from the five-factor model.* Unpublished doctoral dissertation, University of Kentucky, Lexington.

Costa, P. T., Jr., & McCrae, R. R. (1990). Personality disorders and the five-factor model of personality. *Journal of Personality Disorders, 4*, 362-371.

Costa, P. T., Jr., & McCrae, R. R. (1992a). The five-factor model of personality and its relevance to personality disorders. *Journal of Personality Disorders, 6*, 360-359.

Costa, P. T., Jr., & McCrae, R. R. (1992b). *Revised NEO Personality Inventory (NEO PI-R) and NEO Five-Factor Inventory (NEO-FFI) professional manual.* Odessa, FL: Psychological Assessment Resources.

Costa, P. T., Jr., & McCrae, R. R. (1993, September). Some implications of longitudinal personality research for the study of personality disorders. In T. McGlashan (Moderator), *Longitudinal studies.* Symposium conducted at the 3rd International Congress on the Disorders of Personality, Cambridge, MA.

Costa, P. T., Jr., McCrae, R. R., & Dye, D .A. (1991). Facet scales for agreeableness and conscientiousness: A revision of the NEO Personality Inventory. *Personality and Individual Differences, 12*, 887-898.

Costa, P. T., Jr., & Widiger, T. A. (Eds). (1994). *Personality disorders and the five-factor model of personality*. Washington, DC: American Psychological Association.

Digman, J. M. (1990). Personality structure: Emergence of the five-factor model. *Annual Review of Psychology, 41*, 417-44.

Dubro, A. (1988). [Diagnostic efficiency statistics for borderline personality disorder]. Unpublished raw data.

Eckblad, M., & Chapman, L. J. (1983). Magical ideation as a measure of schizotypy. *Journal of Consulting and Clinical Psychology, 51*, 215-225.

Fabrega, H., Ulrich, R., Pilkonis, P., & Mezzich, J. (1991). On the homogeneity of personality disorder clusters. *Comprehensive Psychiatry, 32*, 373-386.

Fahy, T. (1988). The diagnosis of multiple personality disorder: A critical review. *British Journal of Psychiatry, 153*, 597-606.

Feighner, J. P., Robins, E., Guze, S. B., Woodruff, R. A., Winokur, G., & Munoz, R. (1972). Diagnostic criteria for use in psychiatric research. *Archives of General Psychiatry, 26*, 57-63.

Fenichel, O. (1945). *The psychoanalytic theory of neurosis*. New York: Norton.

First, M. B., & Spitzer, R. L. (1989). [Co-occurrence and diagnostic efficiency statistics]. Unpublished raw data.

Ford, M. R., & Widiger, T. A. (1989). Sex bias in the diagnosis of histrionic and antisocial personality disorders. *Journal of Consulting and Clinical Psychology, 57*, 301-305.

Frances, A. J. (1980). The *DSM-III* personality disorders section: A commentary. *American Journal of Psychiatry, 137*, 1050-1054.

Frances, A. J., & Cooper, A. M. (1981). Descriptive and dynamic psychiatry: A perspective on *DSM-III. American Journal of Psychiatry, 138*, 1198-1202.

Frances, A. J., Pincus, H. A., Widiger, T. A., Davis, W. W., & First, M. B. (1990). *DSM-IV*: Work in progress. *American Journal of Psychiatry, 147*, 1439-1448.

Frances, A. J., & Widiger, T. A. (1986). The classification of personality disorders: An overview of problems and solutions. In A. Frances & R. Hales (Eds.), *Psychiatry update* (Vol. 5., pp. 240-257). Washington, DC: American Psychiatric Press.

Frances, A. J., & Widiger, T. A. (1987). A critical review of four *DSM-III* personality disorders: Borderline, avoidant, dependent, and passive-aggressive. In G. Tischler (Ed.), *Diagnosis and classification in psychiatry* (pp. 269-289). New York: Cambridge University Press.

Frances, A. J., Widiger, T. A., & Pincus, H. A. (1989). The development of *DSM-IV. Archives of General Psychiatry, 46*, 373-375.

Frances, A. J., Widiger, T. A., & Sabshin, M. (1991). Psychiatric diagnosis and normality. In D. Offer & M. Sabshin (Eds.), *The diversity of normal behavior* (pp. 3-38). New York: Basic Books.

Frankel, F. H. (1990). Hypnotizability and dissociation. *American Journal of Psychiatry, 147*, 823-829.

Freiman, K., & Widiger, T. A. (1989). [Co-occurrence and diagnostic efficiency statistics]. Unpublished raw data.

Freud, S. (1908). *Character and anal erotism*. London: Hogarth Press.

Fyer, M. R., Frances, A. J., Sullivan, T., Hurt, S. W., & Clarkin, J. (1988). Comorbidity of borderline personality disorder. *Archives of General Psychiatry, 45*, 348-352.

Garamoni, G. L., & Schwartz, R. M. (1986). Type A behavior pattern and compulsive personality: Toward a psychodynamic-behavioral integration. *Clinical Psychology Review, 6*, 311-336.

Gay, M. (in press). Sadistic personality disorder in a child-abusing population. *Child Abuse and Neglect.*

Gerstley, L. J., Alterman, A. I., McLellan, A., & Woody, G. E. (1990). Antisocial personality disorder in patients with substance abuse disorders: A problematic diagnosis? *American Journal of Psychiatry, 147*, 173-178.

Goldberg, L. R. (1990). An alternative "description of personality": The Big-Five factor structure. *Journal of Personality and Social Psychology, 59*, 1216-1229.

Goldberg, L. R. (1993). The structure of phenotypic personality traits. *American Psychologist, 48*, 26-34.

Goodman, A. (1990). Addiction: Definition and implications. *British Journal of Addiction, 85*, 1403-1408.

Goodman, S. H., & Kohlsdorf, B. (1994). The developmental psychopathology of conduct problems: Gender issues. In D. C. Fowles, P. Sutker, & S. H. Goodman (Eds.), *Progress in experimental personality & psychopathology research* (pp. 121-161). New York: Springer.

Gorman, J. M., Liebowitz, M. R., & Shear, M. K. (1992). Panic and anxiety disorders. In R. Michels (Ed.), *Psychiatry* (Chap. 32). Philadelphia: J. B. Lippincott.

Grove, W. M., & Tellegen, A. (1991). Problems in the classification of personality disorders. *Journal of Personality Disorders, 5*, 31-41.

Gunderson, J. G. (1983). *DSM-III* diagnoses of personality disorders. In J. Frosch (Ed.), *Current perspectives on personality disorders* (pp. 20-39). Washington, DC: American Psychiatric Press.

Gunderson, J. G. (1984). *Borderline personality disorder.* Washington, DC: American Psychiatric Press.

Gunderson, J. G. (1987). Interfaces between psychoanalytic and empirical studies of borderline personality. In J. Grotstein, M. Solomon, & J. Lang (Eds.), *The borderline patient* (Vol. 1, pp. 37-59). Hillsdale, NJ: Analytic Press.

Gunderson, J. G. (1992). Diagnostic controversies. In A. Tasman & M. B. Riba (Eds.), *Review of psychiatry* (Vol. 11, pp. 9-24). Washington, DC: American Psychiatric Press.

Gunderson, J. G. (in press-a). *DSM-IV* personality disorders. In T. A. Widiger, A. J. Frances, H. A. Pincus, M. B. First, M. Kline, R. Ross, & W. W. Davis (Eds.), *DSM-IV sourcebook* (Vol. 5). Washington, DC: American Psychiatric Press.

Gunderson, J. G. (in press-b). Introduction to the *DSM-IV* personality disorder literature reviews. In T. A. Widiger, A. J. Frances, H. A. Pincus, M. B. First, R. Ross, & W. W. Davis (Eds.), *DSM-IV sourcebook* (Vol. 2). Washington, DC: American Psychiatric Press.

Gunderson, J. G., & Elliott, G. (1985). The interface between borderline personality disorder and affective disorder. *American Journal of Psychiatry, 142*, 277-288.

Gunderson, J. G., & Kolb, J. (1978). Discriminating features of borderline patients. *American Journal of Psychiatry, 135*, 792-796.

Gunderson, J. G., Kolb, J., & Austin, V. (1981). The diagnostic interview for borderline patients. *American Journal of Psychiatry, 132*, 1-10.

Gunderson, J. G., & Phillips, K. (1991). Borderline personality disorder and depression: A current overview of the interface. *American Journal of Psychiatry, 148*, 967-975.

Gunderson, J. G., & Pollack, W. S. (1985). Conceptual risks of the Axis I-II division. In H. Klar & L. J. Siever (Eds.), *Biologic response styles: Clinical implications* (pp. 81-95). Washington, DC: American Psychiatric Press.

Gunderson, J. G., Ronningstam, E., & Bodkin, A. (1990). The diagnostic interview for narcissistic patients. *Archives of General Psychiatry, 47*, 676-680.

Gunderson, J. G., Ronningstam, E., & Smith, L. (1991). Narcissistic personality disorder: A review of data on *DSM-III-R* descriptions. *Journal of Personality Disorders, 5*, 167-177.

Gunderson, J. G., & Sabo, A. N. (1993). The phenomenological and conceptual interface between borderline personality disorder and PTSD. *American Journal of Psychiatry, 150*, 19-27.

Gunderson, J. G., & Shea, M. T. (1991). *DSM-IV* reviews of the personality disorders: Introduction to the second part of the special series. *Journal of Personality Disorders, 5*, 337-339.

Gunderson, J. G., & Singer, M. T. (1975). Defining borderline patients: An overview. *American Journal of Psychiatry, 132*, 1-10.

Gunderson, J. G, & Zanarini, M. C. (1987). Current overview of the borderline diagnosis. *Journal of Clinical Psychiatry, 48*(Suppl.), 5-11.

Gunderson, J. G., Zanarini, M. C., & Kisiel, C. L. (1991). Borderline personality disorder: A review of data on *DSM-III-R* descriptions. *Journal of Personality Disorders, 5*, 340-352.

Guntrip, H. (1968). *Schizoid phenomena, object relations, and the self.* New York: International Universities Press.

Hamilton, S., Rothbart, M., & Dawes, R. M. (1986). Sex bias, diagnosis, and *DSM-III. Sex Roles, 15*, 269-274.

Hamlin, W. T. (1990). Racism is a personality disorder. *The chains of psychological slavery: The mental illness of racism.* Baltimore: ICFP.

Hare, R. D. (1980). A research scale for the assessment of psychopathy in criminal populations. *Personality and Individual Differences, 1*, 111-117.

Hare, R. D. (1992). *Hare Psychopathy Checklist–Revised.* Toronto, Canada: Multi-Health.

Hare, R. D., Hart, S. D., Forth, A., Harpur, T. (in press). Development of an abbreviated version of the psychopathy checklist. In T. A. Widiger, A. J. Frances, H. A. Pincus, M. B. First, R. Ross, & W. W. Davis (Eds.), *DSM-IV sourcebook* (Vol. 4). Washington, DC: American Psychiatric Press.

Hare, R. D., Hart, S. D., & Harpur, T. J. (1991). Psychopathy and the *DSM-IV* criteria for antisocial personality disorder. *Journal of Abnormal Psychology, 100*, 391-398.

Hart, S. D., & Hare, R. D. (1989). Discriminant validity of the psychopathy checklist in a forensic psychiatric population. *Psychological Assessment, 1*, 211-218.

Herbert, J. D., Hope, D. A., & Bellack, A. S. (1992). Validity of the distinction between generalized social phobia and avoidant personality disorder. *Journal of Abnormal Psychology, 101*, 332-339.

Hertzig, M. E. (1992). Personality disorders in children and adolescents. In R. Michels (Ed.), *Psychiatry* (Vol 1., pp. 1-11). Philadelphia: J.B. Lippincott.

Hilbrand, M., & Hirt, M. (1987). The borderline syndrome: An empirically developed prototype. *Journal of Personality Disorders, 1*, 299-306.

Hirschfeld, R. M. A. (1993). Personality disorders: Definition and diagnosis. *Journal of Personality Disorders, 7*(Suppl.), 9-17.

Hirschfeld, R. M. A., & Goodwin, F. K. (1988). Mood disorders. In J. A. Talbott, R. E. Hales, & S. C. Yudofsky (Eds.), *Textbook of psychiatry* (pp. 403-441). Washington, DC: American Psychiatric Press.

Hirschfeld, R. M., Klerman, G. L., Lavori, P., Keller, M., Griffith, P., & Coryell, W. (1989). Premorbid personality assessments of first onset of major depression. *Archives of General Psychiatry, 46*, 345-350.

Hirschfeld, R. M. A., Shea, M. T., Holzer, C. E., & Scott, R. (1992). *Depressive personality disorder. A proposal for DSM-IV*. Unpublished manuscript, Department of Psychiatry and Behavioral Sciences, University of Texas Medical Branch, Galveston.

Hirschfeld, R. M. A., Shea, M. T., & Weise, R. (1991). Dependent personality disorder: Perspectives for *DSM-IV*. *Journal of Personality Disorders, 5*, 135-149.

Holt, C. S., Heimberg, R. G., & Hope, D. A. (1992). Avoidant personality disorder and the generalized subtype of social phobia. *Journal of Abnormal Psychology, 101*, 318-325.

Hyler, S. E., & Rieder, R. O. (1987). *Personality Diagnostic Questionnaire–Revised* (PDQ-R). New York: Authors.

Jacobson, A., & Richardson, B. (1987). Assault experiences of 100 psychiatric inpatients: Evidence of the need for routine inquiry. *American Journal of Psychiatry, 144*, 900-913.

John, O. P. (1990). The "Big Five" factor taxonomy: Dimensions of personality in the natural language and in questionnaires. In L.A. Pervin (Ed.), *Handbook of personality: Theory and research* (pp. 66-100). New York: Guilford.

Kaelber, C. T., & Maser, J. D. (1992). Challenges of personality disorder assessment. *Journal of Personality Disorders, 6*, 279-286.

Kalus, O., Bernstein, D. P., & Siever, L. J. (1993). Schizoid personality disorder: A review of current status and implications for *DSM-IV*. *Journal of Personality Disorder, 7*, 43-52.

Kaplan, M. (1983). A woman's view of *DSM-III*. *American Psychologist, 38*, 786-792.

Kass, F., Skodol, A. E., Charles, E., Spitzer, R. L., & Williams, J. B. W. (1985). Scaled ratings of *DSM-III* personality disorders. *American Journal of Psychiatry, 142*, 627-630.

Keller, M. (1989). Current concepts in affective disorders. *Journal of Clinical Psychiatry, 50*, 157-162.

Kendler, K. S. (1991). Mood-incongruent psychotic affective illness. *Archives of General Psychiatry, 48*, 362-369.

Kernberg, O. F. (1984a). Problems in the classification of personality disorders. *Severe personality disorders* (pp. 77-94). New Haven, CT: Yale University Press.

Kernberg, O. F. (1984b). Structural diagnosis. *Severe personality disorders* (pp. 3-26). New Haven, CT: Yale University Press.

Kernberg, O. F. (1989). The narcissistic personality disorder and the differential diagnosis of antisocial behavior. *Psychiatric Clinics of North America, 12*, 553-570.

Kernberg, P. F. (1990). Resolved: Borderline personality exists in children under twelve: Affirmative. *Journal of the American Academy of Child and Adolescent Psychiatry, 29*, 478-479.

Kiesler, D. (1991). Interpersonal methods of assessment and diagnosis. In C. Snyder & D. Forsyth (Eds.), *Handbook of social and clinical psychology* (pp. 327-349). New York: Pergamon.

Kirmayer, L. J. (1994). Is the concept of mental disorder culturally relative? In S. A. Kirk & S. D. Einbinder (Eds.), *Controversial issues in mental health* (pp. 1-8). Boston: Allyn & Bacon.

Klein, D. N. (1990). Depressive personality: Reliability, validity, and relations to dysthymia. *Journal of Abnormal Psychology, 99*, 412-421.

Klein, D. N., & Miller, G. A. (1993). Depressive personality in a nonclinical sample. *American Journal of Psychiatry, 150*, 1718-1724.

Klein, M. H. (1993). Issues in the assessment of personality disorders, *Journal of Personality Disorders, 7*(Suppl.), 18-33.

Klein, M. H., Benjamin, L. S., Rosenfeld, R., Treece, C., Justed, J., & Greist, J. H. (1993). The Wisconsin Personality Disorders Inventory: Development, reliability, and validity. *Journal of Personality Disorders, 7*, 285-303.

Koenigsberg, H. W., Kaplan, R. D., Gilmore, M. M., & Cooper, A. M. (1985). The relationship between syndrome and personality disorder in *DSM-III*: Experience with 2,462 patients. *American Journal of Psychiatry, 142*, 207-212.

Kohut, H. (1971). *The analysis of the self.* New York: International Universities Press.

Kohut, H. (1984). *How does analysis cure?* Chicago: University of Chicago Press.

Koss, M. P. (1990). The women's mental health research agenda. Violence against women. *American Psychologist, 45*, 374-380.

Kramer, P. D. (1993). *Listening to prozac*. New York: Viking.

Kwawer, J. S., Lerner, H. D., Lerner, P. M., & Sugarman, A. (Eds). (1980). *Borderline phenomena and the Rorschach test.* New York: International Universities Press.

Lachar, D. (1982). *Personality Inventory for Children revised format manual supplement*. Los Angeles: Western Psychological Services.

Landrine, H. (1992). Clinical implications of cultural differences: The referential versus the indexical self. *Clinical Psychology Review, 12*, 401-415.

Lazare, A., Klerman, G., & Armor, D. (1966). Oral, obsessive, and hysterial personality patterns. *Archives of General Psychiatry, 14*, 624-630.

Lerner, P. M. (1991). *Psychoanalytic theory and the Rorschach*. Hillsdale, NJ: Analytic Press.

Levy, L. (1983). Trait approaches. In M. Hersen, A. Kazdin, & A. Bellack (Eds.), *The clinical psychology handbook* (pp. 123-142). New York: Plenum.

Liebowitz, M. R. (1992). Diagnostic issues in anxiety disorders. In A. Tasman & M. B. Riba (Eds.), *Review of psychiatry* (Vol. 11, pp. 247-259). Washington, DC: American Psychiatric Press.

Liebowitz, M. R., & Klein, D. F. (1981). Interrelationship of hysteroid dysphoria and borderline personality disorder. *Psychiatric Clinics of North America, 4*, 67-87.

Lilienfeld, S. O., Waldman, I. D., & Israel, A. C. (1994). A critical examination of the use of the term and concept of "comorbidity" in psychopathology research. *Clinical Psychology: Science and Practice, 1*, 71-83.

Livesley, W. J. (1990). *Dimensions of Personality Pathology–Basic Questionnaire*. Unpublished manuscript, University of British Columbia, Canada.

Livesley, W. J. (1991). Classifying personality disorders: Ideal types, prototypes, or dimensions? *Journal of Personality Disorders, 5*, 52-59.

Livesley, W. J. (Ed.). (in press). *DSM-IV personality disorders*. New York: Guilford.

Livesley, W. J., Reiffer, L., Sheldon, A., & West, M. (1987). Prototypicality ratings of *DSM-III* criteria for personality disorders. *Journal of Nervous and Mental Disease, 175*, 395-401.

Livesley, W. J., Schroeder, M. L., & Jackson, D. N. (1990). Dependent personality disorder and attachment problems. *Journal of Personality Disorders, 4*, 232-240.

Livesley, W. J., Schroeder, M. L., Jackson, D. N., & Jang, K. L. (1994). Categorical distinctions in the study of personality disorder: Implications for classification. *Journal of Abnormal Psychology, 103*, 6-17.

Livesley, W. J., & West, M. (1986). The *DSM-III* distinction between schizoid and avoidant personality disorders. *American Journal of Psychiatry, 31*, 59-61.

Livesley, W. J., West, M., & Tanney, A. (1985). Historical comment on *DSM-III* schizoid and avoidant personality disorders. *American Journal of Psychiatry, 142*, 1344-1347.

Loftus, E. F. (1993). The reality of repressed memories. *American Psychologist, 48*, 518-537.

Loftus, E. F. (1994). The repressed memory controversy. *American Psychologist, 49*, 443-445.

Loranger, A. W. (1988). *Personality Disorder Examination (PDE) manual*. Yonkers, NY: DV Communications.

Loranger, A. W. (1990). The impact of *DSM-III* on diagnostic practice in a university hospital. *Archives of General Psychiatry, 47*, 672-675.

Loranger, A. W. (1992). Are current self-report and interview measures adequate for epidemiological studies of personality disorders? *Journal of Personality Disorders, 6*, 313-325.

Loranger, A. W., Hirschfeld, R. M. A., Sartorius, N., & Regier, D. A. (1991). The WHO/ADAMHA international pilot study of personality disorders: Background and purpose. *Journal of Personality Disorders, 5*, 296-306.

Loranger, A. W., Lenzenweger, M. F., Gartner, A. F., Susman, V. L., Herzig, J., Zammit, G. K., Gartner, J. D., Abrams, R. C., & Young, R. C. (1991). Trait-state artifacts and the diagnosis of personality disorders. *Archives of General Psychiatry, 48*, 720-728.

Loranger, A. W., Sartorius, N., Andreoli, A., Berger, P., Buchheim, P., Channabasavanna, S. M., Coid, B., Dahl, A., Diekstra, R. F. W., Ferguson, B., Jacobsberg, L. B., Mombour, W., Pull, C., Ono, J., & Regier, D. A. (1994). The International Personality Disorder Examination. The World Health Organization/Alcohol, Drug Abuse, and Mental Health Administration international pilot study of personality disorders. *Archives of General Psychiatry, 51*, 215-224.

Loranger, A. W., Susman, V., Oldham, J., & Russakoff, L. M. (1987). The Personality Disorder Examination: A preliminary report. *Journal of Personality Disorders, 1*, 1-13.

Loring, M., & Powell, B. (1988). Gender, race, and *DSM-III*: A study of the objectivity of psychiatric diagnostic behavior. *Journal of Health and Social Behavior, 29*, 1-22.

Malinow, K. (1981). Passive-aggressive personality. In J. Lion (Ed.), *Personality disorders* (2nd ed., pp. 121-132). Baltimore: Williams & Wilkins.

Malow R., & Donnelly, J. (1988). [Diagnostic efficiency statistics for borderline personality disorder]. Unpublished raw data.

Matarazzo, J. D. (1983). The reliability of psychiatric and psychological diagnosis. *Clinical Psychology Review, 3*, 103-145.

McCann, J. (1988). Passive-aggressive personality disorder: A review. *Journal of Personality Disorders, 2*, 170-179.

McCrae, R. R., & Costa, P. T. (1989). The structure of interpersonal traits: Wiggins' circumplex and the five-factor model. *Journal of Personality and Social Psychology, 56*, 586-595.

McCrae, R. R., & Costa, P. T. (1990). *Personality in adulthood*. New York: Guilford.

McGlashan, T., & Fenton, W. (1988). [Diagnostic efficiency statistics for borderline and schizotypal personality disorders]. Unpublished raw data.

Meehl, P. E. (1964). *Manual for use with checklist of schizotypic signs.* (Unpublished report #PR-73-5). Minneapolis: University of Minnesota Medical School.

Millon, T. (1969). *Modern psychopathology: A biosocial approach to maladaptive learning and functioning*. Philadelphia: W. B. Saunders.

Millon, T. (1981). *Disorders of personality. DSM-III: Axis II.* New York: Wiley.

Millon, T. (1983). *Millon Clinical Multiaxial Inventory manual* (3rd ed.). Minneapolis, MN: National Computer Systems.

Millon, T. (1986). Personality prototypes and their diagnostic criteria. In T. Millon & G. Klerman (Eds.), *Contemporary directions in psychopathology* (pp. 671-712). New York: Guilford.

Millon, T. (1987). *Manual for the MCMI-II* (2nd ed.). Minneapolis, MN: National Computer Systems.

Millon, T. (1991a). Avoidant personality disorder: A brief review of issues and data. *Journal of Personality Disorders*, *5*, 353-362.

Millon, T. (1991b). Classification in psychopathology: Rationale, alternatives, and standards. *Journal of Abnormal Psychology*, *100*, 245-261.

Millon, T. (1993). Negativistic (passive-aggressive) personality disorder. *Journal of Personality Disorders*, *7*, 78-85.

Millon, T., & Tringone, R. (1989). [Co-occurrence and diagnostic efficiency statistics]. Unpublished raw data.

Mischel, W. (1984). Convergences and challenges in the search for consistency. *American Psychologist*, *39*, 351-364.

Mishlove, M., & Chapman, L. J. (1985). Social anhedonia in the prediction of psychosis proneness. *Journal of Abnormal Psychology*, *94*, 384-396.

Morey, L. C. (1988a). A psychometric analysis of the *DSM-III-R* personality disorder criteria. *Journal of Personality Disorders*, *2*, 109-124.

Morey, L. C. (1988b). Personality disorders under *DSM-III* and *DSM-III-R*: An examination of convergence, coverage, and internal consistency. *American Journal of Psychiatry*, *145*, 573-577.

Morey, L. C. (1991). *The Personality Assessment Inventory professional manual.* Odessa, FL: Psychological Assessment Resources.

Morey, L. C., & Goodman, R. (1989) [Diagnostic efficiency statistics]. Unpublished raw data.

Morey, L. C., & Heumann, K. (1988). [Co-occurrence and diagnostic efficiency statistics]. Unpublished raw data.

Morey, L. C., Waugh, M. H., & Blashfield, R. K. (1985). MMPI scales for *DSM-III* personality disorders: Their derivation and correlates. *Journal of Personality Assessment*, *49*, 245-251.

Nikelly, A. G. (1992). The pleonexic personality: A new provisional personality disorder. *Individual Psychology*, *48*, 253-260.

Nurnberg, H. G., Raskin, M., Levine, P. E., Pollack, S., Siegel, O., & Prince, R. (1991a). The comorbidity of borderline personality disorder and other *DSM-III-R* Axis II personality disorders. *American Journal of Psychiatry*, *148*, 1371-1377.

Nurnberg, H. G., Raskin, M., Levine, P. E., Pollack, S., Siegel, O., & Prince, R. (1991b). Hierarchy of *DSM-III-R* criteria efficiency for the diagnosis of borderline personality disorder. *Journal of Personality Disorders*, *5*, 211-224.

O'Boyle, M., & Self, D. (1990). A comparison of two interviews for *DSM-III-R* personality disorders. *Psychiatry Research*, *32*, 85-92.

Oldham, J. M. (1987). *DSM-III* personality disorders: Assessment problems. *Journal of Personality Disorders, 1*, 241-247.

Oldham, J. M., & Skodol, A. E. (1992). Personality disorders and mood disorders. In A. Tasman & M. B. Riba (Eds.), *Review of psychiatry* (Vol. 11, pp. 418-435). Washington, DC: American Psychiatric Press.

Oldham, J. M., Skodol, A. E., Kellman, H. D., Hyler, S. E., Rosnick, L., & Davies, M. (1992). Diagnosis of *DSM-III-R* personality disorders by two structured interviews: Patterns of comorbidity. *American Journal of Psychiatry, 149*, 213-220.

Orford, J. (1985). *Excessive appetites: A psychological view of addiction*. Chichester, England: Wiley.

Pantony, K., & Caplan, P. J. (1991). Delusional dominating personality disorder: A modest proposal for identifying some consequences of rigid masculine socialization. *Canadian Psychology, 32*, 120-133.

Perry, J. C. (1990). Challenges in validating personality disorders: Beyond description. *Journal of Personality Disorders, 4*, 273-289.

Perry, J. C. (1992). Problems and considerations in the valid assessment of personality disorders. *American Journal of Psychiatry, 149*, 1645-1653.

Perry, J. C., & Cooper, A. (1989). An empirical study of defense mechanisms: I. Clinical interview and life vignette ratings. *Archives of General Psychiatry, 46*, 444-452.

Perry, J. C., Lavori, P. W., Cooper, S. H., Hoke, L., & O'Connell, M. E. (1987). The Diagnostic Interview Schedule and *DSM-III* antisocial personality disorder. *Journal of Personality Disorders, 1*, 121-131.

Pfohl, B. (1991). Histrionic personality disorder: A review of available data and recommendations for *DSM-IV*. *Journal of Personality Disorders, 5*, 150-166.

Pfohl, B., & Blum, N. (1990). *Internal consistency statistics for the DSM-III-R personality disorder criteria*. Iowa City: University of Iowa College of Medicine.

Pfohl, B., & Blum, N. (1991). Obsessive-compulsive personality disorder: A review of available data and recommendations for *DSM-IV*. *Journal of Personality Disorders, 5*, 363-375.

Pfohl, B., Blum, N., Zimmerman, M., & Stangl, D. (1989). *Structured Interview for DSM-III-R Personality. SIDP-R*. Iowa City, IA: University of Iowa College of Medicine.

Pfohl, B., Coryell, W., Zimmerman, M., & Stangl, D. (1986). *DSM-III* personality disorders: Diagnostic overlap and internal consistency of individual *DSM-III* criteria. *Comprehensive Psychiatry, 27*, 21-34.

Pfohl, B., Stangl, D., & Zimmerman, M. (1984). The implications of *DSM-III* personality disorders for patients with major depression. *Journal of Affective Disorders, 7*, 309-318.

Phillips, K. A., & Gunderson, J. G. (1990). *Diagnostic Interview for Depressive Personality*. Unpublished manuscript, McLean Hospital, Belmont, MA.

Phillips, K. A., Gunderson, J. G., Hirschfeld, R. M. A., & Smith, L. (1990). A review of the depressive personality. *American Journal of Psychiatry, 147*, 830-837.

Phillips, K. A., Hirschfeld, R. M. A., Shea, M. T., & Gunderson, J.G. (1993). Depressive personality disorder: Perspectives for *DSM-IV*. *Journal of Personality Disorders, 7*, 30-42.

Pilkonis, P. A. (1984). Avoidant and schizoid personality disorders. In H. E. Adams & P. B. Sutker (Eds.), *Comprehensive handbook of psychopathology* (pp. 479-494). New York: Plenum.

Pilkonis, P. A. (1988). Personality prototypes among depressives: Themes of dependency and autonomy. *Journal of Personality Disorders, 2*, 144-152.

Pope, H., & Hudson, J. (1989). Are eating disorders associated with borderline personality disorder? A critical review. *International Journal of Eating Disorders, 8*, 1-9.

Regier, D. A., Boyd, J. H., Burke, J. D., Rae, D. S., Myers, J. K., Kramer, M., Robins, L. N., George, L. K., Karno, M., & Locke, B. Z. (1988). One-month prevalence of mental disorders in the United States. *Archives of General Psychiatry, 45*, 977-986.

Reich, J. H. (1985). Measurement of *DSM-III* Axis II. *Comprehensive Psychiatry, 26*, 352-363.

Reich, J. H. (1987). Instruments measuring *DSM-III* and *DSM-III-R* personality disorders. *Journal of Personality Disorders, 1*, 220-240.

Reich, J. (1988). [Diagnostic efficiency statistics for personality disorders]. Unpublished raw data.

Reich, J. H. (1989). Update on instruments to measure *DSM-III* and *DSM-III-R* personality disorders. *Journal of Nervous and Mental Disease, 177*, 366-370.

Ricciardi, J. N., Baer, L., Jenike, M. A., Fischer, S.C., Sholtz, D., & Buttolph, M. L. (1992). Changes in DSM-III-R Axis II diagnoses following treatment of obsessive-compulsive disorder. *American Journal of Psychiatry, 149*, 829-831.

Robins, L. N. (1966). *Deviant children grown up*. Baltimore: Williams & Wilkins.

Robins, L. N., Helzer, J. E., Croughan, J., & Ratcliff, K. S. (1981). The NIMH Diagnostic Interview Schedule: Its history, characteristics, and validity. *Archives of General Psychiatry, 38*, 381-389.

Robins, L. N., Tipp, J., & Przybeck, T. (1991). Antisocial personality. In L. N. Robins & D. A. Regier (Eds.). *Psychiatric disorders in America* (pp. 258-290). New York: Free Press.

Rogers, R., Bagby, R. M., & Dickens, S. E. (1993). *Structured Interview of Reported Symptoms professional manual*. Odessa, FL: Psychological Assessment Resources.

Rogler, L. H. (1993). Culturally sensitizing psychiatric diagnosis. *Journal of Nervous and Mental Disease, 181*, 401-408.

Ronningstam, E., & Gunderson, J. G. (1988). Comparing three systems for diagnosing narcissistic personality disorder. *Psychiatry, 51*, 300-311.

Ronningstam, E., & Gunderson, J. G. (1989). Descriptive studies on narcissistic personality disorder. *Psychiatric Clinics of North America, 12*, 585-601.

Ronningstam, E., & Gunderson, J. G. (1990). Identifying criteria for narcissistic personality disorder. *American Journal of Psychiatry, 147*, 585-601.

Ronningstam, E., & Gunderson, J. G. (1991). Differentiating borderline personality disorder from narcissistic personality disorder. *Journal of Personality Disorders, 5*, 225-232.

Rorer, L. G., & Widiger, T. A. (1983). Personality structure and assessment. *Annual Review of Psychology, 34*, 431-464.

Rounsaville, B. J., Spitzer, R. L., & Williams, J. B. W. (1986). Proposed changes in *DSM-III* substance use disorders: Description and rationale. *American Journal of Psychiatry, 143*, 463-468.

Sartorius, N. (1988). International perspectives of psychiatric classification. *British Journal of Psychiatry, 152*(Suppl.), 9-14.

Sartorius, N., Kaelber, C. T., Cooper, J. E., Roper, M., Rae, D. S., Gulbinat, W., Ustun, T. B., & Regier, D. A. (1993). Progress toward achieving a common language in psychiatry. *Archives of General Psychiatry, 50*, 115-124.

Schmideberg, M. (1959). The borderline patient. In S. Arieti (Ed.), *American handbook of psychiatry*. New York: Basic.

Schneider, K. (1959). *Clinical psychopathology*. London: Grune & Stratton.

Schneier, F. R., Liebowitz, M. R., Beidel, D. C., Fyer, A. J., George, M. S., Heimberg, R. G., Holt, C. S., Klein, D., Levin, A. P., Lydiard, R. B., Mannuzza, S., Martin, L. Y., Martin, L. Y., Nardi, A. E., Roscow, D. B., Spitzer, R. L., Turner, S. M., Uhde, T. W., Vasconcelos, I. L., & Versiani, M. (in press). *DSM-IV* social phobia. In T. A. Widiger, A. J. Frances, H. A. Pincus, M. B. First, R. Ross, & W. W. Davis (Eds.), *DSM-IV sourcebook* (Vol. 2). Washington, DC: American Psychiatric Press.

Schopp, L. H., & Trull, T. J. (1993). Validity of the *DSM-III-R* personality disorder clusters. *Journal of Psychopathology and Behavioral Assessment, 15*, 219-237.

Schroeder, M. L., Wormworth, J. A., & Livesley, W. J. (1992). Dimensions of personality disorder and their relationships to the Big Five dimensions of personality. *Psychological Assessment, 4*, 47-53.

Shapiro, D. (1965). *Neurotic styles*. New York: Basic.

Shapiro, T. (1990). Resolved: Borderline personality exists in children under twelve: Negative. *Journal of the American Academy of Child and Adolescent Psychiatry, 29*, 480-481.

Shea, M. T. (1992). Some characteristics of the Axis II criteria sets and their implications for assessment of personality disorders. *Journal of Personality Disorders, 6*, 377-381.

Shea, M. T. (1993). *DSM-IV* reviews of the personality disorders: Introduction to the third part of the special series. *Journal of Personality Disorders, 7*, 28-29.

Shea, M. T. (in press). Enduring personality change after catastrophic experience. In T. A. Widiger, A. J. Frances, H. A. Pincus, M. B. First, R. Ross, & W. W. Davis (Eds.), *DSM-IV sourcebook* (Vol. 2). Washington, DC: American Psychiatric Press.

Shea, M. T., Glass, D. R., Pilkonis, P. A., Watkins, J., & Docherty, J. P. (1987). Frequency and implications of personality disorders in a sample of depressed outpatients. *Journal of Personality Disorders, 1*, 27-42.

Shopshire, M. S., & Craik, K. H. (1994). The five factor model of personality and the *DSM-III-R* personality disorders: Correspondence and differentiation. *Journal of Personality Disorders, 8*, 41-52.

Siegman, A. W., & Dembroski, T. M. (Eds.). (1989). *In search of coronary-prone behavior. Beyond Type A*. Hillsdale, NJ: Erlbaum.

Siever, L. J. (1992). Schizophrenia spectrum personality disorders. In A. Tasman & M. B. Riba (Eds.), *Review of psychiatry* (Vol. 11, pp. 25-42). Washington, DC: American Psychiatric Press.

Siever, L. J., Bernstein, D. P., & Silverman, J. M. (1991). Schizotypal personality disorder: A review of its current status. *Journal of Personality Disorders, 5*, 178-193.

Siever, L. J., & Davis, K. L. (1991). A psychobiological perspective on the personality disorders. *American Journal of Psychiatry, 148*, 1647-1658.

Siever, L. J., & Gunderson, J. G. (1979). Genetic determinants of borderline conditions. *Schizophrenia Bulletin, 5*, 49-86.

Siever, L. J., & Klar, H. (1986). A review of *DSM-III* criteria for the personality disorders. In A. Frances & R. Hales (Eds.), *Psychiatry update* (Vol. 5, pp. 279-314). Washington, DC: American Psychiatric Press.

Silverman, J. M., Pinkham, L., Horvath, T. B., Coccaro, E. F., Klar, H., Schear, S., Apter, S., Davidson, M., Mohs, R. C., & Siever, L. J. (1991). Affective and impulsive personality disorder traits in the relatives of patients with borderline personality disorder. *American Journal of Psychiatry, 148*, 1378-1385.

Silverman, J. M., Siever, L. J., Bernstein, D., & Zanarini, M. (in press). Field trial of *DSM-IV* criteria for schizotypal personality disorder. In T. A. Widiger, A. J. Frances, H. A. Pincus, M. B. First, R. Ross, & W. W. Davis (Eds.), *DSM-IV sourcebook* (Vol. 4). Washington, DC: American Psychiatric Press.

Singer, J. L. (Ed.) (1991). *Repression and dissociation: Implications for personality theory, psychopathology, and health*. Chicago: University of Chicago Press.

Skodol, A. E. (1989a). [Co-occurrence and diagnostic efficiency statistics]. Unpublished raw data.

Skodol, A. E. (1989b). *Problems in differential diagnosis: From DSM-III to DSM-III-R in clinical practice*. Washington, DC: American Psychiatric Press.

Skodol, A. E., Oldham, J. M., Rosnick, L., Kellman, H. D., & Hyler, S. E. (1991). Diagnosis of *DSM-III-R* personality disorders: A comparison of two structured interviews. *International Journal of Methods in Psychiatric Research, 1*, 13-26.

Skodol, A. E., Rosnick, L., Kellman, D., Oldham, J., & Hyler, S. (1988). Validating structured *DSM-III-R* personality disorder assessments with longitudinal data. *American Journal of Psychiatry, 145*, 1297-1299.

Soldz, S., Budman, S., Demby, A., & Merry, J. (1993). Representation of personality disorders in circumplex and five-factor space: Explorations with a clinical sample. *Psychological Assessment, 5*, 41-52.

Spitzer, R. L. (1983). Psychiatric diagnosis: Are clinicians still necessary? *Comprehensive Psychiatry, 24*, 399-411.

Spitzer, R. L., Davies, M., & Barkley, R. A. (1990). The *DSM-III-R* field trials of disruptive behavior disorders. *Journal of the American Academy of Child and Adolescent Psychiatry, 29*, 690-697.

Spitzer, R., Endicott, J., & Gibbon, M. (1979). Crossing the border into borderline personality and borderline schizophrenia. *Archives of General Psychiatry, 36*, 17-24.

Spitzer, R. L., Endicott, J., & Robins, E. (1975). Clinical criteria for psychiatric diagnosis and *DSM-III*. *American Journal of Psychiatry, 132*, 1187-1192.

Spitzer, R. L., Endicott, J., & Robins, E. (1978). Research diagnostic criteria. Rationale and reliability. *Archives of General Psychiatry, 35*, 773-782.

Spitzer, R. L., Fiester, S. J., Gay, M., & Pfohl, B. (1991). Results of a survey of forensic psychiatrists on the validity of the sadistic personality disorder diagnosis. *American Journal of Psychiatry, 148*, 875-879.

Spitzer, R. L., & Williams, J. B. W. (1982). The definition and diagnosis of mental disorder. In W. Gove (Ed.), *Deviance and mental illness* (pp. 15-31). Beverly Hills, CA: Sage.

Spitzer, R. L., & Williams, J. B. W. (1985). Proposed revisions in the *DSM-III* classification of anxiety disorders based on research and clinical experience. In A. H. Tuma & J. Maser (Eds.), *Anxiety and the anxiety disorders* (pp. 759-773). Hillsdale, NJ: Erlbaum.

Spitzer, R. L., Williams, J. B. W., Gibbon, M., & First, M. B. (1990). *User's guide for the Structured Clinical Interview for DSM-III-R. SCID*. Washington, DC: American Psychiatric Press.

Spitzer, R. L., Williams, J. B. W., & Skodol, A. E. (1980). *DSM-III*: The major achievements and an overview. *American Journal of Psychiatry, 137*, 151-164.

Sprock, J., Blashfield, R. K., & Smith, B. (1990). Gender weighting of *DSM-III-R* personality disorder criteria. *American Journal of Psychiatry, 147*, 586-590.

Standage, K. (1989). Structured interviews and the diagnosis of personality disorders. *Canadian Journal of Psychiatry, 34*, 906-912.

Stangl, D., Pfohl, B., Zimmerman, M., Bowers, W., & Corenthal, W. (1985). A structured interview for *DSM-III* personality disorder. *Archives of General Psychiatry, 42*, 591-596.

Sternbach, S., Judd, A., Sabo, A., McGlashan, T., & Gunderson, J. G. (1992). Cognitive and perceptual distortions in borderline personality disorder and schizotypal personality disorder in a vignette sample. *Comprehensive Psychiatry, 3*, 186-189.

Stone, M. (1990). Treatment of borderline patients: A pragmatic approach to psychotherapy and psychopharmacology. *Psychiatric Clinics of North America, 13*, 265-285.

Stone, M. (1992). Treatment of severe personality disorders. In A. Tasman & M. B. Riba (Eds.), *Review of psychiatry* (Vol. 11, pp. 98-115). Washington, DC: American Psychiatric Press.

Stone, M. (1993). *Abnormalities of personality. Within and beyond the realm of treatment.* New York: W. W. Norton.

Strack, S., & Lorr, M. (Eds.). (in press). *Differentiating normal and abnormal personality*. New York: Springer.

Strube, M. J. (1988). The decision to leave an abusive relationship: Empirical evidence and theoretical issues. *Psychological Bulletin, 104*, 236-250.

Stuart, S., Simons, A. D., Thase, M. E., & Pilkonis, P. (1992). Are personality disorders valid in acute major depression? *Journal of Affective Disorders, 24*, 281-290.

Sutker, P. B. (1994). Psychopathy: Traditional and clinical antisocial concepts. In D. Fowles, P. Sutker, & S. H. Goodman (Eds.), *Progress in experimental personality & psychopathology research* (pp. 73-120). New York: Springer.

Task Force on *DSM-IV*. (1991, September). *DSM-IV options book: Work in progress*. Washington, DC: American Psychiatric Association.

Task Force on *DSM-IV*. (1993, March). *DSM-IV draft criteria*. Washington, DC: American Psychiatric Association.

Task Force on Nomenclature and Statistics. (1978, January). *DSM-III draft*. Washington, DC: American Psychiatric Association.

Triebwasser, J., & Shea, M. T. (in press). Enduring personality change after mental disorder. In T. A. Widiger, A. J. Frances, H. A. Pincus, M. B. First, R. Ross, & W. W. Davis (Eds.), *DSM-IV sourcebook* (Vol. 2). Washington, DC: American Psychiatric Press.

Trull, T. J. (1992). *DSM-III-R* personality disorders and the five-factor model of personality: An empirical comparison. *Journal of Abnormal Psychology, 101*, 553-560.

Trull, T. J., Widiger, T. A., & Frances, A. J. (1987). Covariation of avoidant, schizoid, and dependent personality disorder criteria sets. *American Journal of Psychiatry, 144*, 767-771.

Turner, S. M., Beidel, D. C., Dancu, C. V., & Keys, D. J. (1986). Psychopathology of social phobia and comparison to avoidant personality disorder. *Journal of Abnormal Psychology, 95*, 389-394.

Turner, S. M., Beidel, D. C., & Townsley, R. M. (1992). Social phobia: A comparison of specific and generalized subtypes and avoidant personality disorder. *Journal of Abnormal Psychology*, *101*, 326-331.

Tyrer, P. (1988). What's wrong with *DSM-III* personality disorders. *Journal of Personality Disorders*, *2*, 281-291.

Wakefield, J. C. (1992). The concept of mental disorder. On the boundary between biological facts and social values. *American Psychologist*, *47*, 373-388.

Wakefield, J. C. (1993). Limits of operationalization: A critique of Spitzer and Endicott's (1978) proposed operational criteria for mental disorder. *Journal of Abnormal Psychology*, *102*, 160-172.

Wakefield, J. C. (1994). Is the concept of mental disorder culturally relative? In S. A. Kirk & S. D. Einbinder (Eds.), *Controversial issues in mental health* (pp. 11-17). Boston: Allyn & Bacon.

Waldinger, R. J., & Gunderson, J. G. (1987). *Effective psychotherapy with borderline patients*. New York: MacMillan.

Walker, L. E. A. (1984). *The battered woman syndrome*. New York: Springer.

Walker, L. E. A. (1987). Inadequacies of the masochistic personality disorder diagnosis for women. *Journal of Personality Disorders*, *1*, 183-189.

Walker, L. E. A. (1994). Are personality disorders gender biased? In S. A. Kirk & S. D. Einbinder (Eds.), *Controversial issues in mental health* (pp. 22-29). New York: Allyn & Bacon.

Widiger, T. A. (1985). *Personality Interview Questions*. Unpublished manuscript, University of Kentucky, Lexington, KY.

Widiger, T. A. (1987). *Personality Interview Questions–II*. Unpublished manuscript, University of Kentucky, Lexington.

Widiger, T. A. (1989). The categorical distinction between personality and affective disorders. *Journal of Personality Disorders*, *3*, 77-91.

Widiger, T. A. (1991). *DSM-IV* reviews of the personality disorders: Introduction to special series. *Journal of Personality Disorders*, *5*, 122-134.

Widiger, T. A. (1992a). Generalized social phobia versus avoidant personality disorder: A commentary on three studies. *Journal of Abnormal Psychology*, *101*, 340-343.

Widiger, T. A. (1992b). Review of the NEO-PI. In J. J. Kramer & J. C. Conoley (Eds.), *The eleventh mental measurements yearbook* (pp. 606-607). Lincoln, NE: Buros Institute of Mental Measurements.

Widiger, T. A. (1993a). The *DSM-III-R* categorical personality disorder diagnoses: A critique and an alternative. *Psychological Inquiry*, *4*, 75-90.

Widiger, T. A. (1993b). Personality and depression: Assessment issues. In M. H. Klein, D. J. Kupfer, & M. T. Shea (Eds.), *Personality and depression* (pp. 77-118). New York: Guilford.

Widiger, T. A. (in press). Deletion of the self-defeating and sadistic personality disorder diagnoses. In W. J. Livesley (Ed.), *DSM-IV personality disorders*. New York: Guilford.

Widiger, T. A., Cadoret, R., Hare, R. D., Hare, L., Rutherford, M., Zanarini, M., Alterman, A., Apple, M., Corbitt, E. M., Forth, A., Hart, S., Kulterman, J., Woody, G., & Frances, A. (in press). *DSM-IV* antisocial personality disorder field trial. In T. A. Widiger, A. J. Frances, H. A. Pincus, M. B. First, M. Kline, R. Ross, & W. Davis (Eds.), *DSM-IV sourcebook* (Vol. 5). Washington, DC: American Psychiatric Press.

Widiger, T. A., & Corbitt, E. M. (1993). Antisocial personality disorder: Proposals for *DSM-IV*. *Journal of Personality Disorders*, *7*, 63-77.

Widiger, T. A., & Corbitt, E. M. (in press-a). Antisocial personality disorder in *DSM-IV*. In W. J. Livesley (Ed.), *DSM-IV personality disorders*. New York: Guilford.

Widiger, T. A., & Corbitt, E. M. (in press-b). Normal versus abnormal personality from the perspective of the *DSM*. In S. Strack & M. Lorr (Eds.), *Differentiating normal and abnormal personality*. New York: Springer.

Widiger, T. A., Corbitt, E. M., Ellis, C. G., & Thomas, G. V. (1992). *Personality Interview Questions–III*. Unpublished manuscript, University of Kentucky, Lexington.

Widiger, T. A., Corbitt, E. M., & Funtowicz, M. (1994). Are the *DSM-III-R* personality disorders sex-biased? In S. A. Kirk & S. D. Einbender (Eds.), *Controversial issues in mental health* (pp. 32-37). New York: Allyn & Bacon.

Widiger, T. A., & Costa, P. T. (1994). Personality and personality disorders. *Journal of Abnormal Psychology*, *103*, 78-91

Widiger, T. A., & Frances, A. J. (1985). The *DSM-III* personality disorders: Perspectives from psychology. *Archives of General Psychiatry*, *42*, 615-623.

Widiger, T. A., & Frances, A. J. (1987). Interviews and inventories for the measurement of personality disorders. *Clinical Psychology Review*, *7*, 49-74.

Widiger, T. A., & Frances, A. J. (1988). Personality disorders. In J. Talbott, R. Hales, & S. Yudofsky (Eds.), *Textbook of psychiatry* (pp. 621-648). Washington, DC: American Psychiatric Press.

Widiger, T. A., & Frances, A. J. (1989a). Controversies concerning the self-defeating personality disorder. In R. Curtis (Ed.), *Self-defeating behaviors: Experimental research, clinical impressions, and practical implications* (pp. 289-309). New York: Plenum.

Widiger, T. A., & Frances, A. J. (1989b). Epidemiology, diagnosis, and comorbidity of borderline personality disorder. In A. Tasman, R. Hales, & A. Frances (Eds.), *Review of psychiatry* (Vol. 8, pp. 8-24). Washington, DC: American Psychiatric Press.

Widiger, T. A., Frances, A. J., Pincus, H. A., & Davis, W. W. (1990). *DSM-IV* literature reviews: Rationale, process, and limitations. *Journal of Psychopathology and Behavioral Assessment*, *12*, 189-202.

Widiger, T. A., Frances, A. J., Pincus, H. A., Davis, W. W., & First, M. B. (1991). Toward an empirical classification for the *DSM-IV*. *Journal of Abnormal Psychology*, *100*, 280-288.

Widiger, T. A., Frances, A. J., Spitzer, R. L., & Williams, J. B. W. (1988). The *DSM-III-R* personality disorders: An overview. *American Journal of Psychiatry*, *145*, 786-795.

Widiger, T. A., Frances, A. J., & Trull, T. J. (1987). A psychometric analysis of the social-interpersonal and cognitive-perceptual items for the schizotypal personality disorder. *Archives of General Psychiatry*, *44*, 741-745.

Widiger, T. A., Frances, A. J., & Trull, T. J. (1989). Personality disorders. In R. Craig (Ed.), *Clinical and diagnostic interviewing* (pp. 221-236). Northvale, NJ: Jason Aronson.

Widiger, T. A., Frances, A. J., Warner, L., & Bluhm, C. (1986). Diagnostic criteria for the borderline and schizotypal personality disorders. *Journal of Abnormal Psychology*, *95*, 43-51.

Widiger, T. A., & Freiman, K. (1988, November). *Personality Interview Questions–II: Reliability and methodological issues*. Paper presented at the NIMH Workshop on Assessment of Personality Disorders, Bethesda, MD.

Widiger, T. A., Freiman, K., & Bailey, B. (1990). Convergent and discriminant validity of personality disorder prototypic acts. *Psychological Assessment*, *3*, 418-423.

Widiger, T. A., Hurt, S., Frances, A. J., Clarkin, J., & Gilmore, M. (1984). Diagnostic efficiency and *DSM-III. Archives of General Psychiatry, 41*, 1005-1012.

Widiger, T. A., Miele, G. M., & Tilly, S. M. (1992). Alternative perspectives on the diagnosis of borderline personality disorder. In J. F. Clarkin, E. Marziali, & H. Munroe-Blum (Eds.), *Borderline personality disorder. Clinical and empirical perspectives* (pp. 89-115). New York: Guilford.

Widiger, T., & Rogers, J. (1989). Prevalence and comorbidity of personality disorders. *Psychiatric Annals, 19*, 132-136.

Widiger, T. A., & Sanderson, C. J. (in press-a). Effective procedures for assessing personality disorders. In J. N. Butcher (Ed.), *Practical considerations in clinical personality assessment.* New York: Oxford University Press.

Widiger, T. A., & Sanderson, C. J. (in press-b). Towards a dimensional model of personality disorders in *DSM-IV* and *DSM-V.* In W. J. Livesley (Ed.), *DSM-IV personality disorders.* New York: Guilford.

Widiger, T. A., & Shea, T. (1991). Differentiation of Axis I and Axis II disorders. *Journal of Abnormal Psychology, 100*, 399-406.

Widiger, T. A., & Smith, G. T. (1994). Substance use disorder: Abuse, dependence, and dyscontrol. *Addiction, 89*, 287-302.

Widiger, T. A., & Spitzer, R. L. (1991). Sex bias in the diagnosis of personality disorders. *Clinical Psychology Review, 11*, 1-22.

Widiger, T. A., & Trull, T. J. (1987). Behavioral indicators, hypothetical constructs, and personality disorders. *Journal of Personality Disorders, 1*, 82-87.

Widiger, T. A., & Trull, T. J. (1991). Diagnosis and clinical assessment. *Annual Review of Psychology, 42*, 109-133.

Widiger, T. A., & Trull, T. J. (1992). Personality and psychopathology: An application of the five-factor model. *Journal of Personality, 60*, 363-393.

Widiger, T. A., & Trull, T. J. (1993). Personality disorders and violence. In J. Monahan & H. Steadman (Eds.), *Violence and mental disorder: Developments in risk assessment* (pp. 203-226). Chicago: University of Chicago Press.

Widiger, T. A., & Trull, T. J. (in press). Performance characteristics of the *DSM-III-R* personality disorder criteria sets. In T. A. Widiger, A. J. Frances, H. A. Pincus, M. B. First, R. Ross, & W. W. Davis (Eds.), *DSM-IV sourcebook* (Vol. 4). Washington, DC: American Psychiatric Press.

Widiger, T. A., Trull, T. J., Clarkin, J. F., Sanderson, C. J., & Costa, P. T. (1994). A description of the *DSM-III-R* and *DSM-IV* personality disorders with the five-factor model of personality. In P. T. Costa & T. A. Widiger (Eds.), *Personality disorders and the five-factor model of personality* (pp. 41-56). Washington, DC: American Psychological Association.

Widiger, T. A., Trull, T. J., Hurt, S., Clarkin, J., & Frances, A. (1987). A multidimensional scaling of the *DSM-III* personality disorders. *Archives of General Psychiatry, 44*, 557-563.

Wiens, A. N. (1990). Structured clinical interviews for adults. In G. Goldstein & M. Hersen (Eds.), *Handbook of psychological assessment* (2nd ed., pp. 324-341). New York: Pergamon.

Wiggins, J. S., & Pincus, A. L. (1989). Conceptions of personality disorders and dimensions of personality. *Psychological Assessment: A Journal of Consulting and Clinical Psychology, 1*, 305-316.

Wiggins, J. S., & Pincus, A. L. (1992). Personality: Structure and assessment. *Annual Review of Psychology, 43*, 473-504.

Williams, J. B. W., & Spitzer, R. L. (1983). The issue of sex bias in *DSM-III.* A critique of "A woman's view of *DSM-III*" by Marcie Kaplan. *American Psychologist, 38*, 793-798.

Wirt, R. D., Lachar, D., Klinedinst, J. K., & Seat, P. D. (1984). *Multidimensional description of child personality: A manual for the Personality Inventory for Children.* Los Angeles: Western Psychological Services.

Work Group to Revise *DSM-III.* (1985, October). *Draft. DSM-III-R in development.* Washington, DC: American Psychiatric Association.

Work Group to Revise *DSM-III.* (1986, August). *Second draft. DSM-III-R in development.* Washington, DC: American Psychiatric Association.

World Health Organization. (1992). *The ICD-10 classification of mental and behavioural disorders. Clinical descriptions and diagnostic guidelines.* Geneva, Switzerland: Author.

Zanarini, M. C. (1993). Borderline personality disorder as an impulse spectrum disorder. In J. Paris (Ed.), *Borderline personality disorder. Etiology and treatment* (pp. 67-85). Washington, DC: American Psychiatric Press.

Zanarini, M. C., Frankenburg, F. R., Chauncey, D. L., & Gunderson, J. G. (1987). The Diagnostic Interview for Personality Disorders: Interrater and test-retest reliability. *Comprehensive Psychiatry, 28*, 467-480.

Zanarini, M. C., Frankenburg, F. R, Chauncey, D. L, & Gunderson, J. G. (1989). [Co-occurrence and diagnostic efficiency statistics]. Unpublished raw data.

Zanarini, M. C., Gunderson, J. G., & Frankenburg, F. R. (1990). Cognitive features of borderline personality disorder. *American Journal of Psychiatry, 147*, 57-63.

Zanarini, M. C., Gunderson, J. G., Frankenburg, F. R., & Chauncey, D. L. (1989). The Revised Diagnostic Interview for Borderlines: Discriminating BPD from other Axis II disorders. *Journal of Personality Disorders, 3*, 10-18.

Zimmerman, M. (1993a, September). Interstudy rater variance: A major problem in diagnosing personality disorders. In R. Weinryb (Moderator), *Assessment of personality disorders I.* Symposium conducted at the 3rd International Congress on the Disorders of Personality, Cambridge, MA.

Zimmerman, M. (1993b, September). *Review of issues and research methods in diagnosing personality disorders. I and II.* Posters presented at the 3rd International Congress on the Disorders of Personality, Cambridge, MA.

Zimmerman, M. (1994). Diagnosing personality disorders. A review of issues and research methods. *Archives of General Psychiatry, 51*, 225-245.

Zimmerman, M., & Coryell, W. H. (1989). *DSM-III* personality disorder diagnoses in a nonpatient sample. *Archives of General Psychiatry, 46*, 682-689.

Zimmerman, M., Pfohl, B., Coryell, W., Stangl, D., & Corenthal, C. (1988). Diagnosing personality disorders in depressed patients. A comparison of patient and informant interviews. *Archives of General Psychiatry, 45*, 733-737.